READY, SET, GO!

WITH DONATELLE, HEALTH: THE BASICS, 12E
The MasteringHealth Edition

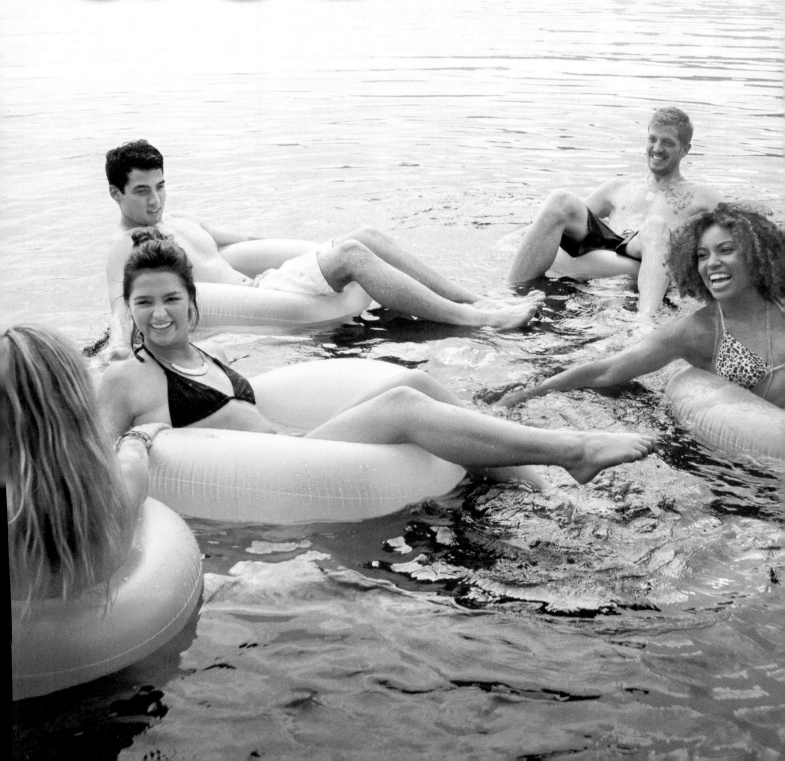

GET YOUR STUDENTS READY!

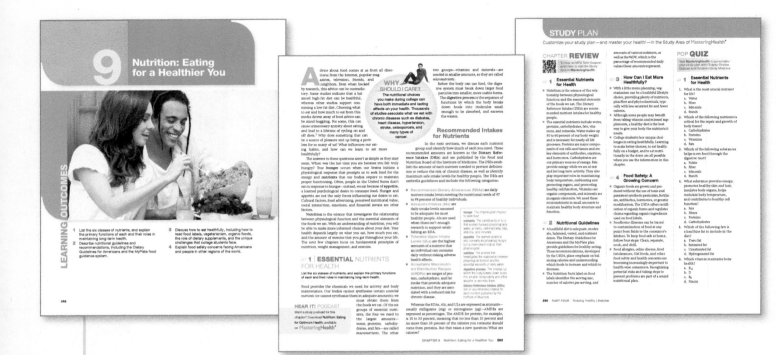

NEW! Study Plan Tied to Learning Outcomes

Numbered learning outcomes now introduce every chapter and mini-chapter, giving students a roadmap for their reading. Each chapter concludes with a Study Plan, which summarizes key points of the chapter and provides review questions and critical thinking questions to check understanding, all tied to the chapter's learning outcomes and assignable in MasteringHealth.

NEW! *ABC News* Lecture Launchers

New videos from *ABC News* bring personal health to life and spark discussion with up-to-date hot topics such as stress among millennials, hate crimes, and rates of heroin use. Assignable multiple-choice questions available in MasteringHealth provide wrong-answer feedback to redirect students to the correct answer.

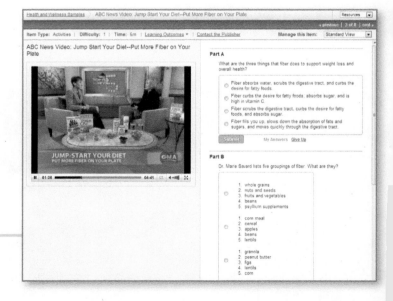

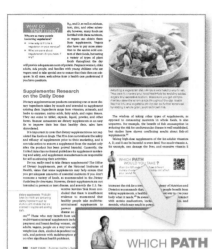

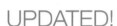

WHICH **PATH** WOULD YOU TAKE ?

Scan the QR code to see how different dietary choices YOU make today can affect your overall health tomorrow.

NEW! Interactive Behavior Change Activities— Which Path Would You Take?

By scanning QR codes with their mobile devices, students gain access to an exploration of various health choices through an engaging, interactive, low-stakes, and anonymous experience. These activities show students the possible consequences of various choices they make today on their future health through a choose-your-own-adventure style interface.

UPDATED!

A new mini-chapter, Focus On: Sexuality, has been pulled from the previously titled Healthy Relationships and Understanding Sexuality chapter, making it easier to assign the sexuality material in connection with the Reproductive Choices chapter (contraception). Additional information on social connections is now included in the Relationships chapter.

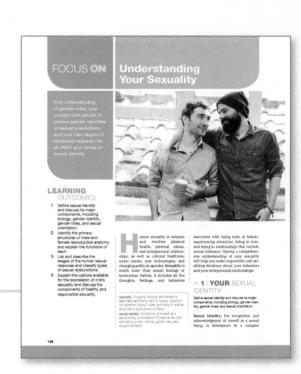

UPDATED!

Current Health Topics Straight from the Headlines

Current health issues are covered throughout the new edition, speaking to students' questions and concerns. New and updated material covers such areas as

- the heritability of well-being
- suicide risk factors
- the psychological and physiological effects of meditation
- technostress
- the relationship between media violence and actual violence
- social network use
- the abuse of heroin, khat, and salvia

- the characteristics of successful weight losers
- orthorexia nervosa
- CrossFit and high-intensity interval training (HIIT)
- the global burden of disease
- safe oral sex
- the human impact on the existence or extinction of other species

UPDATED!

Focus On: Financial Health mini-chapter has been streamlined to focus more on the connection between wealth and health.

GET YOUR **STUDENTS GOING**
WITH MasteringHealth™

Mastering is the most effective and widely used online homework, tutorial, and assessment system for the sciences and now includes content specifically for health courses. Mastering delivers self-paced tutorials that focus on your course objectives, provides individualized coaching, and responds to each student's progress.

BEFORE CLASS — Dynamic Study Modules and eText 2.0 Provide Students with a Preview of What's to Come

NEW! **Dynamic Study Modules** help students study effectively on their own by continuously assessing their activity and performance in real time. Students complete a set of questions with a unique answer format that also asks them to indicate their confidence level. Questions repeat until the student can answer them all correctly and confidently. Once completed, Dynamic Study Modules explain the concept using materials from the text.

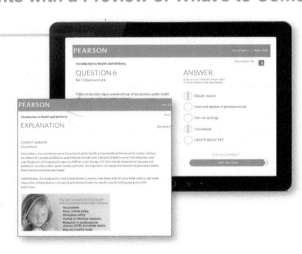

NEW! **Interactive eText 2.0,** complete with embedded media, is mobile friendly and ADA accessible.

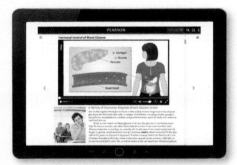

- Now available on smartphones and tablets
- Seamlessly integrated videos and other rich media
- Accessible (screen-reader ready)
- Configurable reading settings, including resizable type and night reading mode
- Instructor and student note-taking, highlighting, bookmarking, and search

DURING CLASS — Engage Students with Learning Catalytics™

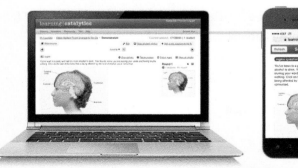 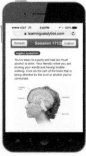

Learning Catalytics, a "bring your own device" student engagement, assessment, and classroom intelligence system, allows students to use their smartphones, tablets, or laptops to respond to questions in class.

AFTER CLASS

Easy-to-Assign, Customizable, and Automatically Graded Assignments

The breadth and depth of content available to you to assign in MasteringHealth is unparalleled, allowing you to quickly and easily assign homework to reinforce key concepts.

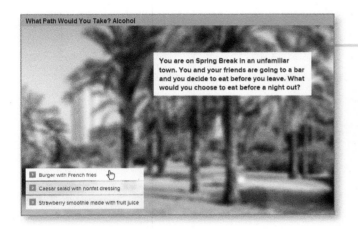

NEW! **Interactive Behavior Change Activities—Which Path Would You Take?—** allow students to explore various health choices through an engaging, interactive, low-stakes, and anonymous experience.

In activities covering topics such as alcohol, smoking, nutrition, and fitness, students receive specific feedback on the choices they make today and the possible consequences on their future health.

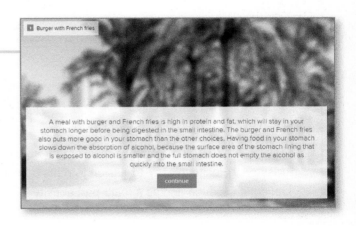

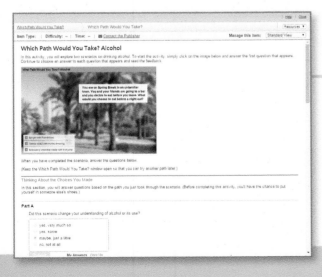

These activities are linked out to Mastering from the book and made assignable in Mastering with follow-up questions.

AFTER CLASS

Other Automatically Graded Health and Fitness Activities Include . . .

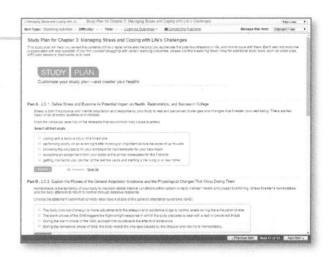

NEW! **Study Plans** tie all end-of-chapter material (including chapter review, pop quiz, and Think About It! questions) to specific numbered learning outcomes and Mastering assets. Assignable Study Plan items contain at least one multiple-choice question per learning outcome and wrong-answer feedback.

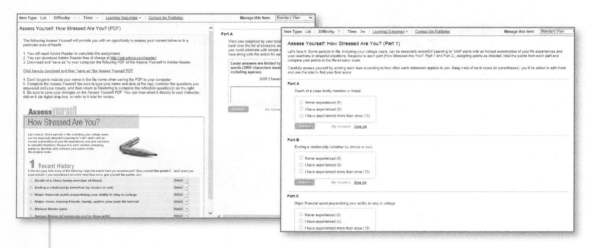

UPDATED! **Self-Assessments** from the text are available within MasteringHealth in easy-to-assign formats both in PDF format with a self-reflection section and as a multi-part activity that speaks to your gradebook.

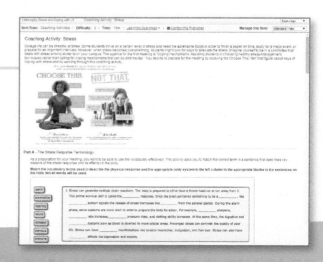

Coaching Activities guide students through key health and fitness concepts with interactive mini-lessons that provide hints and feedback.

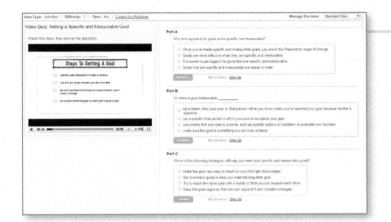

Behavior Change Videos are concise whiteboard-style videos that help students with the steps of behavior change, covering topics such as setting SMART goals, identifying and overcoming barriers to change, planning realistic timelines, and more. Additional videos review key fitness concepts such as determining target heart rate range for exercise. All videos include assessment activities and are assignable in MasteringHealth.

NutriTools Coaching Activities in the nutrition chapter allow students to combine and experiment with different food options and learn firsthand how to build healthier meals.

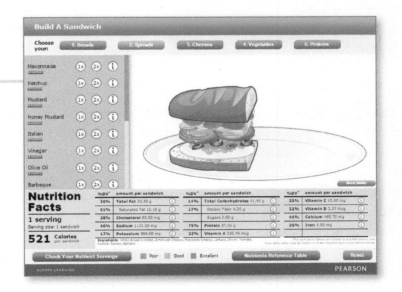

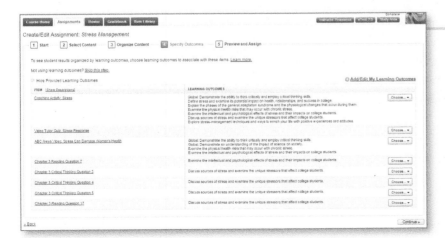

Learning Outcomes

All of the MasteringHealth assignable content is tagged to book content and to Bloom's Taxonomy. You also have the ability to add your own outcomes, helping you track student performance against your learning outcomes. You can view class performance against the specified learning outcomes and share those results quickly and easily by exporting to a spreadsheet.

EVERYTHING YOU NEED TO TEACH **IN ONE PLACE**

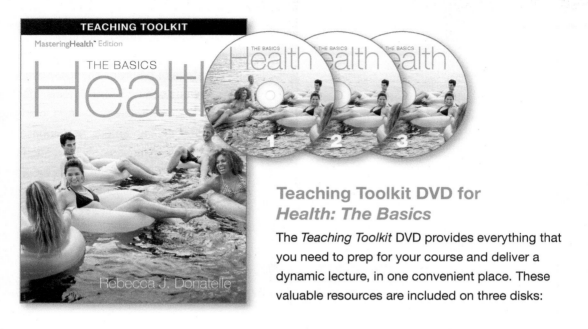

Teaching Toolkit DVD for *Health: The Basics*

The *Teaching Toolkit* DVD provides everything that you need to prep for your course and deliver a dynamic lecture, in one convenient place. These valuable resources are included on three disks:

DISK 1
Robust Media Assets for Each Chapter

- *ABC News* Lecture Launcher videos
- Behavior Change videos
- PowerPoint Lecture Outlines
- PowerPoint clicker questions and Jeopardy-style quiz show questions
- Files for all illustrations and tables and selected photos from the text

DISK 2
Comprehensive Test Bank

- Test Bank in Microsoft Word, PDF, and RTF formats
- Computerized Test Bank, which includes all the questions from the printed test bank in a format that allows you to easily and intuitively build exams and quizzes

DISK 3
Additional Innovative Supplements for Instructors and Students

For Instructors

- *Instructor Resource and Support Manual* in Microsoft Word and PDF formats
- Step-by-step MasteringHealth tutorials
- Video introduction to Learning Catalytics™
- *Great Ideas in Teaching Health & Wellness*
- *Teaching with Student Learning Outcomes*
- *Teaching with Web 2.0*

For Students

- Take Charge Self-Assessment Worksheets
- *Behavior Change Log Book and Wellness Journal*
- *Live Right! Beating Stress in College and Beyond*
- *Eat Right! Healthy Eating in College and Beyond*
- *Food Composition Table*

User's Quick Guide for *Health: The Basics*

This easy-to-use printed supplement accompanies the Teaching Toolkit and offers easy instructions for both experienced and new faculty members to get started with the rich Toolkit content and MasteringHealth.

Rebecca J. Donatelle

Health
The Basics

Fifth Custom Edition for Green River Community College

Taken from:
Health: The Basics, Twelfth Edition
by Rebecca J. Donatelle

Cover Art: Courtesy of Stockbyte/Getty Images and Corbis.

Taken from:

Health: The Basics, Twelfth Edition
by Rebecca J. Donatelle
Copyright © 2017, 2015, 2013 by Pearson Education, Inc.
New York, New York 10013

This special edition published in cooperation with Pearson Learning Solutions.

Pearson Education, Inc. 330 Hudson Street, New York, New York 10013
A Pearson Education Company
www.pearsoned.com

Printed in the United States of America

0002000102720Z2678

HG

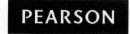
ISBN 10: 1-323-50463-X
ISBN 13: 978-1-323-50463-5

BRIEF CONTENTS

CONTENTS

FOCUS ON Minimizing Your Risk for Diabetes 386

FEATURE BOXES

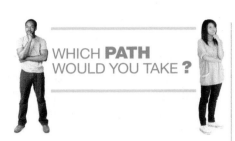
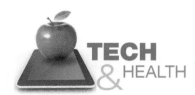
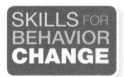
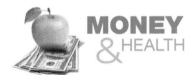

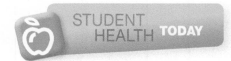

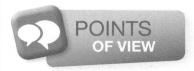

PREFACE

Today, threats to our health and the health of our planet dominate the media and affect our daily lives on a regular basis. Looming water shortages, poor air quality, food safety concerns, violence and the threat of terrorism, chronic and infectious diseases, and other concerns have us wondering about our ability to survive and thrive. We are advised to watch what we eat, lose weight, exercise more, reduce our stress, sleep more, have healthier relationships, be vigilant against a host of threats, and do our part to protect ourselves, our communities, our resources, and our planet. The issues often seem so huge, so far-reaching and overwhelming, that you may wonder if there is anything you can do to make a difference—to ensure a life that is healthy and long and a planet that is preserved for future generations. You are not alone! Getting healthy and staying healthy is a challenge for many, but the good news is that you *can* do things to improve your health and the health of others. Regardless of your age, sex, race, the environment you live in, or the challenges you face, you can be an agent for healthy change for you, your loved ones, and the greater community. It can start now, and it can start with you!

After years of teaching and working with students of all ages and stages of life and careers, I am encouraged by the fact that so many young adults are working hard to change their own health futures and the health of their families and communities. The problem is that with so much "talk" about health on so many platforms, sifting through the "junk information" and making the right choices based on *good science* and *good sense*, can be difficult.

My goal in writing *Health: The Basics,* the MasteringHealth™ Edition, is to build upon the strengths of past editions; to utilize the most current, scientifically valid research, to examine some of the important issues and controversies about health today, and motivate students to become "actively engaged in health" at all levels. As part of the process, we have worked hard to provide students with essential tools and technologically sound resources to empower them to take a careful and realistic look at their health risks, to examine their behaviors and the factors that contribute to those behaviors, and take the steps necessary to prioritize *health* in their lives. Although prioritizing individual and community health is a priority of this text, it is important to recognize that our health is increasingly connected to the health of the global community and our planet. As such, my aim is to challenge students to think globally as they consider health risks and seek creative solutions, both large and small, to address complex health problems. There is no *one-size-fits-all recipe* for health. You can do it your way— whether that means starting slow with "baby steps" designed to change deeply engrained behaviors or gearing up for major changes that all happen at once. Remember, we didn't develop our behaviors overnight. Being patient but persistent with ourselves is often part of the process.

This book is designed to help students quickly grasp the information, focusing on key objectives that have relevance to their own lives, both now and in the future. We provide the most current, comprehensive, concise, and scientifically valid information about each health topic, put a wealth of technological tools and resources at students' fingertips to assist in decision making, encourage students to think about the issues, and help students answer these questions: What is the issue and why should I care? What are my options for action? When and how do I get started?

With each new edition of *Health: The Basics,* I am gratified by the overwhelming success that this book has enjoyed. I am excited about making this edition the best yet—more timely, more relevant, and more interesting for students. Let's face it: Our world faces unprecedented challenges to individual and community health. Understanding these challenges and having a personal plan to preserve, protect, and promote health will help ensure our *healthful* future!

NEW TO THIS EDITION

Health: The Basics, the MasteringHealth Edition, maintains many features that the text has become known for, while incorporating several major revisions, exciting new features, and a more explicit connection between the text and multimedia resources in MasteringHealth. **MasteringHealth** is an online homework, tutorial, and assessment product designed to improve and assess results by helping students quickly master concepts. Students benefit from self-paced tutorials that feature immediate wrong-answer feedback and hints that emulate the office-hour experience to help keep students on track. With a wide range of interactive, engaging, and assignable activities, students are encouraged to actively learn and retain tough course concepts and apply them to real-world changes.

The multimedia created for the MasteringHealth Edition is more innovative and interactive than ever, and a tighter text and MasteringHealth integration provides students the opportunity to master course content using a variety of resources on and off the page, reflecting the manner in which students study today.

The most noteworthy changes to the text and multimedia as a whole include the following.

- **NEW! Interactive Behavior Change Activities—Which Path Would You Take?** Allow students to explore various health choices through an engaging, interactive, low-stakes, and anonymous experience. These choose-your-own-adventure-style activities show students the possible consequences of various choices they make today on their future health; these activities are accessible via the QR code from the book and made assignable in MasteringHealth™ with follow-up questions.
- **NEW! *ABC News* Videos** bring health to life and spark discussion with up-to-date hot topics from 2012 to 2015. MasteringHealth activities tied to the videos include multiple-choice questions that provide wrong-answer feedback to redirect students to the correct answer.
- **NEW! Study Plans** tie all end-of-chapter material (including Chapter Review, Pop Quiz, and Think About It questions) to specific, numbered Learning Outcomes. Assignable Study Plan items in MasteringHealth contain at least one multiple-choice question per Learning Outcome and include wrong-answer feedback.
- **NEW! eText 2.0** complete with embedded *ABC News* videos and Health Video Tutors; eText 2.0 is mobile friendly and ADA accessible.

  - Now available on smartphones and tablets.
  - Seamlessly integrated videos.
  - Accessible (screen-reader ready).
  - Configurable reading settings, including resizable type and night reading mode.
  - Instructor and student note taking, highlighting, bookmarking, and search.

- **NEW! Focus On: Sexuality mini-chapter** has been pulled from the previously titled Healthy Relationships and Understanding Sexuality chapter, and includes expanded coverage of topics such as sexual identity, sexual response and dysfunctions, and variant sexual behavior. This new Focus On makes it easier to assign the sexuality material in connection with the Reproductive Choices chapter (contraception).
- **UPDATED! Chapter 5, Connecting and Communicating in the Modern World** (formerly titled Healthy Relationships and Understanding Sexuality), now includes more information on social connections and how we interact and relate to others, including new research on social network use, addiction and social media meanness.
- **UPDATED! Focus On: Financial Health mini-chapter** has been streamlined to focus more on the connection between money and health and includes updated coverage of college students' financial issues and how these can affect both success in college and future health.

Chapter-by-Chapter Revisions

The MasteringHealth Edition has been thoroughly updated to provide students with the most current information and references for further exploration and includes a tighter integration between the text and multimedia resources in MasteringHealth. Learning outcomes are now explicitly tied to chapter sections and the end-of-chapter Study Plan to create a clear learning path for students. Portions of chapters have been reorganized to improve the flow of topics, and figures, tables, feature boxes, and photos have all been added, improved on, and updated. Throughout the text, all data, statistics, and references have been updated to the most recent possible. The following is a chapter-by-chapter listing of some of the most noteworthy changes, updates, and additions.

Chapter 1: Accessing Your Health

- New and updated coverage of relapse and recovery
- Updated research on health disparities
- New info on the Affordable Care Act

Focus On: Improving Your Financial Health

- Updated material on the link between health and wealth
- Updated coverage of financial struggles in college
- New chapter summaries and Pop Quiz

Chapter 2: Promoting and Preserving Your Psychological Health

- Updated coverage of emotional intelligence
- New research on heritability of well-being
- Updated material on risk factors for mental illness, as well as cost and stigma
- Updated research on mood disorders
- New research on suicide and risks in the United States and abroad

Focus On: Cultivating Your Spiritual Health

- New research on the psychological and physiological effects of meditation
- Updated research on the spiritual tendencies of undergraduates
- New coverage of the relationship between spirituality and stress reduction
- New chapter summaries and Pop Quiz

Chapter 3: Managing Stress and Coping with Life's Challenges

- Updated research on stress in America
- Updated material on massage therapy
- New material on technostress
- New app suggestions for help relaxing

Focus On: Improving Your Sleep

- Updated research on students and sleep
- New Student Health Today box on caffeine, sleep, and your health
- New Skills for Behavior Change on ditching blue-light devices
- New chapter summaries and Pop Quiz

Chapter 4: Preventing Violence and Injury

- Updated research on rates of violent crime in the United States and globally
- Updated research on violence and relationship violence on U.S. college campuses
- New info on the relationship between media violence and actual violence
- Updated research on the relationship between substance abuse and violence
- Updated Skills for Behavior Change with tips for men and women on reducing dating violence

Chapter 5: Connecting and Communicating in the Modern World

- Updated coverage of social support
- Updated discussions of social networks and social capital
- New material on relational connectedness and collective connectedness
- New research surrounding social network use, real-world connection, and addiction
- New Skills for Behavior Change on social media meanness

Focus On: Understanding Your Sexuality

- New Focus On, "Understanding Your Sexuality," with coverage of:
    - Sexual identity and its components
    - Male and female anatomy
    - Sexual response cycles and dysfunctions
    - Varieties of sexual expression
    - Makeup of healthy and responsible sexuality
- New chapter summaries and Pop Quiz

Chapter 6: Considering Your Reproductive Choices

- Updated statistics on contraception use and unintended pregnancy
- Coverage of new diaphragms
- Updated information on IUDs available
- Updated information on ECP availability
- Updated information on maternal health and pregnancy
- New Money & Health box on health care reform and contraceptives
- New Student Health Today box on men's involvement in birth control

Chapter 7: Recognizing and Avoiding Addiction and Drug Abuse

- Updated research regarding the prevalence of gambling addiction in the United States
- New coverage of khat
- New information on heroin use spreading to suburban areas
- New coverage of salvia
- Updated research regarding the prevalence of drug use in college students
- Updated information on the legalization of marijuana and its surrounding debate

Chapter 8: Drinking Alcohol Responsibly and Ending Tobacco Use

- Updated research on drinking rates
- Updated research on the dangers of alcohol use during pregnancy
- New coverage of alcohol use disorder
- New coverage of tobacco use disorder
- Updated information on e-cigarettes

Chapter 9: Nutrition: Eating for a Healthier You

- New Health Headlines on coconut oil
- Updated information on the *Dietary Guidelines for Americans*
- Updated data on the prevalence of vegetarianism
- Updated information on food-borne pathogens

Chapter 10: Reaching and Maintaining a Healthy Weight

- Updated statistics on overweight and obesity in the United States and globally
- New Student Health Today box on characteristics of successful weight losers
- Updated coverage and reviews of major diets and their effectiveness
- Updated coverage of prescription weight-loss drugs

Focus On: Enhancing Your Body Image

- New Student Health Today box on "thinspiration"
- Updated statistics regarding prevalence of eating disorders in the United States
- New discussion of orthorexia nervosa
- New chapter summaries and Pop Quiz

Chapter 11: Improving Your Personal Fitness

- Updated statistics regarding Americans meeting guidelines for aerobic exercise
- Updated research regarding physical activity and cognitive functions
- Updated research regarding physical activity and extended life span
- New coverage of Crossfit and other HIIT exercise plans

Chapter 12: Reducing Your Risk of Cardiovascular Disease and Cancer

- New and updated coverage of the global burden of disease
- Updated statistics regarding prevalence of cancer and heart disease
- Updated coverage of disease disparity and chronic disease across communities
- New guidelines for the management and treatment of high blood pressure
- Updated research on nonmodifiable risk factors for heart disease
- Updated discussion of the role of inflammation and infectious diseases in CVD and cancer risks

- Updated information about risks of prediabetes and strategies for prevention
- Updated research on the importance of prevention for CVD, cancer, and diabetes

Focus On: Minimizing Your Risk for Diabetes

- Updated statistics regarding the prevalence of diabetes
- Updated statistics on the economic burden of diabetes
- New chapter summaries and Pop Quiz

Chapter 13: Protecting against Infectious Diseases and Sexually Transmitted Infections

- Updated research on environmental conditions and the spread of disease
- Updated discussion of antibiotics and superbugs
- Updated coverage of MRSA
- Updated coverage of meningitis and college students, and its prevention
- Updated research on the prevalence of STIs
- Updated discussion of vaccination and opting out
- New Student Health Today box on making oral sex safe

Focus On: Reducing Risks for Chronic Diseases and Conditions

- Updated statistics regarding rates of bronchitis across populations
- Updated statistics regarding the prevalence of asthma and emphysema
- Updated information regarding the prevalence of migraines
- Updated discussion of IBS, IBD, Crohn's disease, and other conditions
- New chapter summaries and Pop Quiz

Chapter 14: Preparing for Aging, Death, and Dying

- Updated statistics on health care costs for older Americans
- Updated information regarding living arrangements of older Americans
- Updated coverage of the legality and controversy surrounding physician-assisted suicide

Chapter 15: Promoting Environmental Health

- Updated statistics on population growth and projections for the future
- Updated discussion of ecological footprints
- New coverage of the impact of human actions on the existence or extinction of other species
- Discussion of carbon tax and cap and trade policies to curb pollution
- Updated information on water use and access
- New tables on indoor air and water pollutants and their health and ecosystem effects

Chapter 16: Making Smart Health Care Choices

- Updated coverage of the ACA, with a special emphasis on young adults/college students
- New coverage of the diverse options for health care, including independent practice associations, HMOs, and others
- New and expanded coverage of Medicare Part A, B, and D, as well as Advantage plans and Medigap plans
- Updated stats on costs of healthcare, strategies for reducing health care and future issues

Focus On: Understanding Complementary and Integrative Health

- Updated coverage of alternative/integrative health approaches, rates of use, and considerations when making decisions about complementary and integrative health
- Updated coverage of complementary medical systems and specific methods of care
- Updated discussion of "natural" supplements
- New chapter summaries and Pop Quiz

TEXT FEATURES AND LEARNING AIDS

Health: The Basics includes the following special features, all of which have been revised and improved upon for this edition:

- **Chapter Learning Outcomes** summarize the main competencies students will gain from each chapter and alert students to the key concepts and are now explicitly tied to chapter sections. Focus On mini-chapters now also include learning outcomes.
- **Study Plans** tie all end-of-chapter material (including Chapter Review, Pop Quiz, and Think About It questions) to specific numbered Learning Outcomes and MasteringHealth™ assets.
- **What Do You Think?** critical-thinking questions appear throughout the text, encouraging students to pause and reflect on material they have read.
- **Why Should I Care?** features present information on the effects poor health habits have on students in the here and now.
- **Assess Yourself** boxes help students evaluate their health behaviors. The **Your Plan for Change** section within each box provides students with targeted suggestions for ways to implement change.
- **Skills for Behavior Change** boxes focus on practical strategies that students can use to improve health or reduce their risks from negative health behaviors.
- **Tech & Health** boxes cover the new technology innovations that can help students stay healthy.
- **Money & Health** boxes cover health topics from the financial perspective.

- **Points of View** boxes present viewpoints on a controversial health issue and ask students *Where Do You Stand?* questions, encouraging them to critically evaluate the information and consider their own opinions.
- **Health Headlines** boxes highlight new discoveries and research, as well as interesting trends in the health field.
- **Student Health Today** boxes focus attention on specific health and wellness issues that relate to today's college students.
- **Health in a Diverse World** boxes expand discussion of health topics to diverse groups within the United States and around the world.
- A **running glossary** in the margins defines terms where students first encounter them, emphasizing and supporting understanding of material.
- A **Behavior Change Contract** for students to fill out is included at the back of the book.

SUPPLEMENTARY MATERIALS

Instructor Supplements

- **MasteringHealth** (www.masteringhealthandnutrition.com or www.pearsonmastering.com). MasteringHealth coaches students through the toughest health topics. A variety of **Coaching Activities** guide students through key health concepts with interactive mini-lessons, complete with hints and wrong-answer feedback. **Reading Quizzes** (20 questions per chapter) ensure students have completed the assigned reading before class. *ABC News* videos stimulate classroom discussions and include multiple-choice questions with feedback for students. Assignable **Behavior Change Video Quiz** and **Which Path Would You Take?** activities ensure students complete and reflect on behavior change and health choices. **NutriTools** in the nutrition chapter allow students to combine and experiment with different food options and learn firsthand how to build healthier meals. **MP3 Tutor Sessions** relate to chapter content and come with multiple-choice questions that provide wrong-answer feedback. **Learning Catalytics** provides open-ended questions students can answer in real time. **Dynamic Study Modules** enable students to study effectively in an adaptive format. Instructors can also assign these for completion as a graded assignment prior to class.
- **Teaching Toolkit DVD.** The Teaching Toolkit DVD includes everything instructors need to prepare for their course and deliver a dynamic lecture in one convenient place. Resources include *ABC News* videos, Health Video Tutor videos, clicker questions, Quiz Show questions, PowerPoint lecture outlines, all figures and tables from the text, PDF and and Microsoft Word files of the *Instructor Resource and Support Manual,* PDF, RTF, and Microsoft Word files of the Test Bank, the Computerized Test Bank, the User's Quick Guide, *Teaching with Student Learning Outcomes, Teaching with Web 2.0, Great Ideas! Active Ways to Teach Health and Wellness, Behavior Change Log Book and Wellness Journal, Eat Right!, Live Right!,* and *Take Charge of Your Health* worksheets.
- ***ABC News* Videos** and **Health Video Tutors.** New *ABC News* videos, each 3 to 8 minutes long, and 27 Health Video Tutors accessible via QR codes in the text help instructors stimulate critical discussion in the classroom. Videos are embedded within PowerPoint lectures on the Teaching Toolkit DVD and through MasteringHealth.
- ***Instructor Resource and Support Manual***. This teaching tool provides chapter summaries, outlines, integrated *ABC News* video discussion questions, tips and strategies for managing large classrooms, ideas for in-class activities, and suggestions for integrating MasteringHealth and MyDietAnalysis into your course.
- **Test Bank.** The Test Bank incorporates Bloom's Taxonomy, or the higher order of learning, to help instructors create exams that encourage students to think analytically and critically. Test Bank questions are tagged to global and book-specific student learning outcomes.

Student Supplements

- **The Study Area of MasteringHealth™** is organized by learning areas. *Read It* houses the Pearson eText 2.0 as well as the Chapter Objectives and up-to-date health news. *See It* includes *ABC News* videos and the Behavior Change videos. *Hear It* contains MP3 Tutor Session files and audio-based case studies. *Do It* contains the choose-your-own-adventure-style Interactive Behavior Change Activities—Which Path Would You Take?, interactive NutriTools activities, critical-thinking Points of View questions, and Web links. *Review It* contains Practice Quizzes for each chapter, Flashcards, and Glossary. *Live It* will help jump-start students' behavior change projects with interactive Assess Yourself Worksheets and resources to plan change.
- **eText 2.0** comes complete with embedded *ABC News* videos and Health Video Tutors. eText 2.0 is mobile friendly and ADA accessible, available on smartphones and tablets, and includes instructor and student note taking, highlighting, bookmarking, and search functions.
- ***Behavior Change Log Book and Wellness Journal.*** This assessment tool helps students track daily exercise and nutritional intake and suggests topics for journal-based activities.
- ***Eat Right! Healthy Eating in College and Beyond.*** This booklet provides students with practical nutrition guidelines, shopper's guides, and recipes.
- ***Live Right! Beating Stress in College and Beyond.*** This booklet gives students tips for coping with stress during college and for the rest of their lives.
- **Digital 5-Step Pedometer.** This pedometer measures steps, distance (miles), activity time, and calories, and provides a time clock.
- **MyDietAnalysis** (www.mydietanalysis.com). Powered by ESHA Research, Inc., MyDietAnalysis features a database of nearly 20,000 foods and multiple reports. It allows students to track their diet and activity using up to three profiles and to generate and submit reports electronically.

ACKNOWLEDGMENTS

It is hard for me to believe that *Health: The Basics* is in its 12th edition! Who would have envisioned the evolution of these health texts even a decade ago? With the nearly limitless resources of the Internet, social networking sites, instantaneous access to national databases for statistics, and a myriad of interesting videos and late-breaking news reports, there is a media blitz of information to communicate with students. Each step along the way in planning, developing, and translating that information to students and instructors requires a tremendous amount of work from many dedicated people, and I cannot help but think how fortunate I have been to work with the gifted publishing professionals at Pearson. Through time constraints, decision making, and computer meltdowns, this group handled every issue, every obstacle with patience, professionalism, and painstaking attention to detail.

Susan Malloy, program manager, used her years of experience organizing and developing major health-related textbooks to direct the planning, implementing, and producing of this text. Her guidance was invaluable in making sure that the book continues to be a market-leading text. In particular, Susan's past experience in the successes of *Access to Health* and *Health: the Basics* over the years and her above-and-beyond the call of duty efforts have been greatly appreciated.

Kari Hopperstead, development editor, has worked on several editions of these books as well. Her attention to detail, fabulous work ethic, and knowledge of the health marketplace (and my books!) were invaluable in creating the structure and plan as well as providing creative direction during the pre-editorial phase.

In addition to Kari, Nic Albert did a fantastic job of providing guidance and editorial assistance in reining in an often "overzealous" author in streamlining page length and fine-tuning the many aspects of each chapter so that I didn't end up with a 1,000-page manuscript! He clearly has a solid grasp of what is important and did an excellent job of putting the pieces together in a concise and easy-to-understand manuscript.

Lastly, I would like to provide a special thank you to Lauren Beebe who has worked tirelessly and efficiently on both *Access to Health*, 14e, and *Health: The Basics*, 12e! Not only is Lauren a creative, highly skilled, and well-organized project manager; she has the temperament and professionalism to help move a project through time constraints, deadlines, and challenges, and to make sure that all of the great work from so many people comes to fruition in a top-notch product. Her skills in navigating production pitfalls, keeping the author and contributors on task, and meeting production deadlines were truly exemplary.

Further praise and thanks go to the highly skilled and hard-working, creative, and charismatic Senior Acquisitions Editor Michelle Cadden, who has helped to catapult this book into a competitive twenty-first century. From searching out and procuring cutting-edge technology to meet the demands of an increasingly savvy student to having her finger on the pulse of what instructors and students need in their classrooms today, Michelle's fresh approach and enthusiasm for the work were much appreciated, and Pearson is fortunate to have a new acquisitions editor with her experience and competence at the helm! Michelle has consistently been a key figure in moving the college/university health text to the next level.

Although these individuals were key contributors to the finished work, there were many other people who worked on this revision of *Health: The Basics*. At every level, I was extremely impressed by the work of key individuals. Thanks also to Jeanine Furino and the hard-working staff at Cenveo Publisher Services who put everything together to make a polished finished product. The talented artists at Lachina deserve many thanks for making our innovative art program a reality. Aimee Pavy, Senior Content Producer, put together our most innovative and comprehensive media package yet. Additional thanks go to the rest of the team at Pearson, especially Editorial Assistant Heidi Arndt, Development Manager Cathy Murphy, and Director of Development Barbara Yien.

The editorial and production teams are critical to a book's success, but I would be remiss if I didn't thank another key group who ultimately helps determine a book's success: the textbook representative and sales group and their hard-working, top-notch marketing leader, Executive Product Marketing Manager Neena Bali. From directing an outstanding marketing campaign to the everyday tasks of being responsive to instructor needs, Neena does a superb job of making sure that *Health: The Basics* gets into instructors' hands and that adopters receive the service they deserve. In keeping with my overall experiences with Pearson, the marketing and sales staffs are among the best of the best. I am very lucky to have them working with me on this project, and I want to extend a special thanks to all of them!

CONTRIBUTORS
TO THE 12TH EDITION

Many colleagues, students, and staff members have provided the feedback, reviews, extra time, assistance, and encouragement that have helped me meet the rigorous demands of publishing this book over the years. Whether acting as reviewers, generating new ideas, providing expert commentary, or revising chapters, each of these professionals has added his or her skills to our collective endeavor.

I would like to thank specific contributors to chapters in this edition. In order to make a book like this happen on a relatively short timeline, the talents of many specialists in the field must be combined. Whether contributing creative skills in writing, envisioning areas that will be critical to the current and future health needs of students, using their experiences to make topics come alive for students, or utilizing their professional expertise to ensure scientifically valid information, each of these individuals was carefully selected to help make this text the best that it can be. I couldn't do it without their help! As always, I would like to give particular thanks to Dr. Patricia Ketcham (Oregon State University), who has helped with the *Health: The Basics* series since its earliest beginnings. As associate director of health promotion in Student Health Services on campus, with specialties in health promotion and health behavior and substance abuse, Dr. Ketcham provides a unique perspective on the key challenges facing today's students. She contributed to revisions of Chapter 7, Recognizing and Avoiding Addiction and Drug Abuse; Chapter 8, Drinking Alcohol Responsibly and Ending Tobacco Use; Focus On: Enhancing Your Body Image; Chapter 14, Preparing for Aging, Death, and Dying; and Chapter 16, Making Smart Health Care Choices. Dr. Susan Dobie, associate professor in the School of Health, Physical Education, and Leisure Services at University of Northern Iowa, used her background in health promotion and health behavior and in teaching a diverse range of students to provide a fresh approach to revisions of Chapter 5, Connecting and Communicating in the Modern World; Focus On: Understanding Your Sexuality; and Chapter 6, Considering Your Reproductive Choices. Dr. Erica Jackson, associate professor in the Department of Public & Allied Health Sciences at Delaware State University, applied her wealth of fitness knowledge to update and enhance Chapter 11, Improving Your Personal Fitness. Deborah Landforce, instructor at Lane Community College, utilized her extensive background in counseling, relationships, and spirituality to provide a fresh and engaging update to Focus On: Cultivating Your Spiritual Health. With her outstanding background in nutrition science and applied dietary behavior, Dr. Kathy Munoz, professor in the Department of Kinesiology and Recreation Administration at Humbolt State University, provided an extensive revision and updating of Chapter 9, Nutrition: Eating for a Healthier You. Laura Bonazzoli, who has been a key part of developing and refining many aspects of this book over the last editions, used her considerable knowledge and skills in providing major revisions of Chapter 1, Accessing Your Health; Focus On: Improving Your Financial Health; and Focus On: Understanding Complementary and Alternative Medicine.

REVIEWERS FOR THE 12TH EDITION

With each new edition of *Health: The Basics*, we have built on the combined expertise of many colleagues throughout the country who are dedicated to the education and behavioral changes of students. We thank the many reviewers who have made such valuable contributions to the past 11 editions of *Health: The Basics*. For the 12th edition, reviewers who have helped us continue this tradition of excellence include the following:

Tia Bennett, Northeastern State University
Daniel Czech, Georgia Southern University
Andy Harcrow, University of Alabama
Sylvette La Touche-Howard, University of Maryland
Theodore Murray, Monroe Community College
Adam Parker, Angelo State University
Carole Sloan, Henry Ford College
Glenda Warren, University of the Cumberlands
Brian Witkov, Salem State University
Sharon Woodard, Wake Forest University

REVIEWERS FOR MASTERINGHEALTH™

We continue to thank the following members of the Faculty Advisory Board, who offered us valuable insights that helped develop MasteringHealth for the previous edition: Steve Hartman (Citrus College), William Huber (County College of Morris), Kris Jankovitz (Cal Poly), Stasi Kasaianchuk (Oregon State University), Lynn Long (University of North Carolina Wilmington), Ayanna Lyles (California University of Pennsylvania), Steven Namanny (Utah Valley University), Karla Rues (Ozarks Technical Community College), Debra Smith (Ohio University), Sheila Stepp (SUNY Orange), and Mary Winfrey-Kovell (Ball State University). For the 12th edition the following people contributed content:

Laura Bonazzoli
Lorin Hawley
Melanie Healy
John Murdzek
Dena Pistor
Karla Rues
Bruce Turchetta

Many thanks to all!
Rebecca J. Donatelle, PhD

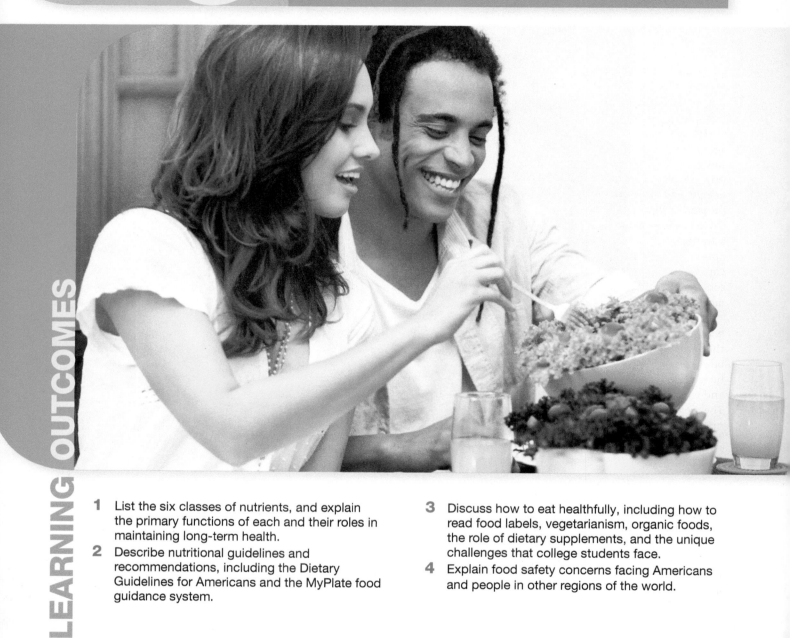

9 Nutrition: Eating for a Healthier You

LEARNING OUTCOMES

1 List the six classes of nutrients, and explain the primary functions of each and their roles in maintaining long-term health.

2 Describe nutritional guidelines and recommendations, including the Dietary Guidelines for Americans and the MyPlate food guidance system.

3 Discuss how to eat healthfully, including how to read food labels, vegetarianism, organic foods, the role of dietary supplements, and the unique challenges that college students face.

4 Explain food safety concerns facing Americans and people in other regions of the world.

Advice about food comes at us from all directions: from the Internet, popular magazines, television, friends, and neighbors. Even when backed by research, this advice can be contradictory. Some studies indicate that a balanced high-fat diet can be healthful, whereas other studies support consuming a low-fat diet. Choosing what to eat and how much to eat from this media-driven array of food advice can be mind-boggling. For some, this can cause unnecessary anxiety about eating and lead to a lifetime of cycling on and off diets.[1] Why does something that can be a source of pleasure end up being a problem for so many of us? What influences our eating habits, and how can we learn to eat more healthfully?

The answers to these questions aren't as simple as they may seem. When was the last time you ate because you felt truly hungry? True **hunger** occurs when our brains initiate a physiological response that prompts us to seek food for the energy and **nutrients** that our bodies require to maintain proper functioning. Often, people in the United States don't eat in response to hunger—instead, we eat because of **appetite**, a learned psychological desire to consume food. Hunger and appetite are not the only forces influencing our desire to eat. Cultural factors, food advertising, perceived nutritional value, social interaction, emotions, and financial means are other factors.

Nutrition is the science that investigates the relationship between physiological function and the essential elements of the foods we eat. With an understanding of nutrition, you will be able to make more informed choices about your diet. Your health depends largely on what you eat, how much you eat, and the amount of exercise that you get throughout your life. The next few chapters focus on fundamental principles of nutrition, weight management, and exercise.

LO 1 | ESSENTIAL NUTRIENTS FOR HEALTH

List the six classes of nutrients, and explain the primary functions of each and their roles in maintaining long-term health.

Food provides the chemicals we need for activity and body maintenance. Our bodies cannot synthesize certain *essential nutrients* (or cannot synthesize them in adequate amounts); we must obtain them from the foods we eat. Of the six groups of essential nutrients, the four we need in the largest amounts—water, proteins, carbohydrates, and fats—are called *macronutrients*. The other

WHY SHOULD I CARE?

The nutritional choices you make during college can have both immediate and lasting effects on your health. Thousands of studies associate what we eat with chronic diseases such as diabetes, heart disease, hypertension, stroke, osteoporosis, and many types of cancer.

two groups—vitamins and minerals—are needed in smaller amounts, so they are called *micronutrients*.

Before the body can use food, the digestive system must break down larger food particles into smaller, more usable forms. The **digestive process** is the sequence of functions by which the body breaks down foods into molecules small enough to be absorbed, and excretes the wastes.

Recommended Intakes for Nutrients

In the next sections, we discuss each nutrient group and identify how much of each you need. These recommended amounts are known as the **Dietary Reference Intakes (DRIs)** and are published by the Food and Nutrition Board of the Institute of Medicine. The DRIs establish the amount of each nutrient needed to prevent deficiencies or reduce the risk of chronic disease, as well as identify maximum safe intake levels for healthy people. The DRIs are umbrella guidelines and include the following categories:

- **Recommended Dietary Allowances (RDAs)** are daily nutrient intake levels meeting the nutritional needs of 97 to 98 percent of healthy individuals.
- **Adequate Intakes (AIs)** are daily intake levels assumed to be adequate for most healthy people. AIs are used when there isn't enough research to support establishing an RDA.
- **Tolerable Upper Intake Levels (ULs)** are the highest amounts of a nutrient that an individual can consume daily without risking adverse health effects.
- **Acceptable Macronutrient Distribution Ranges (AMDRs)** are ranges of protein, carbohydrate, and fat intake that provide adequate nutrition, and they are associated with a reduced risk for chronic disease.

hunger The physiological impulse to seek food.

nutrients The constituents of food that sustain humans physiologically: water, proteins, carbohydrates, fats, vitamins, and minerals.

appetite The learned desire to eat; normally accompanies hunger but is more psychological than physiological.

nutrition The science that investigates the relationship between physiological function and the essential elements of foods eaten.

digestive process The process by which the body breaks down foods into smaller components and either absorbs or excretes them.

Dietary Reference Intakes (DRIs) Set of recommended intakes for each nutrient published by the Institute of Medicine.

Whereas the RDAs, AIs, and ULs are expressed as amounts—usually milligrams (mg) or micrograms (µg)—AMDRs are expressed as percentages. The AMDR for protein, for example, is 10 to 35 percent, meaning that no less than 10 percent and no more than 35 percent of the calories you consume should come from proteins. But that raises a new question: What are calories?

Calories

A *kilocalorie* is a unit of measure used to quantify the amount of energy in food. On nutrition labels and in consumer publications, the term is shortened to **calorie.** *Energy* is defined as the capacity to do work. We derive energy from the energy-containing nutrients in the foods we eat. These energy-containing nutrients—proteins, carbohydrates, and fats—provide calories. Vitamins, minerals, and water do not. TABLE 9.1 shows the caloric needs for various individuals.

Water: A Crucial Nutrient

Humans can survive for several weeks without food but only for about 1 week without water. **Dehydration**, a state of abnormal depletion of body fluids, can develop within a single day, especially in a hot climate. Too much water can also pose a serious risk to your health. This condition, *hyponatremia,* is characterized by low sodium levels.

The human body consists of 50 to 70 percent water by weight. The water in our system bathes cells; aids in fluid, electrolyte, and acid-base balance; and helps regulate body temperature. Water is the major component of our blood, which carries oxygen, nutrients, and hormones and other substances to body cells and removes metabolic wastes.

> **calorie** A unit of measure that indicates the amount of energy obtained from a particular food.
>
> **dehydration** Abnormal depletion of body fluids; a result of lack of water.
>
> **proteins** Large molecules made up of chains of amino acids; essential constituents of all body cells.
>
> **amino acids** The nitrogen-containing building blocks of protein.
>
> **essential amino acids** The nine basic nitrogen-containing building blocks of human proteins that must be obtained from foods.

Individual needs for water vary drastically according to dietary factors, age, size, overall health, environmental temperature and humidity levels, and exercise. The general recommendations for women are approximately 9 cups of total water from all beverages and foods each day and for men an average of 13 cups.[2] We usually get the fluids we need each day through the water and other beverages we consume, as well as through the food we eat. In fact, fruits and vegetables are 80 to 95 percent water, meats are more than 50 percent water, and even dry bread and cheese are about 35 percent water! Contrary to popular opinion, caffeinated drinks, including coffee, tea, and soda, also count toward total fluid intake. Consumed in moderation, caffeinated beverages have not been found to dehydrate people whose bodies are used to caffeine.[3]

There are situations in which a person needs additional fluids in order to stay properly hydrated. It is important to drink extra fluids when you have a fever or an illness involving vomiting or diarrhea. Anyone with kidney function problems or who tends to develop kidney stones may need more water, as may people with diabetes or cystic fibrosis. The elderly and very young also may have increased water needs. When the weather heats up, or when you exercise, work,

DO IT! NUTRITOOLS

Complete the **Know Your Protein Sources** activity, available on MasteringHealth™

TABLE 9.1 | Estimated Daily Calorie Needs

	Calorie Range		
	Sedentary[a]		Active[b]
Children			
2–3 years old	1,000	→	1,400
Females			
4–8 years old	1,200	→	1,800
9–13	1,400	→	2,200
14–18	1,800	→	2,400
19–30	1,800	→	2,400
31–50	1,800	→	2,200
51+	1,600	→	2,200
Males			
4–8 years old	1,200	→	2,000
9–13	1,600	→	2,600
14–18	2,000	→	3,200
19–30	2,400	→	3,000
31–50	2,200	→	3,000
51+	2,000	→	2,800

[a] A lifestyle that includes only the light physical activity associated with typical day-to-day life.

[b] A lifestyle that includes physical activity equivalent to walking more than 3 miles per day at 3 to 4 miles per hour, in addition to the light physical activity associated with typical day-to-day life.

Source: U.S. Department of Agriculture and U.S. Department of Health and Human Services, *Dietary Guidelines for Americans, 2010,* 7th ed. (Washington, DC: U.S. Government Printing Office).

or engage in other activities in which you sweat profusely, extra water is needed to keep your body's core temperature within a normal range. If you are an athlete and wonder about water consumption, visit the American College of Sports Medicine's website (www.acsm.org) to download its brochure, "Selecting and Effectively Using Hydration for Fitness."[4]

Proteins

Next to water, **proteins** are the most abundant substances in the human body. Proteins are major components of living cells and are called the "body builders" because of their role in developing and repairing bone, muscle, skin, and blood cells. They are the key elements of antibodies that protect us from disease, enzymes that control chemical activities in the body, and many hormones that regulate body functions. Proteins also supply an alternative source of energy to cells when fats and carbohydrates are not available. Specifically, every gram of protein you eat provides 4 calories. (There are about 28 grams in an ounce by weight.) Adequate protein in the diet is vital to many body functions and ultimately to survival.

Your body breaks down proteins into smaller nitrogen-containing molecules known as **amino acids,** the building blocks of protein. Nine of the 20 different amino acids needed by the body are termed **essential amino acids,** which means the body must obtain them from the diet; the other 11 amino

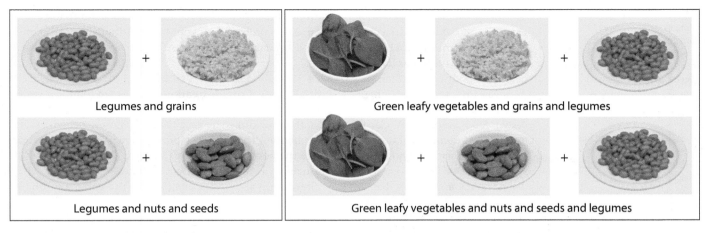

| Legumes and grains | Green leafy vegetables and grains and legumes |
| Legumes and nuts and seeds | Green leafy vegetables and nuts and seeds and legumes |

FIGURE 9.1 **Foods Providing Complementary Amino Acids** Complementary combinations of plant-based foods can provide all essential amino acids. In some cases, you might need to combine three sources of protein to supply all nine; however, the foods do not necessarily have to be eaten in the same meal. Here, two of the limited amino acids in leafy green vegetables are supplied by either grains or nuts and seeds, and the third is found in legumes.

acids are considered nonessential because the body can make them. Dietary protein that supplies all the essential amino acids is called **complete protein.** Typically, protein from animal products is complete.

Nearly all proteins from plant sources are **incomplete proteins** that lack one or more of the essential amino acids. However, it is easy to combine plant foods to produce a complete protein meal (**FIGURE 9.1**). Plant foods rich in incomplete proteins include *legumes* (beans, lentils, peas, peanuts, and soy products); *grains* (e.g., wheat, corn, rice, and oats); and *nuts and seeds.* Certain vegetables, such as leafy green vegetables and broccoli, also contribute valuable plant proteins. Consuming a variety of foods from these categories will provide all the essential amino acids.

Although protein deficiency poses a threat to the global population, few Americans suffer from protein deficiencies. In fact, the average American consumes more than 79 grams of protein daily, much of it from high-fat animal flesh and dairy products.[5] The AMDR for protein is 10 to 35 percent of calories. Adults should consume about 0.8 gram (g) per kilogram (kg) of body weight.[6] To calculate your protein needs, divide your body weight in pounds by 2.2 to get your weight in kilograms, then multiply by 0.8. The result is your recommended protein intake per day. For example, a woman who weighs 130 pounds should consume about 47 grams of protein each day. A 6-ounce steak provides 53 grams of protein—more than she needs!

People who need to eat extra protein include pregnant women and patients fighting a serious infection, recovering from surgery or blood loss, or recovering from burns. In these instances, proteins that are lost to cellular repair and development need to be replaced. Athletes also require more protein to build and repair muscle fibers.[7] In addition, a sedentary person may find it easier to stay in energy balance when consuming a diet with a higher percentage of protein and a lower percentage of carbohydrate. Why? Proteins make a person feel full for a longer period of time because protein takes longer to digest than carbohydrates. Protein also releases certain satiety hormones that contribute to feeling full longer.

Carbohydrates

Carbohydrates supply us with the energy we need to sustain normal daily activity. In comparison to proteins or fats, carbohydrates are broken down more quickly and efficiently, yielding a fuel called glucose. All body cells can burn glucose for fuel; moreover, glucose is the only fuel that red blood cells can use and is the primary fuel for the brain. Carbohydrates are the best fuel for moderate to intense exercise because they can be readily broken down to glucose even when we're breathing hard and our muscle cells are getting less oxygen.

Like proteins, carbohydrates provide 4 calories per gram. The RDA for adults is 130 grams of carbohydrate per day.[8] There are two major types: simple and complex.

Simple Carbohydrates **Simple carbohydrates** or *simple sugars* are found naturally in fruits, many vegetables, and dairy. The most common form of simple carbohydrates is *glucose*. Fruits and berries contain *fructose* (commonly called *fruit sugar*). Glucose and fructose are **monosaccharides.** Eventually, the human body converts all types of simple sugars to glucose to provide energy to cells.

Disaccharides are combinations of two monosaccharides. Perhaps the best-known example is *sucrose* (granulated table sugar). *Lactose* (milk sugar), found in milk and milk products, and

complete proteins Proteins that contain all nine of the essential amino acids.

incomplete proteins Proteins that lack one or more of the essential amino acids.

carbohydrates Basic nutrients that supply the body with glucose, the energy form most commonly used to sustain normal activity.

simple carbohydrates A carbohydrate made up of only one sugar molecule, or of two sugar molecules bonded together; also called simple sugars.

monosaccharides A sugar that is not broken down further during digestion, including fructose and glucose.

disaccharides Combinations of two monosaccharides such as lactose, maltose, and sucrose.

DO IT! NUTRITOOLS

Complete the **Know Your Carbohydrate Sources** activity, available on MasteringHealth™

complex carbohydrates A carbohydrate that can be broken down during digestion into monosaccharides or disaccharides; also called a polysaccharide.

starches Polysaccharides that are the storage forms of glucose in plants.

glycogen The polysaccharide form in which glucose is stored in the liver and, to a lesser extent, in muscles.

fiber The indigestible portion of plant foods that helps move food through the digestive system and softens stools by absorbing water.

whole grains Grains that are milled in their complete form and thus include the bran, germ, and endosperm, with only the husk removed.

maltose (malt sugar) are other examples of common disaccharides. Disaccharides must be broken down into monosaccharides before the body can use them.

Sugar is found in high amounts in a wide range of processed food products. A classic example is the amount of sugar in one can of soda: more than 10 teaspoons per can! Moreover, such diverse items as ketchup, barbecue sauce, and flavored coffee creamers derive 30 to 65 percent of their calories from sugar. Read food labels carefully before purchasing. If *sugar* or one of its aliases (including *high fructose corn syrup* and *cornstarch*) appears near the top of the ingredients list, then that product contains a lot of sugar and is probably not your best nutritional bet. Also, most labels list the amount of sugar as a percentage of total calories.

Complex Carbohydrates: Starches and Glycogen

Complex carbohydrates are found in grains, cereals, legumes, and other vegetables. Also called *polysaccharides,* they are formed by long chains of monosaccharides. Like disaccharides, they must be broken down into simple sugars before the body can use them. *Starches, glycogen,* and *fiber* are the main types of complex carbohydrates.

Starches make up the majority of the complex carbohydrate group and come from flours, breads, pasta, rice, corn, oats, barley, potatoes, and related foods. The body breaks down these complex carbohydrates into glucose, which can be easily absorbed by cells and used as energy or stored in the muscles and the liver as **glycogen.** When the body requires a sudden burst of energy, it breaks down glycogen into glucose.

Complex Carbohydrates: Fiber

Fiber, sometimes referred to as "bulk" or "roughage," is the indigestible portion of plant foods that helps move foods through the digestive system, delays absorption of cholesterol and other nutrients, and softens stools by absorbing water. Dietary fiber is found only in plant foods, such as fruits, vegetables, nuts, and grains.[9]

Fiber is either *soluble* or *insoluble.* Soluble fibers, such as pectins, gums, and mucilages, dissolve in water, form gel-like substances, and can be digested easily by bacteria in the colon. Major food sources of soluble fiber include citrus fruits, berries, oat bran, dried beans, and some vegetables. Insoluble fibers, such as lignins and cellulose, typically do not dissolve in water and cannot be fermented by bacteria in the colon. They are found in most fruits and vegetables and in **whole grains**, such as brown rice, wheat, bran, and whole-grain breads and cereals (see **FIGURE 9.2**). The AMDR for carbohydrates is 45 to

Studies have shown that eating 2.5 servings of whole grains per day can reduce cardiovascular disease risk by as much as 21%. But are people getting the message? One nutrition study showed that only 8% of U.S. adults consume 3 or more servings of whole grains each day, and 42% ate no whole grains at all on a given day.

Source: Huang, T., et al. "Consumption of Whole Grains and Cereal Fiber and Total and Cause-specific Mortality: Prospective Analysis of 367,442 Individuals," *BMC Medicine* 13, no 1(2015): 59, doi: 10.1186/s12916-015-0294-7

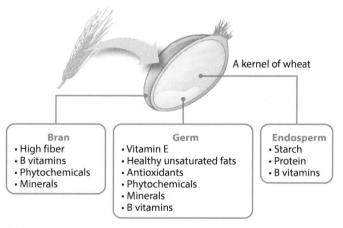

A kernel of wheat

Bran	Germ	Endosperm
• High fiber	• Vitamin E	• Starch
• B vitamins	• Healthy unsaturated fats	• Protein
• Phytochemicals	• Antioxidants	• B vitamins
• Minerals	• Phytochemicals	
	• Minerals	
	• B vitamins	

FIGURE 9.2 Anatomy of a Whole Grain Whole grains are more nutritious than refined grains because they contain the bran, germ, and endosperm of the seed—sources of fiber, vitamins, minerals, and beneficial phytochemicals (chemical compounds that occur naturally in plants).

Source: Adapted from Joan Salge Blake, Kathy D. Munoz, and Stella Volpe, *Nutrition: From Science to You,* 1st ed. © 2010, page 138. Printed and electronically reproduced by permission of Pearson Education, Inc., Upper Saddle River, New Jersey.

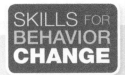
60 percent of total calories, and health experts recommend that the majority of this intake be fiber-rich carbohydrates.

Fiber protects against obesity, colon and rectal cancers, heart disease, constipation, and possibly even type 2 diabetes, so most experts believe that Americans should double their current consumption of dietary fiber—to 25 grams per day for women and 38 grams per day for men.[10] What's the best way to increase your intake of dietary fiber? Eat fewer refined carbohydrates in favor of more fiber-rich carbohydrates, including whole-grain breads and cereals, fresh fruits, legumes and other vegetables, nuts, and seeds. As with most nutritional advice, however, too much of a good thing can pose problems. A sudden increase in dietary fiber may cause flatulence (intestinal gas), cramping, or bloating. Consume plenty of water or other (sugar-free!) liquids to reduce such side effects. Find out more about the benefits of fiber in the Skills for Behavior Change box.

Fats

Fats, perhaps the most misunderstood nutrient, are the most energy dense, providing 9 calories per gram. Fats are a significant source of our body's fuel. Fats also play a vital role in maintaining healthy skin and hair, insulating body organs against shock, maintaining body temperature, and promoting healthy cell function. Fats make foods taste better and carry the fat-soluble vitamins A, D, E, and K to cells. They also make you feel full after eating.

Despite the fact that fats perform all these functions, we are constantly urged to cut back on them, because some fats are less healthy than others and because excessive consumption of fats can lead to weight gain and cardiovascular disease.

Triglycerides make up about 95 percent of total body fat and are the most common form of fat in foods. When we consume too many calories from any source, the liver converts the excess into triglycerides, which are stored in fat cells throughout our bodies. The remaining 5 percent of body fat is composed of substances such as **cholesterol.** The ratio of total cholesterol to a group of compounds called **high-density lipoproteins (HDLs)** is important in determining risk for heart disease. Lipoproteins facilitate the transport of cholesterol in the blood. High-density lipoproteins are capable of transporting more cholesterol than are **low-density lipoproteins (LDLs).** Whereas LDLs transport cholesterol to the body's cells, HDLs transport circulating cholesterol to the liver for metabolism and elimination from the body. Past research has indicated that people with a high percentage of HDLs appear to be at lower risk for developing cholesterol-clogged arteries. However, new research has raised questions about the role of HDL and LDL in cardiovascular health. (See Chapter 12 for information about recent research on cholesterol, inflammation, and other risks for cardiovascular disease.)

fats Basic nutrients composed of carbon and hydrogen atoms; needed for the proper functioning of cells, insulation of body organs against shock, maintenance of body temperature, and healthy skin and hair.

triglycerides The most common form of fat in our food supply and in the body; made up of glycerol and three fatty acid chains.

cholesterol A substance that, like fats, is not soluble in water. It is found in animal-based foods and is synthesized by the body. Although essential to functioning, cholesterol circulating in the blood can accumulate on the inner walls of blood vessels.

high-density lipoproteins (HDLs) Compounds that facilitate the transport of cholesterol in the blood to the liver for metabolism and elimination from the body.

low-density lipoproteins (LDLs) Compounds that facilitate the transport cholesterol in the blood to the body's cells.

saturated fats Fats that are unable to hold any more hydrogen in their chemical structure; derived mostly from animal sources; solid at room temperature.

unsaturated fats Fats that have room for more hydrogen in their chemical structure; derived mostly from plants; liquid at room temperature.

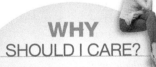

WHY SHOULD I CARE?

Cholesterol can accumulate on the inner walls of arteries and narrow the channels through which blood flows. This buildup, called plaque, is a major cause of *atherosclerosis,* a component of cardiovascular disease.

Types of Dietary Fats Triglycerides contain *fatty acid* chains of oxygen, carbon, and hydrogen atoms. Fatty acid chains that cannot hold any more hydrogen in their chemical structure are called **saturated fats.** They generally come from animal sources, such as meat, dairy, and poultry products, and are solid at room temperature. **Unsaturated fats** have room for additional hydrogen atoms in their chemical structure and are liquid at room temperature. They generally come from plants and include most vegetable oils.

The terms *monounsaturated fatty acids* (*MUFAs*) and *polyunsaturated fatty acids* (*PUFAs*) refer to the relative number of hydrogen atoms that

The AMDR for fats is 20 to 35 percent of calories, with 5 to 10 percent coming from essential fatty acids. Within this range, we should minimize our intake of saturated fats.

Avoiding *Trans* Fatty Acids For decades, Americans shunned butter, cream, and other foods high in saturated fats. What they didn't know is that some processed foods low in animal fats, such as margarine, could be just as harmful. These processed foods contain **trans fatty acids**. Research shows that just a 2 percent caloric intake of these fats is associated with a 23 percent increased risk for heart disease and a 47 percent increased chance of sudden cardiac death.[12]

Although a small amount of *trans* fatty acids do occur in some animal products, the great majority are in processed foods made with partially hydrogenated oils (PHOs).[13] PHOs are produced when food manufacturers add hydrogen to a plant oil, solidifying it, helping it resist rancidity, and giving the food in which it is used a longer shelf life. The hydrogenation process straightens out the fatty acid chain so that it is more like a saturated fatty acid, and it has similar harmful effects, lowering HDLs and raising LDLs. *Trans* fats have been used in margarines, many commercial baked goods, and restaurant deep-fried foods.

In 2013, the U.S. Food and Drug Administration (FDA) issued a preliminary determination that PHOs are no longer recognized as safe for consumption. If it is finalized, foods

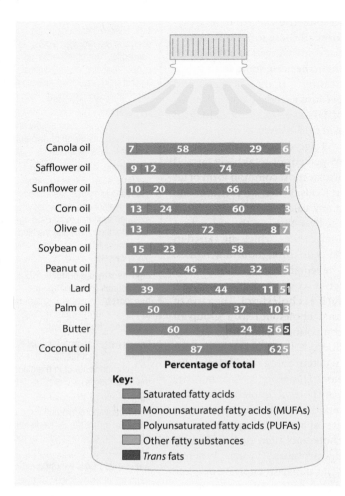

FIGURE 9.3 Percentages of Saturated, Polyunsaturated, Monounsaturated, and *Trans* Fats in Common Vegetable Oils

are missing in a fatty acid chain. Peanut, canola, and olive oils are high in monounsaturated fats, which appear to lower LDL levels and increase HDL levels. Corn, sunflower, and safflower oils are high in polyunsaturated fats. For a breakdown of the types of fats in common vegetable oils, see FIGURE 9.3.

Two specific types of polyunsaturated fatty acids essential to a healthful diet are *omega-3 fatty acids* (found in many types of fatty fish; dark green, leafy vegetables; walnuts; and flaxseeds) and *omega-6 fatty acids* (found in corn, soybean, peanut, sunflower, and cottonseed oils). Both are classified as *essential fatty acids*—that is, those we must receive from our diets—because the body cannot synthesize them yet requires them for functioning. The most important fats within these groups are *linoleic acid*, an omega-6 fatty acid, and *alpha-linolenic acid*, an omega-3 fatty acid. The body needs these to make hormone-like compounds that control immune function, pain perception, and inflammation, to name a few key benefits. You may also have heard of EPA (eicosapentaenoic) and DHA (docosahexaenoic acid). These are derivatives of alpha-linolenic acid that are found abundantly in oily fish such as salmon and tuna and are associated with a reduced risk for heart disease.[11]

trans fats (trans fatty acids) Fatty acids that are produced when polyunsaturated oils are hydrogenated to make them more solid.

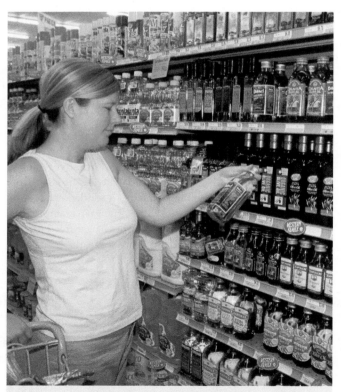

All fats are not the same, and your body needs some fat to function. Try to reduce saturated fats, which are in meat, full-fat dairy, and poultry products, and avoid *trans* fats, which typically come in stick margarines, commercially baked goods, and deep-fried foods. Replace these with unsaturated fats, such as those in plant oils, fatty fish, and nuts and seeds.

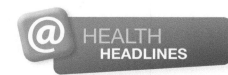
COCONUT OIL
Friend or Foe?

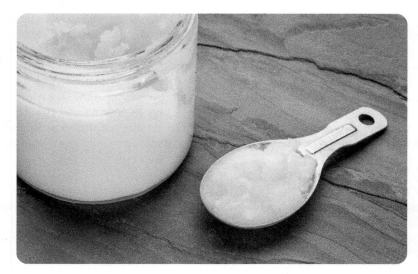

If you're a label reader, you've probably noticed coconut oil on the ingredients list of milk, spreads, and yogurt, or even seen jars filled with a solid milky-white fat on the grocery store shelves. Once thought of as an unhealthy, saturated fat, coconut oil is making a comeback, and is being touted as a healthy alternative to other oils.

The difference between coconut oil and other more commonly used oils is that 87 percent of the fatty acids in coconut oil are mostly saturated. Olive oil, in comparison, is 15 percent saturated. Coconut oil also doesn't contain any polyunsaturated essential fatty acids, but is rich in vitamin E and a variety of phytochemicals. Does coconut oil provide unique health benefits beyond those nutrients?

Some have touted coconut oil may reduce the risk of heart disease, improve weight loss, cure Alzheimer's disease, or protect against infections. The original study that started this craze was observing Polynesian people who have little heart disease but ingest mostly fat from coconuts. The researchers did not explore whether consuming coconut oil reduced the risk of heart disease. There is also no scientific evidence that switching to coconut oil from polyunsaturated oils improves weight loss, cures Alzheimer's disease, or protects against infections.

Health professionals are divided over whether to recommend replacing heart-healthy polyunsaturated vegetable oils with coconut oil. There is a larger body of research in humans that monounsaturated and polyunsaturated fatty acids lower blood cholesterol levels and reduce the risk of heart disease, but little evidence that coconut oil is beneficial for heart health, weight loss, or Alzheimer's. At this point, most health professionals advise against adding coconut oil to your diet.

Sources: Tropical Traditions, "What is Virgin Coconut Oil?," Accessed April 2015, www.tropical-traditions.com/what_is_virgin_coconut_oil.htm; F. Hamam, "Specialty Lipids in Health and Disease," *Food and Nutrition Sciences* 4 (2013): 63–70; American Heart Association, "Fats and Oils: AHA Recommendations," Accessed April 2015, Available at www.heart.org.

---

containing PHOs will no longer be sold legally in the United States.[14] In the meantime, *trans* fats are being removed from most foods, and if they are present, they must be clearly indicated on food packaging. If you see the words *partially hydrogenated oils, fractionated oils, shortening, lard,* or *hydrogenation* on a food label, then *trans* fats are present.

New Fat Advice: Is More Fat Ever Better?

Some researchers worry that we have gone too far in our anti-fat frenzy. In fact, some studies have shown that balanced high-fat diets produce significant improvements in weight loss, blood fat, and blood glucose measures.[15] Balance is the key. No more than 7 to 10 percent of your total calories should come from saturated fat, and no more than 35 percent should come from all forms of fat.[16] Follow these guidelines to add more healthy fats to your diet:

■ Eat fatty fish (herring, mackerel, salmon, sardines, or tuna) at least twice weekly.
■ Use olive, peanut, soy, and canola oils instead of butter or lard. See **Health Headlines** for more information on coconut oil.

■ Add healthy amounts of green leafy vegetables, walnuts, walnut oil, and ground flaxseed to your diet.

Follow these guidelines to reduce your overall intake of less-healthy fats:

■ Read the Nutrition Facts on food labels to find out how much fat is in your food.
■ Chill meat-based soups and stews, scrape off any fat that hardens on top, and then reheat to serve.
■ Fill up on fruits and vegetables.
■ Hold the creams and sauces.
■ Avoid all products with *trans* fatty acids. For healthy toppings on your bread, try vegetable spreads, bean spreads, nut butters, sugar-free jams, fat-free cheese, etc.
■ Choose lean meats, fish, or skinless poultry. Broil or bake whenever possible. Drain off fat after cooking.

DO IT! NUTRITOOLS

Complete the **Know Your Fat Sources** activity, available on **MasteringHealth™**

- Choose fewer cold cuts, bacon, sausages, hot dogs, and organ meats.
- Select nonfat and low-fat dairy products.

Vitamins

Vitamins are organic compounds that promote growth and are essential to life and health. Every minute of every day, vitamins help maintain nerves and skin, produce blood cells, build bones and teeth, heal wounds, and convert food energy to body energy—and they do all this without adding any calories to your diet.

Vitamins are classified as either *fat soluble,* which means they are absorbed through the intestinal tract with the help of fats, or *water soluble,* which means they are dissolved easily in water. Vitamins A, D, E, and K are fat soluble; B-complex vitamins and vitamin C are water soluble. Fat-soluble vitamins tend to be stored in the body, and toxic levels can accumulate if people regularly consume more than the UL. Excesses of water-soluble vitamins generally are excreted in the urine and rarely cause toxicity problems. See TABLE 9.2 for functions, recommended intake amounts, and food sources of specific vitamins.

Vitamin D Vitamin D, the sunshine vitamin, is formed from a compound in the skin when exposed to the sun's ultraviolet rays. In most people, an adequate amount of vitamin D can be synthesized with 5 to 30 minutes of sun on the face, neck, hands, arms, and legs twice a week, without sunscreen.[17]

TABLE **9.2** | A Guide to Vitamins

Vitamin Name	Primary Functions	Recommended Intake	Reliable Food Sources
Thiamin	Carbohydrate and protein metabolism	Men: 1.2 mg/day Women: 1.1 mg/day	Pork, fortified cereals, enriched rice and pasta, peas, tuna, legumes
Riboflavin	Carbohydrate and fat metabolism	Men: 1.3 mg/day Women: 1.1 mg/day	Beef liver, shrimp, dairy foods, fortified cereals, enriched breads and grains
Niacin	Carbohydrate and fat metabolism	Men: 16 mg/day Women: 14 mg/day	Meat/fish/poultry, fortified cereals, enriched breads and grains, canned tomato products
Vitamin B_6	Carbohydrate and amino acid metabolism	Men and women aged 19–50: 1.3 mg/day	Garbanzo beans, meat/fish/poultry, fortified cereals, white potatoes
Folate	Amino acid metabolism and DNA synthesis	Men: 400 µg/day Women: 400 µg/day	Fortified cereals, enriched breads and grains, spinach, legumes, spinach, liver
Vitamin B_{12}	Formation of blood cells and nervous system	Men: 2.4 µg/day Women: 2.4 µg/day	Shellfish, all cuts of meat/fish/poultry, dairy foods, fortified cereals
Pantothenic acid	Fat metabolism	Men: 5 mg/day Women: 5 mg/day	Meat/fish/poultry, shiitake mushrooms, fortified cereals, egg yolks
Biotin	Carbohydrate, fat, and protein metabolism	Men: 30 µg/day Women: 30 µg/day	Nuts, egg yolks
Vitamin C	Collagen synthesis; iron absorption, and promotes healing	Men: 90 mg/day Women: 75 mg/day Smokers: 35 mg more per day than RDA	Sweet peppers, citrus fruits and juices, broccoli, strawberries, kiwi
Vitamin A	Immune function, maintains epithelial cells, healthy bones and vision	Men: 900 µg Women: 700 µg	Beef and chicken liver, egg yolks, milk Carotenoids found in spinach, carrots, mango, apricots, cantaloupe, pumpkin, yams
Vitamin D	Promotes calcium absorption and healthy bones	Adult aged 19–70: 15 µg/day (600 IU/day)	Canned salmon and mackerel, milk, fortified cereals
Vitamin E	Protects cell membranes, and acts as a powerful antioxidant	Men: 15 mg/day Women: 15 mg/day	Sunflower seeds, almonds, vegetable oils, fortified cereals
Vitamin K	Blood coagulation and bone metabolism	Men: 120 µg/day Women: 90 µg/day	Kale, spinach, turnip greens, Brussels sprouts

Note: RDA: Recommended Dietary Allowance; AI: Adequate Intakes; UL: Tolerable Upper Level Intakes. Values are for all adults aged 19 and older, except as noted. Values increase among women who are pregnant or lactating.

Source: Data from J. Thompson and M. Manore, Nutrition: An Applied Approach, 2nd ed., © 2009; The National Academies, "Dietary Reference Intakes for Calcium and Vitamin D," 2011, www.iom.edu.

However, the sun is not high enough in the sky during late fall to early spring in northern climates to allow for vitamin D synthesis. For people who cannot rely on the sun to meet their daily vitamin D needs, consuming vitamin D–fortified milk, yogurt, soy milk, cereals, and fatty fish, such as salmon, can also supply this vitamin.

Vitamin D is essential for the body's regulation of calcium, the primary mineral component of bone. It also assists in the process of calcification by which bone minerals are crystallized. For these reasons, a deficiency of vitamin D can promote loss of bone density and strength, a condition called *osteoporosis.* Two other bone disorders, *rickets* in children, and its adult version, *osteomalacia,* both of which cause softening and distortion of the bones, can also be prevented with adequate intake of vitamin D.[18] Vitamin D also helps fight infections, lowers blood pressure, reduces the risk of developing diabetes mellitus, and may reduce the growth of cancer cells. Breast and prostate cancer, heart disease, and stroke have also been connected to inadequate vitamin D.

More is not always better, however.[19] Too much vitamin D, generally from excessive intake of vitamin D supplements, can reduce appetite and cause nausea, vomiting, and constipation. Excess vitamin D can also affect the nervous system, cause depression, and deposit calcium in the soft tissues of the kidneys, lungs, blood vessels, and heart.

Folate One of the B vitamins, folate is needed for the production of compounds necessary for DNA synthesis in body cells. It is particularly important for proper cell division during embryonic development; folate deficiencies during the first few weeks of pregnancy, typically before a woman even realizes she is pregnant, can prompt a neural tube defect such as spina bifida, in which the primitive tube that eventually forms the brain and spinal cord fails to close properly. The FDA requires that all bread, cereal, rice, and pasta products sold in the United States be fortified with folic acid, the synthetic form of folate, to reduce the incidence of neural tube defects.

vitamins Essential organic compounds that promote metabolism, growth, and reproduction and help maintain life and health.

minerals Inorganic, indestructible elements that aid physiological processes.

Minerals

Minerals are inorganic, indestructible elements that aid physiological processes within the body. Without minerals, vitamins could not be absorbed. Minerals are readily excreted and, with a few exceptions, are usually not toxic. *Major minerals* are the minerals that the body needs in fairly large amounts: sodium, calcium, phosphorus, magnesium, potassium, sulfur, and chloride. *Trace minerals* include iron, zinc, manganese, copper, fluoride, selenium, chromium, and iodine. Only very small amounts of trace minerals are needed, and serious problems may result if excesses or deficiencies occur (see **TABLE 9.3**).

Sodium Sodium is necessary for the regulation of blood volume and blood pressure, fluid balance, transmission of nerve impulses, heart activity, and certain metabolic functions. It enhances flavors, acts as a preservative, and tenderizes meats, so it's often present in high quantities in the foods

TABLE 9.3 | A Guide to Minerals

Mineral Name	Primary Functions	Recommended Intake	Reliable Food Sources
Sodium	Fluid and acid-base balance; nerve impulses and muscle contraction	Adults: 1.5 g/day (1,500 mg/day)	Table salt, pickles, most canned soups, snack foods, lunch meats, tomato products
Potassium	Fluid balance; nerve impulses and muscle contraction	Adults: 4.7 g/day (4,700 mg/day)	Most fresh fruits and vegetables: potato, banana, tomato juice, orange juice, melon
Phosphorus	ATP, fluid balance and bone formation	Adults: 700 mg/day	Milk/cheese/yogurt, soy milk and tofu, legumes nuts, poultry
Selenium	Regulates thyroid hormones and reduces oxidative stress	Adults: 55 µg/day	Seafood, milk, whole grains, and eggs
Calcium	Part of bone; muscle contraction, acid-base balance, and nerve transmission	Adults 1,000 mg/day	Milk/yogurt/cheese. sardines, collard greens and spinach, calcium-fortified juices
Magnesium	Part of bone; muscle contraction	Men: 400 mg/day Women: 310 mg/day	Spinach, kale, collard greens, whole grains, seeds, nuts, legumes
Iodine	Synthesis of thyroid hormones	Adults: 150 µg/day	Iodized salt, saltwater seafood
Iron	Part of hemoglobin and myoglobin	Men: 8 mg/day Women 18 mg/day	Meat/fish/poultry, fortified cereals, legumes
Zinc	Immune system function; growth and sexual maturation	Men: 11 mg/day Women: 8 mg/day	Meat/fish/poultry, fortified cereals, legumes

Note: Values are for all adults aged 19 and older.

Source: Data from J. Thompson and M. Manore, Nutrition: An Applied Approach, 2nd ed., © 2009; The National Academies, "Dietary Reference Intakes for Calcium and Vitamin D," 2011, www.iom.edu.

we eat. A common misconception is that table salt and sodium are the same thing: Table salt is a compound containing both sodium and chloride. It accounts for only 15 percent of our sodium intake. The majority of sodium in our diet comes from processed foods that are infused with sodium to enhance flavor and for preservation. Pickles, fast foods, salty snacks, processed cheeses, canned and dehydrated soups, frozen dinners, many breads and bakery products, and smoked meats and sausages often contain several hundred milligrams of sodium per serving.

Even if you never use table salt, you still may be getting excess sodium in your diet.

The AI for sodium is just 1,500 milligrams, which is about 0.65 of a teaspoon.[20] The latest National Health and Nutrition Examination Survey (NHANES) estimated that the average American over 2 years of age consumes 3,463 milligrams of sodium per day, or about 1.5 teaspoons.[21]

Both the Institute of Medicine and the American Heart Association recommend consuming no more than the AI for sodium.[22] Why is high sodium intake a concern? Salt-sensitive individuals respond to a high-sodium diet with an increase in blood pressure (hypertension), which contributes to heart disease and strokes. Although the cause of the majority of cases of hypertension is unknown, lowering sodium intake reduces the risk.

Calcium Calcium plays a vital role in building strong bones and teeth, muscle contraction, blood clotting, nerve impulse transmission, heartbeat regulation, and fluid balance within cells. The issue of calcium consumption has gained national attention with the rising incidence of osteoporosis among older adults. Most Americans do not consume the recommended 1,000 to 1,200 milligrams of calcium per day.[23]

Milk is one of the richest sources of dietary calcium. Calcium-fortified orange juice and soymilk are good alternatives if you do not drink dairy milk. Many green leafy vegetables are good sources of calcium, but some contain oxalic acid, which makes their calcium harder to absorb. Spinach, chard, and beet greens are not particularly good sources of calcium, whereas broccoli, cauliflower, and many peas and beans offer good supplies.

It is generally best to take calcium throughout the day, consuming it with foods containing protein, vitamin D, and vitamin C for optimal absorption. Many dairy products are both excellent sources of calcium and fortified with vitamin D, which is known to improve calcium absorption.

Do you consume carbonated soft drinks? Be aware that the added phosphoric acid (phosphate) in these drinks can cause you to excrete extra calcium, which may result in calcium loss from your bones. One study of 2,500 men and women found that in women who consumed at least three cans of cola per week, even diet cola, bone density of the hip was 4 to 5 percent lower than in women who drank fewer than one cola per month. Colas

anemia Condition that results from the body's inability to produce adequate hemoglobin.

did not seem to have the same effect on men.[24] There may also be a "milk displacement" effect, meaning that people who drank soda were not drinking milk, thereby decreasing their calcium intake.

Iron Worldwide, iron deficiency is the most common nutrient deficiency, affecting more than 2 billion people, nearly 30 percent of the world's population.[25] In the United States, iron deficiency is less prevalent, but it is still the most common micronutrient deficiency.[26] Women aged 19 to 50 need about 18 milligrams of iron per day, and men aged 19 to 50 need about 8 milligrams.

Iron deficiency can lead to *iron-deficiency anemia.* **Anemia** results from the body's inability to produce adequate amounts of hemoglobin (the oxygen-carrying component of the blood). Anemia can also result from blood loss, cancer, ulcers, and other conditions. When iron-deficiency anemia occurs, body cells receive less oxygen. As a result, the iron-deficient person feels tired. Iron is also important for energy metabolism, DNA synthesis, and other body functions.

Iron overload or iron toxicity due to ingesting too many iron-containing supplements is the leading cause of accidental poisoning in small children in the United States. Symptoms of toxicity include nausea, vomiting, diarrhea, rapid heartbeat, weak pulse, dizziness, shock, and confusion. Excess iron intake

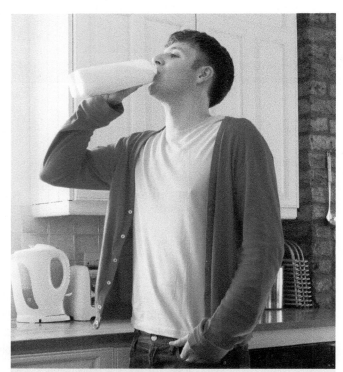

Milk is a great source of calcium and other nutrients. If you don't like milk or can't drink it, make sure to get enough calcium—at least 1,000 milligrams a day—through other sources.

from high meat consumption, iron fortification, and supplementation is also associated with problems such as cardiovascular disease and cancer.[27]

Beneficial Non-Nutrient Components of Foods

Increasingly, nutrition research is focusing on components of foods that interact with nutrients to promote human health rather than solely as sources of macro- and micronutrients.[28] Foods that may confer health benefits beyond the nutrients they contribute to the diet—whole foods, fortified foods, enriched foods, or enhanced foods—are called **functional foods**. When functional foods are included as part of a varied diet, they have the potential to positively impact health.[29]

Some of the most popular functional foods today are those containing **antioxidants.** These substances appear to protect against oxidative stress, a complex process in which *free radicals* (atoms with unpaired electrons) destabilize other atoms and molecules, prompting a chain reaction that can damage cells, cell proteins, or genetic material in the cells. Free radical formation is a natural process that cannot be avoided, but antioxidants combat it by donating their electrons to stabilize free radicals, activating enzymes that convert free radicals to less-damaging substances, or reducing or repairing the damage they cause.

Among the more commonly cited antioxidants are vitamins C and E, as well as the minerals copper, iron, manganese, selenium, and zinc. Other potent antioxidants are **phytochemicals**, compounds that occur naturally in plants and are thought to protect them against ultraviolet radiation, pests, and other threats. Common examples include the *carotenoids,* pigments found in red, orange, and dark green fruits and vegetables. Beta-carotene, the most researched carotenoid, is a precursor of vitamin A, meaning that vitamin A can be produced in the body from beta-carotene. Both vitamin A and beta-carotene have antioxidant properties. Phenolic phytochemicals, which include a group known as flavonoids, are found in an array of fruits and vegetables as well as soy products, tea, and chocolate. Like carotenoids, they are thought to have antioxidant properties that may prevent cardiovascular disease.[30]

To date, many such claims about the health benefits of antioxidant nutrients and phytochemicals have not been fully investigated. However, studies do show that individuals deficient in antioxidant vitamins and minerals have an increased risk for age-related diseases, and that antioxidants consumed in whole foods, mostly fruits and vegetables, may reduce these individuals' risks.[31] In contrast, antioxidants consumed as supplements do not confer such a benefit, and may be harmful. For example, researchers have long theorized that because many cancers

result from DNA damage, and because vitamin E appears to protect against such damage, vitamin E would also reduce cancer risk. Surprisingly, the great majority of studies have demonstrated no effect or, in some cases, a negative effect.[32]

Foods rich in nutrients and phytochemicals are increasingly being referred to as "superfoods." Do they live up to their name? See the **Health Headlines** box on page 274.

> **functional foods** Foods believed to have specific health benefits beyond their basic nutrients.
>
> **antioxidants** Substances believed to protect against oxidative stress and resultant tissue damage.
>
> **phytochemicals** Naturally occurring non-nutrient plant chemicals believed to have beneficial health effects.

LO 2 | NUTRITIONAL GUIDELINES

Describe nutritional guidelines and recommendations, including the Dietary Guidelines for Americans and the MyPlate food guidance system.

Today, Americans consume more calories than ever before. From 1970 to 2010, average calorie consumption increased from 2,169 to 2,614 calories per day (see **FIGURE 9.4**).[33] In general, it isn't the actual amount of food, but rather the number of calories in the foods we choose to eat, that has increased. When these trends are combined with our increasingly sedentary lifestyle, it is not surprising that we have seen a dramatic rise in obesity.[34]

The Center for Nutrition Policy and Promotion at the U.S. Department of Agriculture (USDA) publishes two dietary tools created for consumers to make healthy eating easy: the *2010 Dietary Guidelines for Americans* and the MyPlate food guidance system.

Dietary Guidelines for Americans, 2010

The Dietary Guidelines for Americans are a set of recommendations for healthy eating created by the U.S. Department of Health and Human Services and the USDA. These guidelines are revised every 5 years. New recommendations are currently being reviewed, and final approval is likely in the fall of 2015. The information in *2010 Dietary Guidelines for Americans* was designed to help bridge the gap between the standard American diet and the key recommendations that aim to combat the growing obesity epidemic by balancing calories with adequate physical activity.[35]

Blueberries are a great source of antioxidants.

Balancing Calories to Manage Weight The recommendations in *Dietary Guidelines for Americans* were developed to prevent overnutrition, especially when it comes to kilocalories. People who are successful at maintaining a

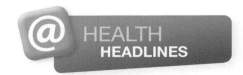
HEALTH CLAIMS OF SUPERFOODS

Functional foods contain both nutrients and other active compounds that may improve overall health, reduce the risk for certain diseases, or delay aging. If the term "functional foods" strikes you as a bit stodgy, you're not alone. In food advertisements, fitness and food magazines, and even among health care organizations, these foods are increasingly being referred to as "superfoods." For instance, Harvard Medical School recently published a list of 12 superfoods, including broccoli, beans, salmon, oatmeal, Greek yogurt, and dark chocolate. Do superfoods live up to their new name? Let's look at a few.

Salmon is a rich source of the omega-3 fatty acids EPA and DHA, which combat inflammation, improve HDL/LDL blood profiles, and reduce the risk for cardiovascular disease. DHA may also promote a healthy nervous system, reducing the risk for age-related dementia.

Yogurt makes it onto most superfood lists because it contains living, beneficial bacteria called probiotics. You will see their genus name, for example, *Lactobacillus* or *Bifidobacterium*, in the

Yogurt and kefir (a fermented milk drink) are dairy products containing beneficial bacteria called *probiotics*.

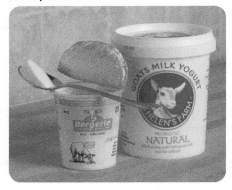

list of ingredients on the product's label. Probiotics colonize the large intestine, where they help complete digestion, produce certain vitamins, and may reduce the risk of diarrhea and other bowel disorders, boost immunity, and help regulate body weight.

Cocoa is particularly rich in a class of chemicals called flavonols that have been shown in many studies to reduce the risk for cardiovascular disease, diabetes, and even arthritis. Dark chocolate has

a higher level of flavonols than milk chocolate.

Given such claims, it's easy to get carried away by the idea that superfoods, like superheros, have superpowers. But eating a square of dark chocolate won't rescue you from the ill effects of a fast-food burger and fries. What matters is your whole diet. Focus on including superfoods as components of a varied diet rich in fresh fruits, legumes and other vegetables, whole grains, lean sources of protein, and nuts and seeds. These are the "everyday heroes" of a super-healthful diet.

Sources: Academy of Nutrition and Dietetics, "Position of the Academy of Nutrition and Dietetics: Functional Foods," *Journal of the Academy of Nutrition and Dietetics* 113 (2013): 1096–1103; D. Swanson, R. Block, and S .A. Mousa, "Omega-3 Fatty Acids EPA and DHA: Health Benefits Throughout Life," *Advances in Nutrition* 3, no. 1 (2012): 1–7; R. Krajmalnik-Brown et al., "Effects of Gut Microbes on Nutrient Absorption and Energy Regulation," *Nutrition in Clinical Practice* 27, no. 2 (2012): 201–14; L. Hooper et al., "Effects of Chocolate, Cocoa, and Flavan-3-ols on Cardiovascular Health: A Systematic Review and Meta-Analysis of Randomized Trials," *American Journal of Clinical Nutrition* 95, no. 3 (2012): 740–53, doi: 10.3945/ajcn.111.023457

healthy body weight do so by controlling their intake of kilocalories and being more active. To decrease the number of kilocalories you eat, avoid oversized portions, switch from whole milk to fat-free or 1 percent milk, fill your plate with vegetables and fruit, and increase your physical activity at each stage of life. Remember to enjoy your food, but eat less of it.

Foods and Food Components to Reduce

The recommendations set forth in *Dietary Guidelines for Americans* promote eating more nutrient dense foods and beverages. A healthy eating pattern limits your intake of saturated fats to 10 percent of total kilocalories by eating less meat and butter and switching from whole-milk products to low-fat or nonfat dairy.[36] Reduce your cholesterol intake to 300 milligrams or less by consuming fewer animal products; reduce foods high in sodium, including processed and canned foods, to 2,300 milligrams, or as low as 1,500 milligrams, if you have high blood pressure.[37] Limit your intake of refined grains, *trans* fats, and added sugars. If you drink alcohol, drink in moderation; limit to one drink per day for women and two drinks per day for men.

Foods and Nutrients to Increase
A healthy diet emphasizes a variety of protein foods including seafood, lean meat and poultry, eggs, beans, peas, soy products, and unsalted nuts and seeds. Protein foods that are higher in solid fats, such as red meat, should be replaced with protein foods that are lower in solid fats. A healthy diet is rich in plant-based foods, including leafy green, red, and orange vegetables, and whole grains.

Building Healthy Eating Patterns
A healthy eating pattern takes time to establish. Set a goal that you can achieve over time. Begin by accounting for all foods and beverages you eat each day; assess how they meet your nutrient goals over time with a healthy balance of kilocalories to maintain your weight. Don't just cut high-sugar, high-fat, and processed foods; focus on adding healthy foods such as fruits, vegetables, and whole grains to your eating patterns. Pack healthy lunches and snacks to take with you to avoid fast foods. Control portions by measuring out your snacks rather than eating from the package. Don't skip meals,

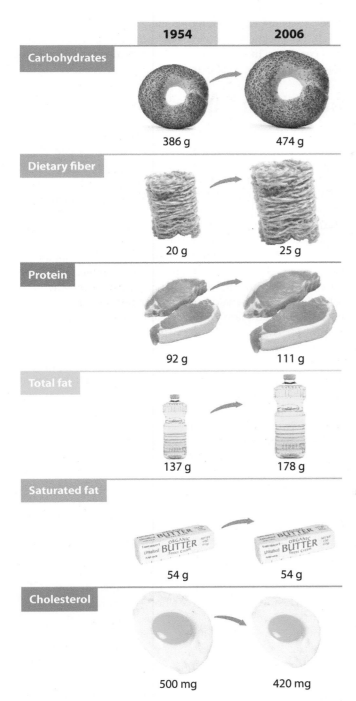

	1954	2006
Carbohydrates	386 g	474 g
Dietary fiber	20 g	25 g
Protein	92 g	111 g
Total fat	137 g	178 g
Saturated fat	54 g	54 g
Cholesterol	500 mg	420 mg

FIGURE 9.4 Trends in Per Capita Nutrient Consumption Since 1954, Americans' daily caloric intake has increased by about 25%, as has daily consumption of carbohydrates, fiber, and protein. Daily total fat intake has increased by 30%.

Source: Data are from USDA/Center for Nutrition Policy and Promotion, Nutrient Availability, updated February 2014, www.ers.usda.gov/data-products/food-availability-(per-capita)-data-system/.aspx#26715.

especially breakfast. Reduce the risk of foodborne illnesses by following good food safety practices. And finally, make eating fun and enjoyable!

MyPlate Food Guidance System

To help consumers understand and implement the Dietary Guidelines, the USDA has developed an easy-to-follow graphic and guidance system called MyPlate, which can be found at www.choosemyplate.gov and is illustrated in **FIGURE 9.5**. The MyPlate food guidance system takes into consideration the dietary and caloric needs for a wide variety of individuals, such as pregnant or breast-feeding women, those trying to lose weight, and adults with different activity levels. The interactive website can create personalized dietary and exercise recommendations based on the individual information you enter.

Eat Nutrient-Dense Foods Although eating the proper number of servings from MyPlate is important, it is also important to recognize that there are large caloric, fat, and energy differences among foods within a given food group. For example, salmon and hot dogs provide vastly different nutrient levels per calorie. Salmon is rich in essential fatty acids and is considered nutrient dense—dense in nutrients compared to kilocalories. Hot dogs, which are not nutrient dense, are loaded with kilocalories, saturated fats, cholesterol, and sodium—all substances we should limit. It is important to eat foods that have a high nutritional value for their caloric content.

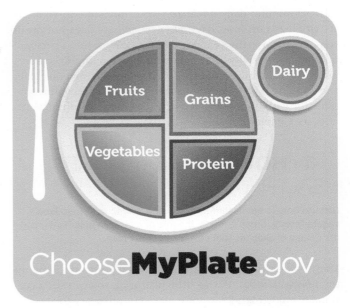

FIGURE 9.5 The MyPlate System The USDA MyPlate food guidance system takes a new approach to dietary and exercise recommendations. Each colored section of the plate represents a food group, and an interactive tool at www.choosemyplate.gov helps you analyze and track your foods and physical activity, and provides helpful tips to personalize your plan.

Source: U.S. Department of Agriculture, 2010, www.choosemyplate.gov.

Reduce Empty Calorie Foods

Avoid *empty calories*, that is, high-calorie foods and drinks with little nutritional value. MyPlate recommends we limit our intake of sugary drinks as well as the following sugar- and fat-laden items:[38]

- **Cakes, cookies, pastries, and donuts.** One slice of chocolate cake contains 77 percent empty calories.
- **Cheese.** Switching from whole milk mozzarella cheese to nonfat mozzarella cheese saves you 76 empty calories per ounce.
- **Pizza.** One slice of pepperoni pizza adds 139 empty calories to your meal.
- **Ice cream.** More than 75 percent of the 275 calories in ice cream are empty calories.
- **Sausages, hot dogs, bacon, and ribs.** Adding a sausage link to your breakfast adds 96 empty calories.
- **Wine, beer, and all alcoholic beverages.** A whopping 155 empty calories are consumed with each 12 fluid ounces of beer.
- **Refined grains, including crackers, cookies, and white rice.** Switching to whole wheat versions can save you 25 fat-laden empty calories per serving.

Physical Activity Strive to be physically active for at least 30 minutes daily, preferably with moderate to vigorous activity levels on most days. Physical activity does not mean you have to go to the gym, jog 3 miles a day, or hire a personal trainer. Any activity that gets your heart pumping counts, including gardening and other yard work, playing basketball, and dancing. MyPlate personalized plans offer recommendations for weekly physical activity. (For more on physical fitness, see Chapter 11.)

LO 3 | HOW CAN I EAT MORE HEALTHFULLY?

Discuss how to eat healthfully, including how to read food labels, vegetarianism, organic foods, the role of dietary supplements, and the unique challenges that college students face.

Many Americans believe eating healthfully means giving up their favorite foods. With a little planning, you can still occasionally enjoy high-kilocalorie, high-fat, or sugary foods. The key to following a healthy eating pattern is to achieve balance between food groups, choose a variety of foods each day, and moderate the amounts of food you eat. A healthful eating plan also includes foods that are nutrient dense and low in energy density or kilocalories.

Whether you follow a vegetarian diet, eat only organic foods, take dietary supplements, or choose to eat locally grown foods, there are ways to improve the nutrient content of your meals. Let's begin with how to read a food label. The information contained in a food label can be useful when it comes to planning a healthy meal plan.

Read Food Labels

How do you know what nutrients the packaged foods you eat are contributing to your diet? To help consumers evaluate the nutritional values of packaged foods, the FDA and the USDA developed the Nutrition Facts label that is typically displayed on the side or back of packaged foods. One of the most helpful items on the label is the **% daily values (%DVs)** list, which tells you how much of an average adult's allowance for a particular substance (fat, fiber, calcium, etc.) is provided by a serving of the food. The %DV is calculated based on a 2,000 calorie per day diet, so your values may be different from those listed on a label. The label also includes information on the serving size and calories. In 2014, the FDA announced plans to make the data on the label more helpful for consumers by identifying the calories per serving in much larger type, and adjusting the serving size so that it better reflects the amount of the food that people typically eat.[39] FIGURE 9.6 walks you through a typical Nutrition Facts label and the proposed label changes. For the latest information on the new label, go to www.FDA.gov and search "Nutrition Facts label."

Food labels contain other information as well, such as the name and manufacturer of the product, an ingredients list, and sometimes claims about the product's contents or effects. The FDA allows three types of claims on the packages of foods and dietary supplements:[40]

- **Health claims** describe a relationship between a food product and health promotion or disease prevention. It cannot claim to diagnose, cure, or treat a disease. When the current scientific evidence supports the risk reduction, the FDA approves the health claim. For example, an approved health claim on a package of whole-grain bread may state, "In a low-fat diet, whole-grain foods like this bread may reduce the risk of heart disease." The FDA can also evaluate whether health claims meet the standard for *significant scientific agreement* (SSA) among experts. If there is agreement that a food may reduce your risk of a disease and experts are confident their opinion won't change with more scientific study, the health claim is approved.
- **Nutrient content claims** indicate a specific nutrient is present at a certain level. For example, a product label might

% daily values (%DVs) Percentages listed as "% DV" on food and supplement labels; identify how much of each listed nutrient or other substance a serving of food contributes to a 2,000 calorie/day diet.

50%

OF ADULTS DRINK AT LEAST ONE **SUGARY** DRINK A DAY.

Sample Label for Macaroni and Cheese

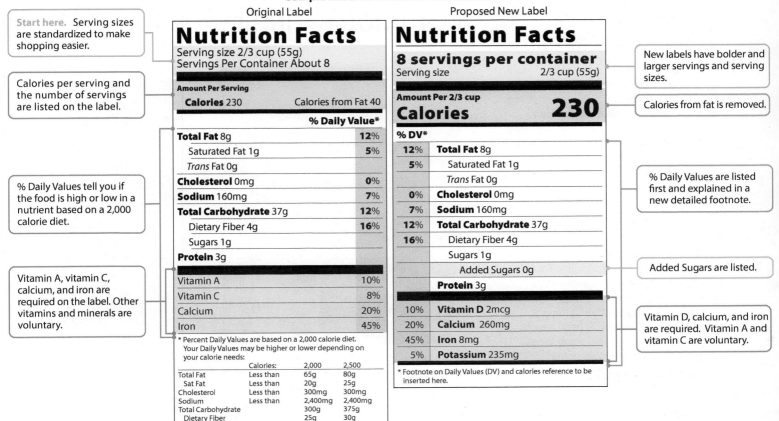

Original Label

Proposed New Label

Start here. Serving sizes are standardized to make shopping easier.

Nutrition Facts
Serving size 2/3 cup (55g)
Servings Per Container About 8

Amount Per Serving
Calories 230   Calories from Fat 40

Calories per serving and the number of servings are listed on the label.

	% Daily Value*
Total Fat 8g	12%
Saturated Fat 1g	5%
Trans Fat 0g	
Cholesterol 0mg	0%
Sodium 160mg	7%
Total Carbohydrate 37g	12%
Dietary Fiber 4g	16%
Sugars 1g	
Protein 3g	
Vitamin A	10%
Vitamin C	8%
Calcium	20%
Iron	45%

% Daily Values tell you if the food is high or low in a nutrient based on a 2,000 calorie diet.

Vitamin A, vitamin C, calcium, and iron are required on the label. Other vitamins and minerals are voluntary.

* Percent Daily Values are based on a 2,000 calorie diet. Your Daily Values may be higher or lower depending on your calorie needs:

		Calories:	2,000	2,500
Total Fat	Less than		65g	80g
Sat Fat	Less than		20g	25g
Cholesterol	Less than		300mg	300mg
Sodium	Less than		2,400mg	2,400mg
Total Carbohydrate			300g	375g
Dietary Fiber			25g	30g

Nutrition Facts
8 servings per container
Serving size   2/3 cup (55g)

Amount Per 2/3 cup
Calories   **230**

% DV*		
12%	**Total Fat** 8g	
5%	Saturated Fat 1g	
	Trans Fat 0g	
0%	**Cholesterol** 0mg	
7%	**Sodium** 160mg	
12%	**Total Carbohydrate** 37g	
16%	Dietary Fiber 4g	
	Sugars 1g	
	Added Sugars 0g	
	Protein 3g	
10%	**Vitamin D** 2mcg	
20%	**Calcium** 260mg	
45%	**Iron** 8mg	
5%	**Potassium** 235mg	

* Footnote on Daily Values (DV) and calories reference to be inserted here.

New labels have bolder and larger servings and serving sizes.

Calories from fat is removed.

% Daily Values are listed first and explained in a new detailed footnote.

Added Sugars are listed.

Vitamin D, calcium, and iron are required. Vitamin A and vitamin C are voluntary.

FIGURE 9.6 Reading a Food Label

Sources: U.S. Food and Drug Administration, "How to Understand and Use the Nutrition Facts Panel," April 2015, www.fda.gov/Food/IngredientsPackagingLabeling/LabelingNutrition/ucm274593.htm; U.S. Food and Administration, "Proposed Changes to the Nutrition Facts Label," August 2014, www.fda.gov/Food/GuidanceRegulation /GuidanceDocumentsRegulatoryInformation/LabelingNutrition/ucm385663.htm

▶ **VIDEO TUTOR** Understanding Food Labels

say "High in fiber" or "Low in fat" or "This product contains 100 calories per serving." Nutrient content claims can use the following words: *more, less, fewer, good source of, free, light, lean, extra lean, high, low, reduced.*

■ Structure and function claims describe the effect that a component in the food product has on the body. For example, the label of a carton of milk is allowed to state, "Calcium builds strong bones."

In addition to food labels, shoppers are increasingly being guided in their food choices by nutritional rating systems. What are these systems, and can they help you make smarter choices? See the **Student Health Today** box on the next page for answers.

Front of Package Labeling The FDA has proposed new guidelines for the nutrition labeling on the front of packages to help consumers choose healthy foods. Currently, the labeling on the front of packages is unregulated and may cause confusion for consumers.

The *Facts Up Front* initiative is a voluntary labeling system that can be used by manufacturers to provide quick, accurate information for the consumer. The most important information from the Nutrition Facts panel is placed on the front of the package. As shown in **FIGURE 9.7**, Facts Up Front illustrates the kilocalories, saturated fat, sodium, and added sugars per serving. If a serving of the food contains more than 10 percent of a vitamin or mineral, the manufacturer can also include

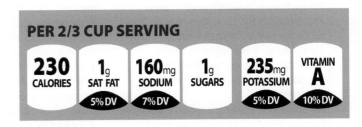

PER 2/3 CUP SERVING

| **230** CALORIES | **1**g SAT FAT 5% DV | **160**mg SODIUM 7% DV | **1**g SUGARS | **235**mg POTASSIUM 5% DV | VITAMIN **A** 10% DV |

FIGURE 9.7 Facts Up Front Information is placed on the front of the package for a quick and accurate picture of the nutritional content of a serving of the food.

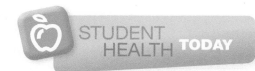

NUTRITION RATING SYSTEMS

Next time you're at the grocery store, take a close look at the tags on the store shelves. Do you see anything different—stars, perhaps, or numbers inside blue hexagons? If so, you're looking at one of several new nutrition rating systems. Nutrition scientists and physicians designed these systems to help consumers quickly locate healthful foods. Four of the most popular systems in American markets are as follows:

- **Guiding Stars.** This system rates the nutritional quality of foods using information from the Nutrition Facts label and the food's ingredients list. Foods are rated with from zero to three stars, with three indicating the highest nutritional quality. A fresh tomato, for example, gets three stars. When the program was implemented, all foods sold by the participating retailers were evaluated, and less than one fourth earned even a single star. What the system lacks in subtlety it makes up for in simplicity—even consumers who haven't been introduced to it can almost instantly understand the basic message behind it: The product with the most stars "wins."

- **NuVal.** The NuVal System uses a scale of 1 to 100. The higher the number, the higher the nutritional quality. In rating each food, the system considers more than 30 dietary components—not just nutrients, but fiber, antioxidants, and other food components known to affect health. In this system, a tomato gets a top score of 100 points. The 100-point rating scale allows consumers to make more subtle distinctions between very similar foods; for example, two brands of whole-grain bread get scores of 48 versus 29. Although the consumer doesn't need to stop and research the food, the ranking suggests real differences, and in fact, the bread with the higher score is lower in calories and sodium, higher in calcium, and has twice the dietary fiber per slice.

- **American Heart Association Heart Check.** The AHA Heart Check is based on foods that contain sufficient

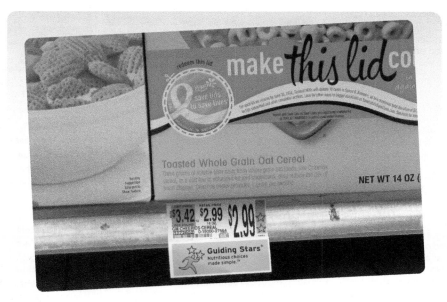

nutrients to promote heart health. To receive a Heart Check rating, the food must meet specific nutrient requirements in six different food categories based on total fat, saturated and *trans* fat, cholesterol, and sodium. For example, to receive a Heart Check rating, a serving of food must not contain more than 20 milligrams of cholesterol. Products that contain partially hydrogenated oils are ineligible to receive a Heart Check rating. Each serving must also contain 10 percent or more of the Daily Value of at least one of these nutrients: dietary fiber, vitamin A, vitamin C, iron, protein, or calcium.

- **Aggregate Nutrient Density Index (ANDI).** This index ranks foods based on the number of micronutrients per calorie and takes into account as many known beneficial phytochemicals as possible. It does not, however, consider macronutrient density, such as the amount of high-quality protein or essential fatty acids in the food. A top score is 1,000. How does this system rate our tomato? It gets just 164 points! In contrast, kale gets a top score of 1,000. Again, the difference is in the calorie/micronutrient ratio: A medium-sized tomato and two thirds of a cup of kale have about the same number of calories, yet the kale has about 7 times

as much vitamin A and 3.5 times as much vitamin C.

Do these ranking systems prompt shoppers to choose more healthful foods? Research suggests they just might. An evaluation in the *American Journal of Clinical Nutrition* found that the systems reduce the time and effort consumers spend in making food choices, as compared with more detailed labels and have the potential to help them choose more healthful foods. That's important because, as an evaluation of the NuVal system from the Harvard School of Public Health found, people who eat food with higher scores have a lower risk of cardiovascular disease and diabetes, and may even enjoy a longer life.

Sources: S. A. Gerrior, "Nutrient Profiling Systems: Are Science and the Consumer Connected?," *American Journal of Clinical Nutrition* 91, no. 4 (2010): 1116S–17S; L. M. Fischer et al., "Development and Implementation of the Guiding Stars Nutrition Guidance Program," *American Journal of Health Promotion* 26, no. 2 (2011): e55–63, doi: 10.4278/ajhp.100709-QUAL-238; S. E. Chiuve, L. Sampson, and W. C. Willett, "The Association between a Nutritional Quality Index and Risk of Chronic Disease," *American Journal of Preventive Medicine* 40, no. 5 (2011): 505–13, doi: 10.1016/j.amepre.2010.11.022. A. H. Lichtenstein et al., "Food-intake Patterns Assessed by Using Front-of-Pack Labeling Program Criteria Associated with Better Diet Quality and Lower Cardiometabolic Risk," *American Journal of Clinical Nutrition* 99 (2013): 454–62, doi:10.3945/ajcn.113.071407

that information on the front of the package.

Understand Serving Sizes

MyPlate presents personalized dietary recommendations based on servings of particular nutrients. But how much is one serving? Is it different from a portion? Although these two terms are often used interchangeably, they actually mean very different things. A *serving* is the recommended amount you should consume, whereas a *portion* is the amount you choose to eat at any one time. The saying "your eyes are bigger than your stomach" is rooted in truth—most of us select portions that are much bigger than recommended servings. See **FIGURE 9.8** for a handy pocket guide with tips on recognizing serving sizes.

Unfortunately, we don't always get a clear picture from food producers and advertisers about what a serving really is. Consider a bottle of chocolate milk: The food label may list one serving size as 8 fluid ounces and 150 calories. However, note the size of the entire bottle. If it holds 16 ounces, drinking the whole thing serves up 300 calories.

Vegetarianism: A Healthy Diet?

The word **vegetarian** means different things to different people. Strict vegetarians, or *vegans*, avoid all foods of animal origin, including dairy products and eggs. Their diet is based on vegetables, grains, fruits, nuts, seeds, and legumes. Far more common are *lacto-vegetarians*, who eat dairy products but avoid flesh foods and eggs. *Ovo-vegetarians* add eggs to a vegan diet, and *lacto-ovo-vegetarians* eat both dairy products and eggs. *Pesco-vegetarians* eat fish, dairy products, and eggs, and *semi-vegetarians* eat chicken, fish, dairy products, and eggs. Some people in the semivegetarian category prefer to call themselves "non–red meat eaters."

According to a poll conducted by the Vegetarian Resource Group, more than 4 percent of U.S. adults, approximately 9 million people, are vegetarians.[41] Other surveys have shown that 5 percent of Americans consider themselves to be "vegetarian" and 2 percent stated they are vegans.[42]

Common reasons for pursuing a vegetarian lifestyle include concern for animal welfare, the environmental costs of meat production, food safety, personal health, weight loss, and weight maintenance. Generally, people who follow a balanced vegetarian diet weigh less and have better cholesterol levels, fewer problems with irregular bowel movements (constipation and diarrhea), and a lower risk of heart disease than do nonvegetari-

ans. A recent analysis of 29 studies involving a total of more than 20,000 participants found that people who follow a vegetarian diet have an average blood pressure several points lower than that of

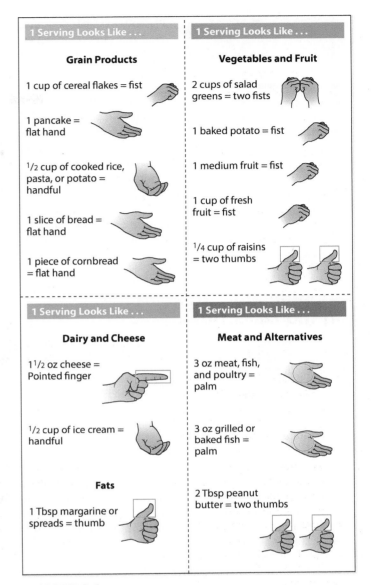

FIGURE 9.8 Serving Size Card One of the challenges of following a healthy diet is judging how big a portion size should be and how many servings you are really eating. The comparisons on this card can help you recall what a standard food serving looks like. For easy reference, photocopy or cut out this card, fold on the dotted lines, and keep it in your wallet. You can even laminate it for long-term use.

Sources: National Heart, Lung and Blood Institute, "Serving Size Card," Accessed April 2015, http://hp2010.nhlbihin.net/portion/servingcard7.pdf; National Dairy Council, "Serving Size Comparison Chart," Accessed April 2015, www.healthyeating.org/Portals/0/Documents/Schools/ Parent%20Ed/Portion_Sizes_Serving_Chart.pdf

nonvegetarians.[43] Some studies suggest that vegetarianism may also reduce the risk of some cancers, particularly colon cancer.[44]

With proper meal planning, vegetarianism provides a healthful alternative to a meat-based diet. Eating a variety of healthful foods throughout the day helps to ensure proper nutrient intake. Vegan diets are of greater concern than diets that include dairy products and eggs. Vegans may be deficient in vitamins B_2 (riboflavin),

vegetarian A person who follows a diet that excludes some or all animal products.

Why are so many people becoming vegetarians?

- How easy is it to be a vegetarian on your campus?
- What concerns about vegetarianism do you have, if any?

B_{12}, and D, as well as calcium, iron, zinc, and other minerals; however, many foods are fortified with these nutrients, or vegans can obtain them from supplements. Vegans also have to pay more attention to the amino acid content of their foods, but eating a variety of types of plant foods throughout the day will provide adequate amounts of protein. Pregnant women, older adults, sick people, and families with young children who are vegans need to take special care to ensure that their diets are adequate. In all cases, seek advice from a health care professional if you have questions.

Supplements: Research on the Daily Dose

Dietary supplements are products containing one or more dietary ingredients taken by mouth and intended to supplement existing diets. Ingredients range from vitamins, minerals, and herbs to enzymes, amino acids, fatty acids, and organ tissues. They can come in tablet, capsule, liquid, powder, and other forms. Because consumers see dietary supplements as an easy fix to improve their less than healthy diets, sales have skyrocketed.

It is important to note that dietary supplements are not regulated like foods or drugs. The FDA does not evaluate the safety and efficacy of supplements prior to their marketing, and it can take action to remove a supplement from the market only after the product has been proved harmful. Currently, the United States has no formal guidelines for supplement marketing and safety, and supplement manufacturers are responsible for self-monitoring their activities.

Do you really need to take dietary supplements? The Office of Dietary Supplements, part of the National Institutes of Health, states that some supplements may help ensure that you get adequate amounts of essential nutrients if you don't consume a variety of foods, as recommended in the *Dietary Guidelines for Americans*. However, dietary supplements are not intended to prevent or treat disease, and recently the U.S. Preventive Services Task Force concluded that there is insufficient evidence to recommend that healthy people take multivitamin/mineral supplements to prevent cardiovascular disease or cancer.[45] Those who may benefit from using multivitamin/mineral supplements include pregnant and breast-feeding women, older adults, vegans, people on a very low-calorie weight-loss diets, alcohol-dependent individuals, and patients with malabsorption problems or other significant health problems.

dietary supplements Products taken by mouth and containing dietary ingredients such as vitamins and minerals that are intended to supplement existing diets.

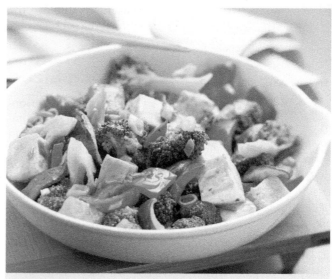

Adopting a vegetarian diet can be a very healthy way to eat. Take care to prepare your food healthfully by avoiding added sugars and excessive sodium. Make sure you get complementary essential amino acids throughout the day. Meals like this tofu and vegetable stir-fry can be further enhanced by adding a whole grain, such as brown rice.

The wisdom of taking other types of supplements, as opposed to consuming nutrients in whole foods, is also unproven. For example, the benefit of fish consumption in reducing the risk for cardiovascular disease is well-established, but studies have shown conflicting results about fish-oil supplements.[46]

Taking high-dose supplements of the fat-soluble vitamins A, D, and E can be harmful or even fatal. Too much vitamin A, for example, can damage the liver, and excessive vitamin E

WHICH **PATH** WOULD YOU TAKE **?**

Scan the QR code to see how different dietary choices YOU make today can affect your overall health tomorrow.

increases the risk for a stroke.[47] The Academy of Nutrition and Dietetics recommends that, though some people benefit from taking supplements, a healthy diet is the best way to give your body what it needs.[48] Be aware that supplements can interact with certain medications, including aspirin, diuretics, and steroids, which may result in potential problems.

If you do decide to take a multivitamin, choose brands that contain the US Pharmacopeia or Consumer Lab seal. This ensures that the supplement has been reviewed, is free of toxic ingredients, and contains the ingredients stated on the label. Store your supplements in a dark, dry place (not the bathroom or other damp

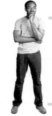

spots), make sure they are out of reach of small children, and check the expiration date.

Eating Well in College

Many college students find it hard to fit a well-balanced meal into the day, but breakfast and lunch are important if you are to keep energy levels up and get the most out of your classes. Eating a complete breakfast that includes fiber-rich carbohydrates, protein, and healthy unsaturated fat (such as a banana, peanut butter and whole-grain bread sandwich or a bowl of oatmeal topped with dried fruit and nuts) is key. If you are short on time, bring a container of yogurt and a handful of almonds to your morning class.

If your campus is like many others, your lunchtime options include a variety of fast-food restaurants. Generally speaking, you can eat more healthfully and for less money if you bring food from home or eat at your campus dining hall. If you must eat fast food, follow the tips below to get more nutritional bang for your buck:

- Ask for nutritional analyses of menu items. Most fast-food chains now have them.
- Order salads, but be careful about what you add to them. Taco salads and Cobb salads are often high in fat, calories, and sodium. Ask for low-fat dressing on the side, and use it sparingly. Stay away from high-fat add-ons, such as bacon bits, croutons, and crispy noodles.
- If you crave french fries, try baked "fries," which may be lower in fat.
- Avoid giant sizes, and refrain from ordering extra sauce, bacon, cheese, and other toppings that add calories, sodium, and fat.
- Limit sodas and other beverages that are high in added sugars.
- At least once per week, swap a vegetable-based meat substitute into your fast-food choices. Most places now offer veggie burgers and similar products, which provide excellent sources of protein and often have less fat and fewer calories.

In the dining hall, try these ideas:

- Choose lean meats, grilled chicken, fish, or vegetable dishes. Avoid fried chicken, fatty cuts of red meat, or meat dishes smothered in creamy or oily sauce.
- Hit the salad bar and load up on leafy greens, beans, tuna, or tofu. Choose items such as avocado or nuts for "good" fat. Go easy on the dressing, or substitute vinaigrette or low-fat dressings.

COLLEGE MALES SPEND AN AVERAGE OF

$99.17

AND COLLEGE FEMALES SPEND AN AVERAGE OF $52.11 ON **FAST FOOD** IN A MONTH.

- When choosing items from a made-to-order food station, ask the preparer to hold the butter or oil, mayonnaise, sour cream, or cheese- or cream-based sauces.
- Avoid going back for seconds and consuming large portions.
- If there is something you'd like but don't see in your dining hall, speak to your food service manager and provide suggestions.
- Pass on high-calorie, low-nutrient foods such as sugary cereals, ice cream, and other sweet treats. Choose fruit or low-fat yogurt to satisfy your sweet tooth.

Between classes, avoid vending machines. Reach into your backpack for an apple, banana, some dried fruit and nuts, a single serving of unsweetened applesauce, or whole-grain crackers spread with peanut butter. Energy bars can be a nutritious option if you choose right. Check the Nutrition Facts label for bars that are below 200 calories and provide at least 3 grams of dietary fiber. Cereal bars usually provide less protein than energy bars; however, they also tend to be much lower in calories and sugar, and high in fiber.

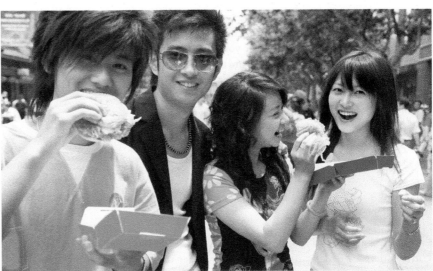

Meals like this one may be convenient, but they are high in saturated fat, sodium, refined carbohydrates, and calories. Even when you are short on time and money, it is possible—and worthwhile—to make healthier choices. If you are ordering fast food, opt for foods prepared by baking, roasting, or steaming; ask for the leanest meat option; and request that sauces, dressings, and gravies be served on the side.

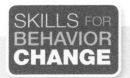

SKILLS FOR BEHAVIOR CHANGE

NATURAL VERSUS ORGANIC FOODS

When you buy foods that state they are "natural" on the label, does that also mean the food is organic? There is no official definition for the term "natural." In fact, because high fructose corn syrup doesn't contain any artificial or synthetic ingredients, it can be deemed "natural" based on a ruling by the FDA. The USDA has a strict definition for the term "organic" on a food label. Here are some key points to remember when buying natural versus organic foods:

▶ Products labeled "100% organic" contain 100 percent organic ingredients.

▶ Products labeled "organic" contain 95 percent organic ingredients, and the other 5 percent contain no GMO's or irradiated ingredients.

▶ Products labeled "Made with organic ingredients" contain a minimum of 70 percent organic ingredients; the remaining 30 percent contain no GMO's or irradiated ingredients.

▶ Products with less than 70 percent of organic ingredients may include the organic ingredients on the ingredients list but may not use the term *organic* on the front of the package.

▶ The USDA allows the word *natural* to describe meal and poultry that contains no artificial ingredients or added color.

Source: Food Marketing Institute, "FMI Backgrounder: Natural and Organic Foods," September 2008, Available at www.fmi.org/docs/media-backgrounder/natural_organic_foods.pdf?sfvrsn=2

Maintaining a nutritious diet within the confines of student life can be challenging. However, if you take the time to plan healthy meals, you will find that you are eating better, enjoying it more, and actually saving money. The Money & Health box examines ways to include fruits and vegetables in your diet without breaking the bank.

LO 4 | FOOD SAFETY: A GROWING CONCERN

Explain food safety concerns facing Americans and people in other regions of the world.

Eating unhealthy food is one thing. Eating food that has been contaminated with a pathogen, toxin, or other harmful substance is quite another. As outbreaks of foodborne illness (commonly called food poisoning) make the news, the food industry has come under fire. The Food Safety Modernization Act, passed into law in 2011, included new requirements for food processors to take actions to prevent contamination of foods. The act gave the FDA greater authority to inspect food-manufacturing facilities and to recall contaminated foods.[49]

organic Grown without use of toxic and persistent pesticides, chemicals, or hormones.

Choosing Organic or Locally Grown Foods

Concerns about the health effects of chemicals used to grow and produce food have led many people to turn to foods that are **organic**—foods and beverages developed, grown, or raised without the use of toxic and persistent pesticides or fertilizers, antibiotics, or hormones. Any food sold in the United States as organic has to meet criteria set by the USDA under the National Organic Rule and can carry a USDA seal verifying products as "certified organic." Under this rule, a product that is certified may carry one of the following terms: "100 percent Organic" (100% compliance with organic criteria), "Organic" (must contain at least 95% organic materials), "Made with Organic Ingredients" (must contain at least 70% organic ingredients), or "Some Organic Ingredients" (contains less than 70% organic ingredients—usually listed individually). To be labeled with any of the above terms, the foods also must be produced without genetic modification or germ-killing radiation. However, reliable monitoring systems to ensure credibility are still under development. See the Skills for Behavior Change box for a breakdown of natural versus organic foods.

The market for organic foods has been increasing faster than food sales in general for many years. Whereas only a small subset of the population once bought organic, 81 percent of all U.S. families are now buying organic foods at least occasionally.[50] In 2012, annual organic food sales were estimated to be $31 billion and are expected to rise to $35 billion in 2014.[51]

Is organic food really more nutritious? That depends on what aspect of the food is being studied and how the research is conducted. Two recent review studies, both of which examined decades of research into the nutrient quality of organic versus traditionally grown foods, reached opposite conclusions: One found organic foods more nutritious, and the other did not.[52] However, we do know that pesticide residues remain on conventionally grown produce. The U.S. Environmental Protection Agency warns that food pesticides can lead to health problems like cancer, nerve damage, and birth defects.[53] In 2013, the USDA reported that 3.7 percent of food samples harvested in 2011 had pesticide residues that exceeded the established tolerance level or had residues of pesticides for which no

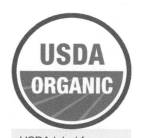

USDA label for organic foods.

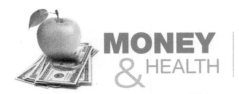

MONEY & HEALTH | ARE FRUITS AND VEGGIES BEYOND YOUR BUDGET?

Many people on a tight budget, including college students, think that fruits and vegetables are beyond their budget. Maybe a carton of orange juice and a package of carrots are affordable, but five to nine servings a day? No way.

If that sounds like you, it's time for some facts. In 2011, the U.S. Department of Agriculture published data showing that the average American family spends more money on food than is necessary to consume a nutritious diet—one that includes the recommended servings of fruits and vegetables. The report concluded that, contrary to popular opinion, people on a tight budget can eat healthfully, including plenty of fruits and vegetables, and spend less on food.

So how do you do it? Here are some tips:

■ **Focus on five fresh favorites.** Throughout the United States, five of the least expensive, perennially available fresh vegetables are carrots, eggplant, lettuce, potatoes, and summer squash. Five fresh fruit options are apples, bananas, pears, pineapple, and watermelon.

■ **Buy small amounts frequently.** Most items of fresh produce keep only a few days, so buy amounts that you know you'll be able to eat or freeze.

■ **Celebrate the season.** From apples to zucchini, when fruits and veggies are in season, they cost less. If you can freeze them, stock up. If not, enjoy them fresh while you can.

■ **Do it yourself.** Avoid prewashed, precut fruits and vegetables, including salad greens. They cost more and often spoil faster. Also choose frozen 100 percent juice concentrate and add the water yourself.

■ **Buy canned or frozen on sale, in bulk.** Canned and frozen produce, especially when it's on sale, may be much less expensive than fresh. Most frozen items are just as nutritious as fresh, and can be even more so, depending on how long ago the fresh food was harvested. For canned items, choose fruits without added sugars and vegetables without added salt or sauces. Bear in mind that beans are legumes and count as a vegetable choice. Low-sodium canned beans are one of the most affordable, convenient, and nutritious foods you can buy. If you can't find low-sodium beans, just rinse them before heating.

■ **Fix and freeze.** Make large batches of homemade soup, vegetable stews, and pasta sauce and store them in single-serving containers in your freezer.

■ **Grow your own.** All it takes is one sunny window, a pot, soil, and a packet of seeds. Lettuce, spinach, and fresh herbs are particularly easy to grow indoors in small spaces.

Sources: U.S. Department of Agriculture, *Eating Healthy on a Budget: The Consumer Economics Perspective*, September 2011, www.choosemyplate.gov/food-groups/downloads/ConsumerEconomicsPerspective.pdf; U.S. Department of Agriculture, Center for Nutrition Policy and Promotion, *Smart Shopping for Veggies and Fruits*, September 2011, www.choosemyplate.gov/food-groups/downloads/TenTips/DGTipsheet9SmartShopping.pdf; U.S. Centers for Disease Control and Prevention, Fruits & Veggies: More Matters, *30 Ways in 30 Days to Stretch Your Fruit & Vegetable Budget*, September 2011, www.fruitsandveggiesmatter.gov/downloads/Stretch_FV_Budget.pdf

---

tolerance level has been established.[54] Both agencies advise consumers to wash fruits and vegetables before cooking or consuming them.

The word **locavore** has been coined to describe people who eat mostly food grown or produced locally, usually within close proximity to their homes. Farmers' markets or homegrown foods or those grown by independent farmers are thought to be fresher and to require far fewer resources to get them to market and keep them fresh for longer periods of time. Locavores believe that locally grown food is preferable to foods produced by large corporations or supermarket-based organic foods, as they make a smaller impact on the environment. The locavore movement is less concerned about foods that are grown organically as they are about buying locally grown foods.

Foodborne Illnesses

Are you concerned that the chicken you are buying doesn't look pleasingly pink or your "fresh" fish smells a little *too* fishy? You may have good reason to be worried. Scientists estimate that foodborne illnesses sicken 1 in 6 Americans (over 48 million people) and cause some 128,000 hospitalizations and 3,000 deaths in the United States annually.[55] Although the incidence of infection with certain microbes has declined, current data from the U.S. Centers for Disease Control and Prevention (CDC) show a lack of recent progress in reducing foodborne infections and highlight the need for improved prevention.[56]

Several common types of bacteria and viruses, including the bacteria salmonella, listeria, and campylobacter and the virus norovirus, cause most foodborne infections and illnesses. Foodborne illnesses can also be caused by a toxin in food that was originally produced by a bacterium or other microbe in the food. These toxins can produce illness even if the microbes that produced them are no longer there. For example, the illness listeriosis is caused by the

locavore A person who primarily eats food grown or produced locally.

SEE IT! VIDEOS

Is organic produce better for you? Watch **Organic Produce,** available on **Mastering**Health™

bacterium *Listeria monocytogenes*, which seriously affects approximately 1,600 individuals in the United States annually, with pregnant women being 10 times more likely than others to become infected.[57] This bacterium is found in the intestinal tracts of humans and animals, milk, soil, and leafy vegetables and can grow slowly at refrigerator temperatures.[58] Potential food sources include ready-to-eat foods such as hot dogs, luncheon meats, cold cuts, fermented or dry sausage, other deli-style meat and poultry, soft cheeses, and unpasteurized milk.[59] Illness from listeria causes fever, chills, headache, abdominal pain and diarrhea; it may later develop into more serious illness in high-risk individuals such as pregnant women.[60]

Signs of foodborne illnesses vary tremendously and usually include one or several symptoms: diarrhea, nausea, cramping, and vomiting. Depending on the amount and virulence of the pathogen, symptoms may appear as early as 30 minutes after eating contaminated food or as long as several days or weeks later. Most of the time, symptoms occur 5 to 8 hours after eating and last only a day or two. For certain populations, such as the very young; older adults; or people with severe illnesses such as cancer, diabetes, kidney disease, or AIDS, foodborne diseases can be fatal.

Several factors contribute to foodborne illnesses. Since fresh foods are not in season much of the year, the United States imports $18 billion in fresh fruits and vegetables from other countries, often from great distances. These countries include Mexico (36% of imports), several Central and South American countries (about 25%), and China (8%).[61] Although we are

CLEAN   SEPARATE   COOK   CHILL

FIGURE 9.9 The Four Core Practices
This logo reminds consumers how to prevent foodborne illness.

Source: Partnership for Food Safety Education, 2919, www.fightbac.org/safe-food-handling

told when we travel to developing and transitioning countries to "boil it, peel it, or don't eat it," we bring these imported foods into our kitchens at home and eat them, often without washing them—or knowing how they were handled or treated during harvest or production.

Food can become contaminated in the field by being watered with tainted water, fertilized with animal manure, or harvested by people who have not washed their hands properly after using the toilet. Food-processing equipment, facilities, or workers may contaminate food, or it can become contaminated if not kept clean and cool during transport or on store shelves. To give you an idea of the implications, studies have shown that the bacterium *Escherichia coli* can survive in cow manure for up to 70 days and can multiply in crops grown with manure unless heat or additives such as salt or preservatives are used to kill the microbes.[62] There are no regulations that prohibit farmers from using animal manure to fertilize crops. In addition, *E. coli* quickly reproduces in summer months as cattle await slaughter in crowded, overheated pens. This increases the chances of meat coming to market already contaminated.

Avoiding Risks in the Home

Part of the responsibility for preventing foodborne illness lies with consumers—more than 30 percent of all foodborne illnesses result from unsafe handling of food at home. Four basic steps reduce the likelihood of contaminating your food (see FIGURE 9.9). Among the most basic precautions are to wash your hands and to wash all produce before eating it. Also, avoid cross-contamination in the kitchen by using separate cutting boards and utensils for meats and produce. Temperature control is also important—refrigerators must be set at 40°F or lower. Cook meats to the recommended temperature to kill contaminants before eating. Keep hot foods hot and cold foods cold to avoid unchecked bacterial growth. Eat leftovers within 3 days, and if you're unsure how long something has been sitting in the fridge, don't take chances. When in doubt, throw it out. See the Skills for Behavior Change box for more tips about reducing risk of foodborne illness.

Food Sensitivities, Allergies, and Intolerances

About 33 percent of people today *think* they have a food allergy; however, it is estimated that only 5 percent of children and 4 percent of adults actually do.[63] Still, the prevalence of

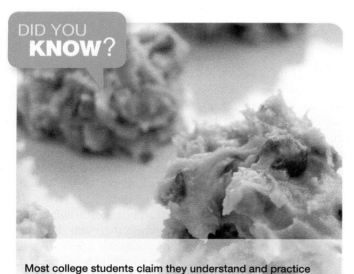

DID YOU KNOW?

Most college students claim they understand and practice food safety guidelines. For instance, in one survey, 88% said they understood the importance of hand washing in preventing foodborne illness. Yet only 49% of those surveyed actually washed their hands always or most of the time before meals.

Source: Data are from B.A. Miko et al., "Personal and Household Hygiene, Environmental Contamination, and Health in Undergraduate Residence Halls in New York City, 2011," *PLoS One* 8, no. 11 (2013): e81460.

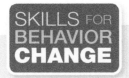

SKILLS FOR BEHAVIOR CHANGE

REDUCE YOUR RISK FOR FOODBORNE ILLNESS

When shopping, put perishable foods in your cart last. Check for cleanliness throughout the store, especially at the salad bar and at the meat and fish counters. Never buy dented cans of food. Check the "sell by" or "use by" date on foods.

▶ Once you get home, put dairy products, eggs, meat, fish, and poultry in the refrigerator immediately. If you don't plan to eat meats within 2 days, freeze them. You can keep an unopened package of hot dogs or luncheon meats for about 2 weeks.

▶ When refrigerating or freezing raw meats, make sure their juices can't spill onto other foods.

▶ Never thaw frozen foods at room temperature. Put them in the refrigerator to thaw or thaw in the microwave, following manufacturer's instructions.

▶ Wash your hands with soap and warm water before preparing food. Wash fruits and vegetables before peeling, slicing, cooking, or eating them—but not meat, poultry, or eggs! Wash cutting boards, countertops, and other utensils and surfaces with detergent and hot water after food preparation.

▶ Use a meat thermometer to ensure that meats are completely cooked. To find out proper cooking temperatures for different types of meat, visit http://foodsafety.gov/keep/charts/mintemp.html

▶ Refrigeration slows the secretion of bacterial toxins into foods. Never leave leftovers out for more than 2 hours. On hot days, don't leave foods out for longer than 1 hour.

reported food allergies is on the rise. Data suggest the prevalence of peanut allergies among children tripled between 1997 and 2008.[64]

A **food allergy,** or hypersensitivity, is an abnormal response to a component—usually a protein—in food that is triggered by the immune system. Symptoms of an allergic reaction vary in severity and may include a tingling sensation in the mouth; swelling of the lips, tongue, and throat; difficulty breathing; skin hives; vomiting; abdominal cramps; and diarrhea. Approximately 100 to 200 deaths per year occur as a result of more severe reactions called *anaphylaxis* that cause widespread inflammation and cardiovascular problems such as a sudden drop in blood pressure.[65] Anaphylaxis may occur within

Peanuts are among the eight most common food allergens.

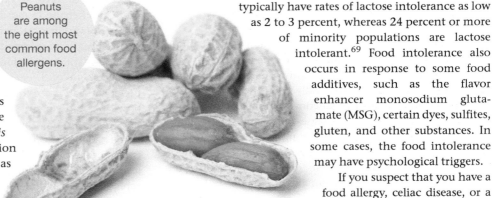

seconds to hours after eating the foods to which one is allergic.

The Food Allergen Labeling and Consumer Protection Act (FALCPA) requires food manufacturers to label foods clearly to indicate the presence of (or possible contamination by) any of the eight major food allergens: milk, eggs, peanuts, wheat, soy, tree nuts (walnuts, pecans, cashews, pistachios, etc.), fish, and shellfish. Al- though over 160 foods have been identified as allergy triggers, these eight foods account for 90 percent of all food allergies in the United States.[66]

Celiac disease is an autoimmune disorder that causes malabsorption of nutrients from the small intestine in genetically susceptible people. It is thought to affect over 2 million Americans, most of whom are undiagnosed.[67] When a person with celiac disease consumes gluten— a protein found in wheat, rye, and barley—the person's immune system responds with inflammation. This degrades the lining of the small intestine and reduces nutrient absorption. Pain, abdominal cramping, often diarrhea, and other symptoms follow in the short term. Untreated, celiac disease can lead to long-term health problems, such as nutritional deficiencies, tissue wasting, osteoporosis, seizures, liver disease, and cancer of the small intestine. Individuals diagnosed with celiac disease are encouraged to consult a dietitian for help designing a gluten-free diet. For more information on gluten-free diets, read Health Headlines: Gluten-Free Diets on the next page.

food allergy Overreaction by the immune system to normally harmless proteins in foods, which are perceived as allergens. In response, the body produces antibodies, triggering allergic symptoms.

celiac disease An inherited immune disorder causing malabsorption of nutrients from the small intestine and triggered by the consumption of gluten, a protein found in certain grains.

food intolerance Adverse effects that result when people who lack the digestive chemicals needed to break down certain substances eat those substances.

Food intolerance can cause you to have symptoms of digestive upset, but the upset is not the result of an immune system response. Probably the best example of a food intolerance is *lactose intolerance,* a problem that affects about 1 in every 10 American adults.[68] Lactase is an enzyme produced by the small intestine that degrades lactose, the sugar in dairy products. If you don't have enough lactase, you cannot digest lactose, and it remains in the gut to be used by bacteria. Gas is formed, and you experience bloating, abdominal pain, and sometimes diarrhea. The prevalence of primary lactose intolerance varies according to race; Americans of European descent typically have rates of lactose intolerance as low as 2 to 3 percent, whereas 24 percent or more of minority populations are lactose intolerant.[69] Food intolerance also occurs in response to some food additives, such as the flavor enhancer monosodium glutamate (MSG), certain dyes, sulfites, gluten, and other substances. In some cases, the food intolerance may have psychological triggers.

If you suspect that you have a food allergy, celiac disease, or a

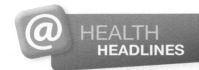

GLUTEN-FREE DIETS

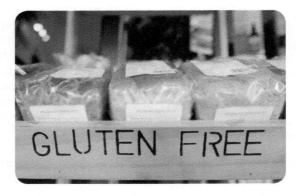

Gluten-free diets have become a fad. The number of individuals consuming a gluten-free diet is fueling a market of gluten-free products. In a 5-year period ending in 2014, gluten-free products grew by more than 34 percent. There are more people following a gluten-free diet than there are diagnosed with celiac disease, a condition that worsens when gluten is consumed. Is this healthy?

A gluten-free diet is an eating plan that leaves out gluten, a protein found in wheat, barley, rye, and triticale, a cross between wheat and rye. Eating a gluten-free diet improves control of the symptoms and complications for those individuals who have celiac disease, Hashimoto's, or who are gluten sensitive.

Going gluten free for people who do not have gluten sensitivities is not necessarily healthier when it means eliminating many common, nutritious foods. Gluten itself doesn't provide any nutritional benefits, but the foods that contain gluten do. These foods are rich in dietary fiber, vitamins, and minerals. Many gluten-free products are made with refined, unenriched gluten-free grains, such as sorghum and rice flours, which are low in essential nutrients and high in fat and kilocalories—not to mention expensive. For this reason, there are no real benefits to eating a gluten-free

diet unless you are gluten sensitive, or have been diagnosed with an autoimmune disorder such as Hashimoto's or celiac disease. In fact, people who follow a gluten-free diet may have low levels of certain vitamins and nutrients in their diets, including iron, calcium, fiber, and the B vitamins riboflavin, thiamin, folate, and niacin.

Switching to a gluten-free diet may seem daunting at first. It's a good idea to consult a dietitian for advice about how to avoid gluten while still eating a healthy, balanced diet. Many healthy foods are naturally free of gluten, including beans, nuts, seeds, legumes, eggs, meats, fish, poultry, fruits, vegetables, and low-fat dairy foods. When buying foods on a gluten-free diet, fresh, unprocessed foods are the best choice.

Certain grains that are naturally gluten free, such as oats, can be contaminated when gluten-free foods come into contact

with gluten-containing foods during manufacturing. You might inadvertently cross-contaminate foods yourself if you prepare gluten-free foods on the same surfaces as wheat breads or other gluten-containing foods. For instance, toasting gluten-free bread in the same toaster you use to toast wheat bread can result in cross-contamination.

Processed foods may also be labeled as "certified gluten-free." The FDA requires that, to use a gluten-free label, the product must contain less than 20 parts per million of gluten. It's best to read the ingredient list before buying. Even if the label states the product is wheat free, it still may contain gluten.

Sources: Packaged Facts, *Gluten-free Foods and Beverages in the US*, 5th ed. (Rockville, MD: Packaged Foods, 2015.) Available from www.packagedfacts.com/Gluten-Free-Foods-8108350/; G. A. Gaesser, and S. S. Angadi, "Gluten-free Diet: Imprudent Dietary Advice for the General Population?," *Journal of the Academy of Nutrition and Dietetics* 112, no. 9 (2012): 1300–1333; S. J. Shepherd and P. R. Gibson, "Nutritional Inadequacies of the Gluten-free Diet in Both Recently-Diagnosed and Long-Term Patients with Celiac Disease," *Journal of Human Nutrition and Dietetics* 26, no. 4 (2013): 349–58, doi: 10.1111/jhn.12018; T. B. Koerner et al., "Gluten Contamination in the Canadian Commercial Oat Supply," *Food Additives and Contaminants Part A, Chemistry, Analysis, Control, Exposure and Risk Assessment*, 28, no. 6 (2013): 705–710, doi: 10.1080/19440049.2011.579626; May Clinic, "Gluten-Free Diet," November 25, 2014, www.mayoclinic.org/healthy-lifestyle/nutrition-and-healthy-eating/in-depth/gluten-free-diet/art-20048530

food intolerance, see your doctor. Because these diseases can have some common symptoms, as well as share symptoms with other gastrointestinal disorders, clinical diagnosis is essential.

Genetically Modified Food Crops

Genetically modified crop farming is expanding rapidly around the world. Genetic modification involves the insertion or deletion of genes into the DNA of an organism. In the case of **genetically modified (GM) foods**, usually this genetic cutting and pasting is done to enhance production, for example, by making disease- or insect-resistant plants, improving yield, or controlling weeds. In addition, GM foods are sometimes created to improve the color and appearance of foods or

genetically modified (GM) foods Foods derived from organisms whose DNA has been altered using genetic engineering techniques.

to enhance specific nutrients. For example, in regions where rice is a staple and vitamin A deficiency and iron-deficiency anemia are leading causes of morbidity and mortality, GM technology has been used to create varieties of rice high in vitamin A and iron. Another use under development is the production and delivery of vaccines through GM foods.

The long-term safety of GM foods—for humans and other species—is still in question. The American Association for the Advancement of Science reports that foods containing GM ingredients are no more a risk than are the same foods composed of crops modified over time with conventional plant breeding techniques, and the World Health Organization states that no adverse effects on human health have been shown from consumption of GM foods in countries that have approved their use.[70] The debate surrounding GM foods is not likely to end soon; see the Points of View box for more on this debate.

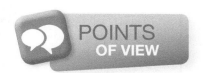

Genetically Modified Foods
Boon or Bane?

Farmers in the United States have widely accepted GM crops. Genetically modified (GM) foods do not occur naturally but have been altered by introducing a gene from a different organism. Soybeans and cotton are the most common GM crops, followed by corn. On supermarket shelves, an estimated 75 percent of processed foods are genetically modified. Even much of the produce you buy in stores has been genetically modified, including tomatoes, corn, potatoes, squash, and soybeans.

State governments, industry, and scientists tout the benefits of genetically modified foods for health, agriculture, and the ecosystem, including feeding the world's population. In contrast, consumer activists, environmental organizations, religious groups, and health advocates warn of unexpected health risks and environmental and socioeconomic consequences. Consumers question whether genetically modified plants are safe to eat. By 2014, two states—Connecticut and Maine—had enacted GMO-labeling laws. However, the legislation doesn't go into effect until nearby states enact similar labeling laws. The FDA continues to evaluate the safety issues of genetically modified foods and future regulations to protect the world's food supply.

Below are some of the main points for and against the development of GM food.

Arguments for the Development of GM Foods

- People have been manipulating food crops—primarily through selective breeding—since the beginning of agriculture. Genetic modification is fundamentally the same thing, just more precise.
- Modified fruits and vegetables produce higher levels of antioxidants, which reduce the risk of heart disease and cancer, and vitamin A to prevent blindness.
- Genetically modified seeds and products are tested for safety, and there has never been a substantiated claim for a human illness resulting from consumption of a GM food.
- Genetically modified crops have the potential to reduce world hunger: They can be created to grow more quickly than conventional crops, increasing productivity and allowing for faster cycling of crops, which means more food yield. In addition, nutrient-enhanced crops can address malnutrition, and crops engineered to resist spoiling or damage can allow for transportation to areas affected by drought or natural disaster.

Arguments against the Development of GM Foods

- Genetic modification may cause an allergic reaction. Allergic reactions occur in humans when their immune system recognizes a protein as a foreign invader. Research in vitro studies suggests that some GM foods may cause allergic reactions.
- GM foods have the potential to reduce absorption of essential nutrients. For example, if the gene inserted to make the new GM food increases the phytate content of the food, which reduces the absorption of certain minerals, such as calcium and iron. Modified soy products may also produce less phytoestrogens known to reduce the risk of heart disease and cancer.
- Plants naturally produce low levels of substances that are toxic to humans. While these toxins do not produce problems for humans, there is a concern that adding a new gene to produce a GM plant may cause the new plant to produce toxins at higher levels that could be dangerous if eaten. For instance, GM potatoes produce higher levels of glycoalkaloids.

WHERE DO YOU STAND?

- Do you think GM foods are more helpful or harmful?
- What are your greatest concerns over GM foods? What do you think are their greatest benefits?
- In what ways could the creators of GM foods address the concerns of those opposed to them?

- What sort of regulation do you think the government should have with regard to the creation, cultivation, and sale of GM foods?
- Currently, there are no GM livestock; however, many livestock are fed GM feed or feed that includes additives and vaccines produced by GM microorganisms. Do you feel any differently about directly consuming GM crops versus eating the flesh, milk, or eggs of an animal that has been fed on GM crops?

Sources: U.S. Department of Agriculture, Economic Research Service, "Adoption of Genetically Engineered Crops in the U.S.," July 2013, www.ers.usda.gov/data-products/adoption-of-genetically-engineered-crops-in-the-us.aspx; Center for Food Safety, "About Genetically Engineered Foods," Accessed March 2014, www.centerforfoodsafety.org/issues/311/ge-foods/about-ge-foods; A. Bakshi, "Potential Adverse Health Effects of Genetically Modified Crops," *Journal of Toxicology and Environmental Health. Part B Critical Reviews* 6, no. 3 (2003): 211–25.

ASSESS | YOURSELF

How Healthy Are Your Eating Habits?

1 Keep Track of Your Food Intake

Keep a food diary for 5 days, writing down everything you eat or drink. Be sure to include the approximate amount or portion size. Add up the number of servings from each of the major food groups on each day and enter them into the chart below.

Number of Servings:	Day 1	Day 2	Day 3	Day 4	Day 5	Average
Fruits						
Vegetables						
Grains						
Protein Foods						
Dairy						
Fats and Oils						
Sweets						

2 Evaluate Your Food Intake

Now compare your consumption patterns to the MyPlate recommendations. Look at **TABLE 9.1** (page 264) and **FIGURE 9.5** (page 275) and visit **www.choosemyplate.gov** to evaluate your daily caloric needs and the recommended consumption rates for the different food groups. How does your diet match up?

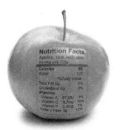

	Less than the Recommended Amount	About Equal to the Recommended Amount	More than the Recommended Amount
1. How does your daily fruit consumption compare to the recommendation for you?	○	○	○
2. How does your daily vegetable consumption compare to the recommendation for you?	○	○	○

	Less than the Recommended Amount	About Equal to the Recommended Amount	More than the Recommended Amount
3. How does your daily grain consumption compare to the recommendation for you?	○	○	○
4. How does your daily protein food consumption compare to the recommendation for you?	○	○	○
5. How does your daily dairy food consumption compare to the recommendation for you?	○	○	○
6. How does your daily calorie consumption compare to the recommendation for your age and activity level?	○	○	○

Scoring 2

If you found that your food intake is consistent with the MyPlate recommendations, congratulations! If you are falling short in a major food group or are overdoing it in certain categories, consider taking steps to adopt healthier eating habits. Following are some additional assessments to help you figure out where your diet is lacking.

Source: J. S. Blake, K. D. Munoz, and S. Volpe, *Nutrition: From Science to You*, 3rd ed., © 2016. Reprinted and electronically reproduced by permission of Pearson Education, Inc., Upper Saddle River, New Jersey.

YOUR PLAN FOR CHANGE

The **ASSESS YOURSELF** activity gave you the chance to evaluate your current nutritional habits. Once you have considered these results, you can decide whether you need to make changes in your daily eating for long-term health.

TODAY, YOU CAN:

☐ Start keeping a more detailed food log. The easy-to-use SuperTracker at www.supertracker.usda.gov can help you keep track of your food intake and analyze what you eat. Take note of the nutritional content of the various foods you eat and write down particulars about the number of calories, grams of saturated fat, grams of sugar, milligrams of sodium, and so on of each food. Try to find specific weak spots: Are you consuming too many calories or too much salt or sugar? Do you eat too little calcium or iron? Use the SuperTracker to plan a healthier food intake to overcome these weak spots.

☐ Take a field trip to the grocery store. Forgo your fast-food dinner and instead spend time in the produce section of the supermarket. Purchase your favorite fruits and vegetables, and try something new to expand your tastes.

WITHIN THE NEXT TWO WEEKS, YOU CAN:

☐ Plan at least three meals that you can make at home or in your dorm room, and purchase the ingredients you'll need ahead of time. Something as simple as a chicken sandwich on whole-grain bread will be more nutritious, and probably cheaper, than heading out for a fast-food meal.

☐ Start reading labels. Be aware of the amount of calories, sodium, sugars, and saturated fats in prepared foods; aim to buy and consume those that are lower in all of these and are higher in micronutrients and fiber.

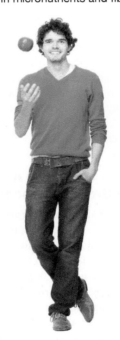

BY THE END OF THE SEMESTER, YOU CAN:

☐ Get in the habit of eating a healthy breakfast every morning. Combine whole grains, proteins, and fruit in your breakfast—for example, eat a bowl of cereal with soy milk and bananas or a cup of low-fat yogurt with granola and berries. Eating a healthy breakfast will jump-start your metabolism, prevent drops in blood glucose levels, and keep your brain and body performing at their best through your morning classes.

☐ Commit to one or two healthful changes to your eating patterns for the rest of the semester. You might resolve to eat five servings of fruits and vegetables every day, to switch to low-fat or nonfat dairy products, to stop drinking soft drinks, or to use only olive oil in your cooking. Use your food diary to help you spot places where you can make healthier choices on a daily basis.

CHAPTER REVIEW

To hear an MP3 Tutor Session, scan here or visit the Study Area in **MasteringHealth**.

LO 1 | Essential Nutrients for Health

- Nutrition is the science of the relationship between physiological function and the essential elements of the foods we eat. The Dietary Reference Intakes (DRIs) are recommended nutrient intakes for healthy people.
- The essential nutrients include water, proteins, carbohydrates, fats, vitamins, and minerals. Water makes up 50 to 60 percent of our body weight and is necessary for nearly all life processes. Proteins are major components of our cells and tissues and are key elements of antibodies, enzymes, and hormones. Carbohydrates are our primary sources of energy. Fats provide energy while we are at rest and for long-term activity. They also play important roles in maintaining body temperature, cushioning and protecting organs, and promoting healthy cell function. Vitamins are organic compounds, and minerals are inorganic elements. We need these micronutrients in small amounts to maintain healthy body structure and function.

LO 2 | Nutritional Guidelines

- A healthful diet is adequate, moderate, balanced, varied, and nutrient dense. The Dietary Guidelines for Americans and the MyPlate plan provide guidelines for healthy eating. These recommendations, developed by the USDA, place emphasis on balancing calories and understanding which foods to increase and which to decrease.
- The Nutrition Facts label on food labels identifies the serving size, number of calories per serving, and amounts of various nutrients, as well as the %DV, which is the percentage of recommended daily values those amounts represent.

LO 3 | How Can I Eat More Healthfully?

- With a little menu planning, vegetarianism can be a healthful lifestyle choice, providing plenty of nutrients, plus fiber and phytochemicals, typically with less saturated fat and fewer calories.
- Although some people may benefit from taking vitamin and mineral supplements, a healthy diet is the best way to give your body the nutrients it needs.
- College students face unique challenges in eating healthfully. Learning to make better choices, to eat healthfully on a budget, and to eat nutritionally in the dorm are all possible when you use the information in this chapter.

LO 4 | Food Safety: A Growing Concern

- Organic foods are grown and produced without the use of toxic and persistent synthetic pesticides, fertilizers, antibiotics, hormones, or genetic modification. The USDA offers certification of organic farms and regulates claims regarding organic ingredients used on food labels.
- Foodborne illnesses can be traced to contamination of food at any point from fields to the consumer's kitchen. To keep food safe at home, follow four steps: Clean, separate, cook, and chill.
- Food allergies, celiac disease, food intolerances, GM foods, and other food safety and health concerns are becoming increasingly important to health-wise consumers. Recognizing potential risks and taking steps to prevent problems are part of a sound nutritional plan.

POP QUIZ

Visit **MasteringHealth** to personalize your study plan with Chapter Review Quizzes and Dynamic Study Modules.

LO 1 | Essential Nutrients for Health

1. What is the most crucial nutrient for life?
   a. Water
   b. Fiber
   c. Minerals
   d. Starch

2. Which of the following nutrients is critical for the repair and growth of body tissue?
   a. Carbohydrates
   b. Proteins
   c. Vitamins
   d. Fats

3. Which of the following substances helps move food through the digestive tract?
   a. Folate
   b. Fiber
   c. Minerals
   d. Starch

4. What substance provides energy, promotes healthy skin and hair, insulates body organs, helps maintain body temperature, and contributes to healthy cell function?
   a. Fats
   b. Fibers
   c. Proteins
   d. Carbohydrates

5. Which of the following fats is a healthier fat to include in the diet?
   a. *Trans* fat
   b. Saturated fat
   c. Unsaturated fat
   d. Hydrogenated fat

6. Which vitamin maintains bone health?
   a. B_{12}
   b. D
   c. B_6
   d. Niacin

LO 2 | Nutritional Guidelines

7. Which of the following foods would be considered a healthy, *nutrient-dense* food?
   a. Nonfat milk
   b. Cheddar cheese
   c. Soft drink
   d. Potato chips

8. The *Dietary Guidelines for Americans 2010* recommend that you
   a. stop smoking and walk daily.
   b. sleep 8 hours a night and jog every other day.
   c. maintain a kilocalorie balance over time and stop smoking.
   d. maintain a kilocalorie balance over time and sustain a healthy body weight.

LO 3 | How Can I Eat More Healthfully?

9. Carrie eats dairy products and eggs, but she does not eat fish, poultry, or meat. Carrie is considered a(n)
   a. vegan.
   b. lacto-ovo-vegetarian.
   c. ovo-vegetarian.
   d. pesco-vegetarian.

LO 4 | Food Safety: A Growing Concern

10. Lucas's doctor diagnoses him with celiac disease. Which of the following foods should Lucas cut out of his diet to eat gluten free?
    a. Shellfish
    b. Eggs
    c. Peanuts
    d. Wheat

Answers to the Pop Quiz can be found on page A-1. If you answered a question incorrectly, review the section tagged by the Learning Outcome. For even more study tools, visit MasteringHealth.

THINK ABOUT IT!

LO 1 | Essential Nutrients for Health

1. Which factors influence a person's dietary patterns and behaviors? What factors have been the greatest influences on your eating behaviors?

2. What are the major types of nutrients that you need to obtain from the foods you eat? What happens if you fail to get enough of some of them? Are there significant differences between men and women in particular areas of nutrition?

LO 2 | Nutritional Guidelines

3. What are the four main recommendations from the *Dietary Guidelines for Americans 2010*? What can you do to balance your kilocalories to maintain a healthy body weight?

4. What are the major food groups in the MyPlate plan? From which groups do you eat too few servings? What can you do to increase or decrease your intake of selected food groups?

LO 3 | How Can I Eat More Healthfully?

5. Distinguish among varieties of vegetarianism. Which types are most likely to lead to nutrient deficiencies? What can be done to ensure that even the most strict vegetarian receives enough of the major nutrients?

6. What are the major problems that many college students face when trying to eat the right foods? List five actions that you and your classmates could take immediately to improve your eating.

LO 4 | Food Safety: A Growing Concern

7. What are the major risks for foodborne illnesses, and what can you do to protect yourself?

8. How does a food intolerance differ from a food allergy?

ACCESS YOUR HEALTH ON THE INTERNET

The following websites explore further topics and issues related to personal health. Visit MasteringHealth for links to the websites and RSS feeds.

Academy of Nutrition and Dietetics. The academy provides information on a full range of dietary topics, including sports nutrition, healthful cooking, and nutritional eating; the site also links to scientific publications and information on scholarships and public meetings. **www.eatright.org**

U.S. Food and Drug Administration (FDA). The FDA provides information for consumers and professionals in the areas of food safety, supplements, and medical devices. There are links to other sources of information about nutrition and food. **www.fda.gov**

Food and Nutrition Information Center. This site offers a wide variety of information related to food and nutrition. **http://fnic.nal.usda.gov**

National Institutes of Health: Office of Dietary Supplements. This is the site of the International Bibliographic Database of Information on Dietary Supplements (IBDIDS), updated quarterly. **http://dietary-supplements .info.nih.gov**

U.S. Department of Agriculture, USDA: Choose MyPlate. The USDA offers a personalized nutrition and physical activity plan based on the MyPlate program, sample menus and recipes, and a full discussion of the *Dietary Guidelines for Americans.* **www.choosemyplate.gov**

U.S. Department of Health and Human Services: Food Safety. This is the official gateway site to food safety information provided by the federal government, including recalls and alerts, news, and tips for reporting problems. **www .foodsafety.gov**

10 Reaching and Maintaining a Healthy Weight

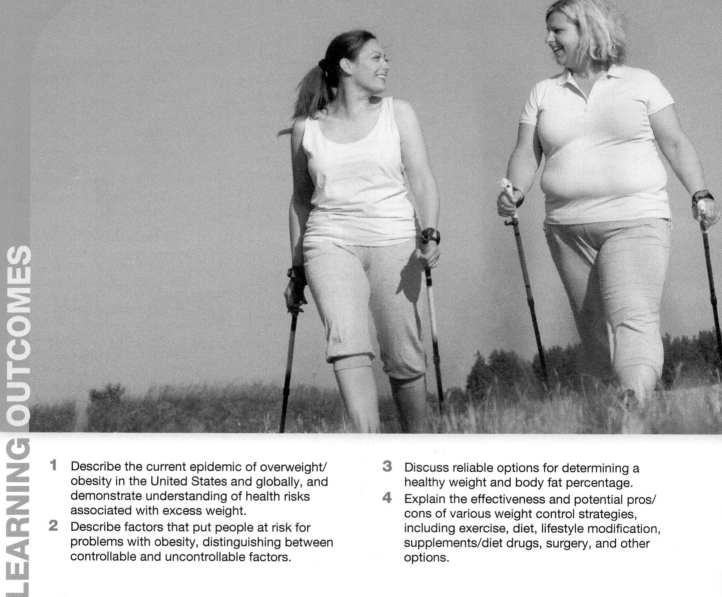

1 Describe the current epidemic of overweight/obesity in the United States and globally, and demonstrate understanding of health risks associated with excess weight.

2 Describe factors that put people at risk for problems with obesity, distinguishing between controllable and uncontrollable factors.

3 Discuss reliable options for determining a healthy weight and body fat percentage.

4 Explain the effectiveness and potential pros/cons of various weight control strategies, including exercise, diet, lifestyle modification, supplements/diet drugs, surgery, and other options.

The United States currently has the dubious distinction of being among the fattest developed nations on Earth. Young and old, rich and poor, rural and urban, educated and uneducated, Americans share one thing in common—they are fatter than virtually all previous generations.[1] The word **obesogenic** refers to environmental conditions that promote obesity, such as the availability and marketing of unhealthy foods, social and cultural norms that lead to high calorie consumption and lack of physical activity—an apt descriptor of our society.

LO 1 | OVERWEIGHT AND OBESITY: A GROWING CHALLENGE

Describe the current epidemic of overweight/obesity in the United States and globally, and demonstrate understanding of health risks associated with excess weight.

Today **obesity** is often categorized by class, reflecting both severity and increasing risks based on percent body fat. *Obesity* refers to a body weight that is more than 20 percent above recommended levels for health or a **body mass index (BMI)** over 30. *Class 1 obesity* refers to those with a BMI ≥30 but less than 35. *Class 2 obesity* includes those with a BMI of ≥35, but less than 40, and *Class 3 obesity* includes those with a BMI ≥40, often referred to as *morbidly obese*.[2] Less extreme, but still damaging, is *overweight*, which is body weight more than 10 percent above healthy levels or a BMI between 25 and 29.

Overweight and Obesity in the United States

FIGURE 10.1 illustrates just how high levels of obesity have risen in the United States, as a percentage of the population, since the 1960s. Indeed, the prevalence of obesity has steadily increased in recent decades, with disproportionate risks among some populations.[3] Children aged 2 to 5 have shown slight decreases overall in prevalence in recent years. Children and adolescents living in low-income, low-education, and higher-unemployment homes are at significantly greater risk of developing obesity, while those from higher income homes with more educated parents have decreasing risk.[4] More than 69 percent of U.S. adults overall (over 178 million people) are overweight or obese.[5] Rates of obesity are 34 percent among men and 36 percent for women, and rates of extreme obesity are on the rise.[6]

HEAR IT! PODCASTS

Want a study podcast for this chapter? Download **Managing Your Weight: Finding a Health Balance**, available on MasteringHealth™

Research points to higher obesity rates and risks among some ethnic groups in the United States. Hispanic men (80 percent) and non-Hispanic white men (73 percent) are more likely to be overweight/obese than are non-Hispanic black men

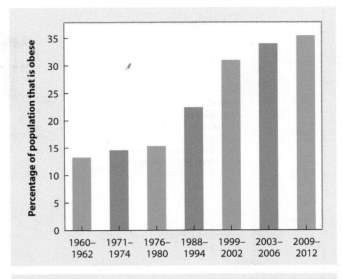

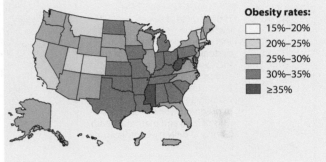

FIGURE 10.1 Obesity in the United States

Sources: Centers for Disease Control and Prevention, "Health, United States, 2013, Table 69. Healthy weight, overweight, and obesity among adults aged 20 and over, by selected characteristics: United States, selected years 1960–1962 through 2009–2012," 2013, www.cdc.gov/nchs/data/hus/2013/069 .pdf; Centers for Disease Control and Prevention, "Obesity Prevalence Maps 2013," www.cdc.gov/obesity/data/prevalence-maps.html

(69 percent). Non-Hispanic black women (82 percent) and Hispanic women (76) percent) are more likely to be overweight or obese than are non-Hispanic white women (61 percent).[7] In sharp contrast, between 51 and 68 percent of Asian populations are at a healthy weight.[8]

An Obesogenic World

The United States is not alone in the obesity epidemic. In fact, obesity has more than doubled globally since 1980, with over 1.9 billion overweight and 600 million obese adults.[9] While obesity was once predominantly a problem in high-income countries, today increasing numbers of low- and middle-income countries have overweight/obesity

obesogenic refers to environmental conditions that promote obesity, such as the availability of unhealthy foods, social and cultural norms that lead to high calorie consumption and lack of physical activity.

obesity Having a body weight more than 20 percent above healthy recommended levels; in an adult, a BMI of 30 or more.

body mass index (BMI) A number calculated from a person's weight and height that is used to assess risk for possible present or future health problems.

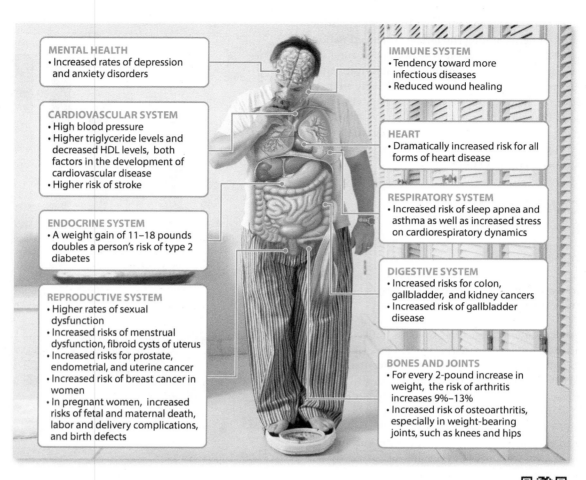

FIGURE 10.2 Potential Negative Health Effects of Overweight and Obesity

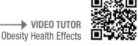
→ VIDEO TUTOR
Obesity Health Effects

globesity Global rates of obesity

problems.[10] The global epidemic of high rates of overweight and obesity in multiple regions of the world has come to be known as **globesity**.

Health Risks of Excess Weight

Although smoking is still the leading cause of preventable death in the United States, obesity is rapidly gaining ground. Cardiovascular disease (CVD), stroke, cancer, hypertension, diabetes, depression, digestive problems, gallstones, sleep apnea, osteoarthritis, certain cancers, and other ailments lead the list of life-threatening, weight-related problems. **FIGURE 10.2** summarizes these and other potential health consequences of obesity.

Consider the following facts about specific risks for obese individuals compared to their nonobese counterparts:[11]

■ They have a 104 percent increase in risk of heart failure.
■ BMI greater than 30 reduces their life expectancy by 2 to 4 years.
■ BMI greater than 40 costs 8 to 10 years of life expectancy—similar to a long-term smoker.

■ Obese adolescents have a 16-times increased risk of becoming severely obese adults, and at current prevalence rates, will result in 1.5 million life years lost.[12]

Diabetes, strongly associated with overweight and obesity, is another major concern. Over 29 million Americans have diabetes, and another 86 million adults have pre-diabetes.[13] **Focus On: Minimizing Your Risk for Diabetes** discusses the devastating effects of obesity on diabetes-related risks and the benefits of prevention. (See the **Money & Health** box for information on the costs of obesity.)

CVD and chronic, killer diseases are not the only risks associated with overweight and obesity. The costs of social isolation, bullying in school, stigmatization, discrimination, and diminished quality of life can also be devastating. Obese individuals suffer more major disability and difficulty with activities of daily living (ADLs) than do their nonobese counterparts. They are also more likely to experience falls and injury, with the exception of morbidly obese individuals—who may fall less—perhaps because they are less active, and seem to be less prone to injury when they fall.[14]

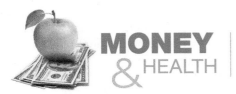

MONEY & HEALTH | "LIVING LARGE" CAN BE INCREASINGLY COSTLY

"The startling economic costs of obesity, often borne by the nonobese, could become the epidemic's second-hand smoke."

—Sharon Begley, "As America's Waistline Expands, Costs Soar," Reuters, April 30, 2012.

A large body of literature points to evidence that as BMI increases, healthcare consumption and associated costs also increase. Consider the following:

- Obesity is believed to be one of the three largest human-generated social burdens in the world.
- More than 2.1 billion people, almost 30 percent of the world's population, are overweight or obese—more than 2.5 times the number of people who are undernourished.
- Obesity is responsible for nearly 5 percent of all the deaths each year globally. Its economic impact hits international gross domestic product hard, costing nearly $2.0 trillion—right up there with smoking ($2.1 trillion), armed violence ($2.1 trillion), war and terrorism ($2.1 trillion), and alcoholism ($1.4 trillion).
- Obese populations have a 36 percent higher annual health care cost than healthy-weight populations. Lifetime medical costs for major diseases increase by over 50 percent for obese individuals—twice that amount for severely obese.
- More than double previous estimates, almost 21 percent of U.S. health care costs can be attributed to obesity. By some estimates, morbidly obese individuals may cost between $6,500 and $15,000 dollars more per year

in additional health care costs when factors such as longer hospital stays, recovery, and increased medications are included.

- Obese populations incur 37 percent higher prescription drug costs than healthy-weight populations
- Obese individuals miss nearly 2 days of work more than their healthy weight counterparts, accounting for between 6.5 to 12.6 percent of total absenteeism costs each year.
- Obese individuals are more likely to suffer from "presenteeism" where they are less likely to be productive and have less stamina than their healthy-weight counterparts.
- Obesity may mean increased transportation costs for more fuel consumption and larger vehicles/seats, bigger ambulances, and other issues.
- A recent study of 150,000 Swedish brothers indicated that *being obese is as costly as not having an undergraduate degree*; an "obesity penalty" is equivalent to earning over 16 percent less than their normal weight counterparts.

Many insurance companies are charging more for people who are overweight and refuse to participate in available "wellness" programs. In fact, the U.S. Patient Protection and Affordable Care Act has a provision that allows employers to charge obese workers significantly higher premiums (between 30 and 50 percent more in some cases!) for their health insurance if they don't make a good faith effort to reduce their health risks and must provide support for services to help them lose weight. Some workplaces offer counseling and

free gym memberships for those struggling with their weight. Are these fair? Many argue that such penalties unfairly reflect a form of obesity stigma and size discrimination, whereas others argue that those within a normal weight range shouldn't have to subsidize excess costs. Still others argue that this is a slippery slope on the way to paying more for factors like eating high-fat foods and having high cholesterol, having too many beers in a week, or even unintended pregnancy.

Currently, there is much debate about these extra costs, even as many insurers and businesses implement policies and programs to motivate employees and members of insurance groups to take action, "or else."

Sources: A. Dee et al., "The Direct and Indirect Costs of Both Overweight and Obesity: A systematic Review," *BMC Research Notes* 7, no. 1 (2014): 242, doi: 10.1186/1756-0500-7-242; R. Hammond and R. Levine, "The Economic Impact of Obesity in the United States," *Diabetes, Metabolic Syndrome and Obesity: Targets and Therapy* 3 (2010): 285–95; T. Andreyeva et al., "State-Level Estimates of Obesity-Attributable Costs of Absenteeism," *Journal of Occupational and Environmental Medicine* 56, no. 11 (2014): 1120–27; P. Lunderg et al., "Body Size, Skills and Income: Evidence from 150,000 Teenage Siblings," *Demography* 51, no. 5 (2014): 1573–96; C. Roberts, et al., "Patchy Progress on Obesity Prevention: Emerging Examples, Entrenched Barriers and New Thinking," *The Lancet* (2015), dx.doi.org/10.1016/S0140-6736(14)61744-x. (Epub ahead of print.); McKinsey & Company, "How the World Could Better Fight Obesity," November 2014, www.mckinsey.com/insights/economic_studies/how_the_world_could_better_fight_obesity; J. Cawley and C. Meyerhoefer, "The Medical Care Costs of Obesity: An Instrumental Variables Approach," *Journal of Health Economics* 31, no. 1 (2012): 219, doi: 10.1016/j.jhealeco.2011.10.003; E. A. Finkelstein et al., "The Costs of Obesity in the Workplace," *Journal of Occupational and Environmental Medicine* 52, no. 10 (2012): 971–76.

LO 2 | FACTORS CONTRIBUTING TO OVERWEIGHT AND OBESITY

Describe factors that put people at risk for problems with obesity, distinguishing between controllable and uncontrollable factors.

The reasons for our soaring rates of overweight and obesity are complex, and not all of them are within easy individual

control. Although diet and exercise are two major contributors, other factors, including genetics and physiology, are also important. Newer thinking regarding reducing obesity risk involves a more ecological approach that seeks to change obesogenic environmental and contextual factors. Learned behaviors in the home; influences at school and in social environments; media influences; and the environments where we live, work, and play are important to our weight profiles.[15]

Genetic and Physiological Factors

Are some people born to be fat? Genes, hormones, and other aspects of your physiology seem to influence whether you become obese or thin.

Genes: A Variety of Theories In spite of decades of research, the exact role of genes in one's predisposition toward obesity remains in question. Countless observational studies back up the theory that fat parents tend to have fat children. Whether that is due to learned eating and exercise behaviors, environmental cues, genes, or a combination is unclear. Early support for a genetic basis for obesity came from twin research. Researchers found that adopted individuals tend to be similar in weight to their biological parents and that identical twins are twice as likely to weigh the same as are fraternal twins, even if they are raised separately.[16] Subsequent research supported this theory, exploring the fact that obesity involves complex gene-gene and gene-environmental interactions: One gene in particular, the *FTO* gene, may be among the most important.[17] Much of this work has centered on the role of genes such as FTO on regulation the hormone ghrelin—a key factor in eating behavior.[18] Specifically, people with certain genetic variations may tend to graze for food more often, eat more meals, and consume more calories every day, as well as display patterns of seeking out high-fat food groups. Also, different genes may influence weight gain at certain periods of life, particularly during adolescence and young adulthood.[19] Rather than acting individually, the effects of the genes may be in clusters, influencing the regulation of food intake through action in the central nervous system, as well as influencing fat cell synthesis and functioning.

So, if your genes play a key role in obesity tendencies, are you doomed to a lifelong battle with your weight? Probably not. A healthy lifestyle may be able to override "obesity" genes. Results of a major European study found that the effects of the *FTO* gene on obesity is over 30 percent less among physically active adults. Those who seemed to be beating their obesity tendencies exercised at least 90 minutes a day compared to those who exercised 30 minutes.[20]

One potential genetic basis for obesity was identified as a result of observational studies of certain Native American and African tribes. Labeled the *thrifty gene theory*, researchers noted higher body fat and obesity levels in some of these tribes than in the general population.[21] Because their ancestors struggled through centuries of famine, members of the tribes appear to have survived by adapting metabolically to periods of famine with slowed metabolism. Over time, ancestors may have passed on a genetic, hormonal, or metabolic predisposition toward fat storage that makes losing fat more difficult. Critics of this theory believe that there are many other factors that influence obesity development, most of which focus on *obesogenic* behaviors and environments.

Metabolic Rates Several aspects of your metabolism also help determine whether you gain, maintain, or lose weight. Each of us has an innate energy-burning capacity called **basal metabolic rate (BMR)**—the minimum rate at which the body uses energy to maintain basic vital functions. A BMR for the average, healthy adult is usually between 1,200 and 1,800 calories per day. Technically, to measure BMR, a person would be awake, but all major stimuli (including stressors to the sympathetic nervous system and digestion) would be at rest. Usually, the best time to measure BMR is after 8 hours of sleep and after a 12-hour fast.

A more practical way of assessing your energy expenditure levels is the **resting metabolic rate (RMR).** Slightly higher than the BMR, the RMR includes the BMR plus any additional energy expended through daily sedentary activities such as food digestion, sitting, studying, or standing. The **exercise metabolic rate (EMR)** accounts for the remaining percentage of all daily calorie expenditures and refers to the energy expenditure that occurs during physical activity. For most of us, these calories come from light daily activities, such as walking, climbing stairs, and mowing the lawn.

Your BMR and RMR fluctuate through life, and are highest during infancy, puberty, and pregnancy. Generally, the younger you are, the higher your BMR, partly because cells undergo rapid subdivision during periods of growth, consuming lots of energy. After age 30, a person's BMR slows down 1 to

---

basal metabolic rate (BMR) The rate of energy expenditure by a body at complete rest in a neutral environment.

resting metabolic rate (RMR) The energy expenditure of the body under BMR conditions plus other daily sedentary activities.

exercise metabolic rate (EMR) The energy expenditure that occurs during exercise.

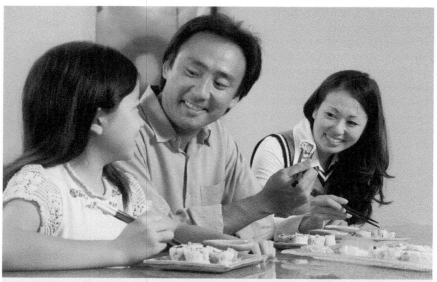

Many factors help determine weight and body type, including heredity and genetic makeup, environment, and learned eating patterns, which are often connected to family habits.

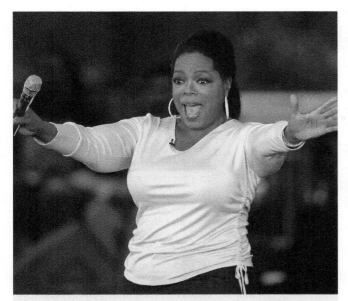

Oprah Winfrey has been candid about her struggles with yo-yo dieting. Such a pattern disrupts the body's metabolism and makes future weight loss more difficult and permanent changes even harder to maintain.

2 percent a year; older people commonly find an extra helping of ice cream harder to burn off. Slower BMR, coupled with less activity, age-related muscle loss, and shifting priorities from fitness to family and career obligations contribute to the weight gain of many middle-aged people.

Anyone who has ever lost weight only to reach a point at which, try as they might, they can't lose another ounce, may be a victim of **adaptive thermogenesis**, whereby the body slows metabolic activity and energy expenditure as a form of defensive protection against possible starvation. With increased weight loss may come increased hunger sensations, slowed energy expenditure, and a tendency to regain weight or make further weight loss more difficult.[22]

Yo-yo diets refer to when people cycle between periods of weight loss and gain. Typically, after weight loss, BMR is lower due to the fact that they body has less muscle mass and weight and requires less energy for basic functioning. When dieters resume eating after their weight loss, due to the related BMR decrease, calories burn more slowly, and they regain weight. Repeated cycles of dieting and regaining weight may actually increase the likelihood of getting heavier over time. Increased age and overall loss of muscle mass through inactivity also tend to result in lowered BMR.

On the other side of the BMR equation is **set point theory**, which suggests that our bodies fight to maintain weight around a narrow range or set point. If we go on a drastic starvation diet or fast, BMR slows to conserve energy. Set point theory, which suggests that our own bodies may sabotage our weight loss efforts by holding on to calories, explaining why people tend to stay near a certain weight threshold and why moving to a different level of weight loss is difficult. The good news is that set points can be changed; however, these changes may take time to be permanent.

Hormonal Influences Obese people may be more likely than thin people to satisfy their appetite and eat for reasons other than nutrition.[23] In some instances, the problem with overconsumption may be related more to **satiety** than it is to appetite or hunger. People generally feel satiated, or full, when they have satisfied their nutritional needs and their stomach signals "no more."

One hormone, produced in the stomach, that researchers suspect may influence satiety and play a role in keeping weight off is *ghrelin,* sometimes referred to as "the hunger hormone." Initial interest in ghrelin was the result of an early study that focused on a small group of obese people who had lost weight over a 6-month period.[24] The researchers noted that ghrelin levels rose before every meal and fell drastically shortly afterward, suggesting that the hormone plays a role in appetite stimulation. Since then, ghrelin has been shown to be an important growth hormone that plays a key role in the regulation of appetite and food intake control, gastrointestinal motility, gastric acid secretion, endocrine and exocrine pancreatic secretions, glucose and lipid metabolism, and cardiovascular and immunological processes.[25]

Another hormone that has gained increased attention and research is *leptin,* an appetite regulator produced by fat cells in mammals. As fat tissue increases, levels of leptin in the blood increase, and when levels of leptin in the blood rise, appetite drops. Scientists believe leptin serves as a form of "adipostat" that signals you are getting full, slows food intake, and promotes energy expenditure.[26] For unknown reasons, obese people seem to have faulty leptin receptors, although it may be that environmental cues are stronger than biological signals in some individuals.

adaptive thermogenesis Theoretical mechanism by which the brain regulates metabolic activity according to caloric intake.

yo-yo diets Cycles in which people diet and regain weight.

set point theory Theory that a form of internal thermostat controls our weight and fights to maintain this weight around a narrowly set range.

satiety The feeling of fullness or satisfaction at the end of a meal.

hyperplastic obesity A condition characterized by an excessive number of fat cells.

hypertrophy The act of swelling or increasing in size, as with cells.

Fat Cells and Predisposition to Fatness

Some obese people may have excessive numbers of fat cells. Where an average-weight adult has approximately 25 to 35 billion fat cells and a moderately obese adult 60 to 100 billion, an extremely obese adult has as many as 200 billion.[27] This condition, **hyperplastic obesity**, usually appears in early childhood and perhaps, due to the mother's dietary habits, even prior to birth. The most critical periods for the development of hyperplasia are the last 2 to 3 months of fetal development, the first year of life, and the period between ages 9 and 13. Central to this theory is the belief that the number of fat cells in a body does not increase appreciably during adulthood. However, the ability of each of these cells to swell (**hypertrophy**) and shrink does carry over into adulthood. People with large numbers of fat cells may be able to lose weight by decreasing the size of each cell in adulthood, but with the next calorie binge, cells swell and sabotage

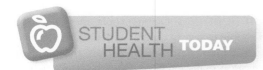
BEWARE OF PORTION INFLATION AT RESTAURANTS

From burgers and fries to meat-and-potato or pasta meals, today's popular restaurant foods dwarf their earlier counterparts. For example, a 25-ounce prime rib dinner served at one local steak chain contains nearly 3,000 calories and 150 grams of fat. That's 1.5 times the calories and two to three times the fat that most adults need in a whole day!

Many researchers believe that the main reason Americans are gaining weight is that people no longer recognize a normal serving size. The National Heart, Lung, and Blood Institute has developed a pair of "Portion Distortion" quizzes that show how today's portions compare with those of 20 years ago. Test your knowledge of portion size online at www.nhlbi.nih.gov/health/educational/wecan/eat-right/portion-distortion.htm.

To make sure you're not overeating when you dine out, follow these strategies:

- Order the smallest size available. Focus on taste and quality, rather than quantity. When you eat huge amounts at the all-you-can-eat buffet, focus on how you feel. Get used to eating less,

Today's bloated portions.

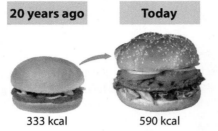

20 years ago	Today
333 kcal	590 kcal

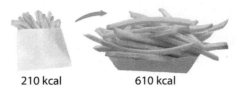

210 kcal	610 kcal

eating slowly, and enjoying what you eat.

- Take your time, and let your fullness indicator have a chance to kick in while there is still time to quit. Chew more, talk more, set your fork down more often between bites.

- Order condiments and dressings on the side and don't use the entire container! Lightly dip your food in dressings or gravies rather than pouring on extra calories.
- Order a healthy, protein-rich appetizer as your main meal, and a small salad or vegetable. Happy hour menus often offer great smaller choices.
- Split an entrée with a friend, and order a side salad for each of you. Alternately, put half of your meal in a takeout box immediately, and finish the rest at the restaurant.
- Avoid buffets and all-you-can-eat establishments. If you go to them, use small plates and fill them with salads, vegetables and other high-protein, low-calorie, low-fat options. Pay careful attention to newly required menu labeling for fast-food restaurants. These can be helpful in making sure you choose the best alternative for healthy dining.

Source: Data are from National Heart, Lung, and Blood Institute, "Portion Distortion," Accessed April 1, 2015, www.nhlbi.nih.gov/health/educational/wecan/eat-right/portion-distortion.htm

weight-loss efforts. Weight gain may be tied to both the number of fat cells in the body and the capacity of individual cells to enlarge.

Environmental Factors

Environmental factors have come to play a large role in weight maintenance. Automobiles, remote controls, desk jobs, and sedentary habits contribute to decreased physical activity and energy expenditure. Coupled with our culture of eating more, it's a recipe for weight gain.

U.S. ADULTS GET

11.3%

OF TOTAL DAILY **CALORIES** FROM FAST FOODS—DOWN FROM 12.8% IN 2007–2008.

Greater Access to High-Calorie Foods More foods that are high in calories and low in nutrients exist today compared to the past. There are many environmental factors that can prompt us to consume them:

- Because of constant advertising, we are bombarded with messages to eat, eat, eat, and taste often trumps nutrition.
- Super-sized portions are now the norm (see the **Student Health Today** box), leading to increased calorie and fat intake.
- Widespread availability of high-calorie coffee and sugary drinks lure people in for a form of break/reward between meals, which really add up in calories over time.
- Families have increased reliance on restaurant and store-bought convenience foods, which tend to be higher in calories than food made from scratch.
- Bottle-feeding infants may increase energy intake relative to breast-feeding.
- Misleading food labels confuse consumers about serving sizes.

Although we still consume about 500 calories per day more today than we did in 1970, daily consumption of some foods

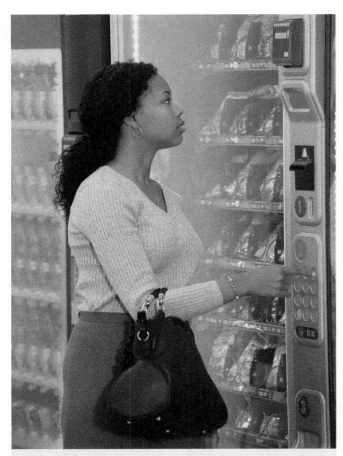

The easy availability of high-calorie foods, such as those found in most vending machines, is one of the environmental factors contributing to the obesity problem in the United States today.

appears to be declining in the last decade. For example, annual consumption of sugars, including *high fructose corn syrup* was 119 pounds per person in 1970, increasing to 151 pounds per person in 1999. Today's consumption has decreased to 139 pounds per person.[28] If we are consuming less, why aren't we seeing major changes in obesity rates? One possibility is that we are exercising less than ever, thereby offsetting potential weight loss.[29]

Lack of Physical Activity Although heredity, metabolism, and environment all have an impact on weight management, the way we live our lives is also responsible. In general, Americans are eating more and moving less than ever before—becoming overfat as a result.

According to data from the 2014 *National Health Interview Survey*, 50 percent of adults 18 and over in the United States met the guidelines for aerobic activity through involvement in leisure time activity. However, a recent Behavioral Risk Factor Surveillance System (*BRFSS*) survey reported that only 21% percent of adults engaged in enough aerobic and muscle strengthening exercise to meet the guidelines.[30]

The above differences in statistics are, in part, a reflection of the fact that data are largely based on self-reporting, and people over-estimate their daily exercise level and intensity. Complicating the problem further is a hodgepodge of terminology for determining activity levels and more than one fitness measure, so defining yourself as "active" can mean very different things for different people.

Psychosocial and Socioeconomic Factors

The relationship of weight problems to emotional insecurities, needs, and wants remains difficult to assess. What we do know is eating tends to be a focal point of people's lives and is in part a social ritual associated with companionship, celebration, and enjoyment. *Comfort food* is also used to help you feel good when other things in life are not going well. Our friends and loved ones are often key influences in our eating behaviors. In fact, according to recent research, young adults who are overweight and obese tend to befriend and date overweight and obese people in much the same way that smokers or exercisers tend to hang out with other smokers or exercisers. People may gain or lose weight based on support for loss or social undermining of weight loss attempts ("Let's go out for ice cream!").[31]

Socioeconomic status can have a significant effect on risk for obesity. When times are tough, people tend to eat more inexpensive, high-calorie processed foods. People living in poverty may have less access to fresh, nutrient-dense foods and have less time to cook nutritious meals due to shiftwork, longer commutes, or multiple jobs.[32] Counselors, fitness center memberships, and other supports for weight loss are often too expensive or unavailable. Additionally, unsafe neighborhoods and poor infrastructure, such as lack of sidewalks or parks, can make it difficult for less-affluent people to exercise.[33]

LO 3 | ASSESSING BODY WEIGHT AND BODY COMPOSITION

Discuss reliable options for determining a healthy weight and body fat percentage.

Everyone has his or her own ideal weight, based on individual variables such as body structure, height, and fat distribution. Traditionally, experts used measurement techniques such as height-weight charts to determine whether an individual was an ideal weight, overweight, or obese. These charts can be misleading because they don't take body composition—a person's

underweight Having a body weight more than 10 percent below healthy recommended levels; in an adult, having a BMI below 18.5.

healthy weight Those with BMIs of 18.5 to 24.9, the range of lowest statistical health risk

overweight Having a body weight more than 10 percent above healthy recommended levels; in an adult, having a BMI of 25 to 29.9.

morbidly obese Having a body weight 100 percent or more above healthy recommended levels; in an adult, having a BMI of 40 or more.

super obese Having a body weight higher than morbid obesity; in an adult, having a BMI of 50 or more.

ratio of fat to lean muscle—or fat distribution into account. More accurate measures of evaluating healthy weight and disease risk focus on a person's percentage of body fat and how that fat is distributed in his or her body.

It's important to remember that body fat isn't all bad. In fact, some fat is essential for healthy body functioning. Fat regulates body temperature, cushions and insulates organs and tissues, and is the body's main source of stored energy. Body fat is composed of two types: essential fat and storage fat. *Essential fat* is the fat necessary for maintenance of life and reproductive functions. *Storage fat,* the nonessential fat that many of us try to shed, makes up the remainder of our fat reserves. Being **underweight,** or having extremely low body fat, can cause a host of problems, including hair loss, visual disturbances, skin problems, a tendency to fracture bones easily, digestive system disturbances, heart irregularities, gastrointestinal problems, difficulties in maintaining body temperature, and loss of menstrual period in women.

Body Mass Index (BMI)

As mentioned in earlier discussion, BMI is a description of body weight relative to height—numbers that are highly correlated with your total body fat. Find your BMI in inches and pounds in FIGURE 10.3, or calculate your BMI now by dividing your weight in kilograms by height in meters squared. The mathematical formula is

$$BMI = weight (kg)/height\ squared\ (m^2)$$

A BMI calculator is also available from the National Heart, Lung, and Blood Institute at www.nhlbi.nih.gov/guidelines/obesity/BMI/bmicalc.htm.

Desirable BMI levels may vary with age and by sex; however, most BMI tables for adults do not account for such variables. **Healthy weight** is defined as having a BMI of 18.5 to 24.9, the range of lowest statistical health risk.[34] A BMI of 25 to 29.9 indicates **overweight** and potentially significant health risks. A BMI of 30 to 39.9 is classified as **obese.** A BMI of 40 to 49.9 is **morbidly obese,** and a new category of BMI of 50 or higher—one increasing in numbers—has been labeled as **super obese.**[35] In 2011–2012, over 6 percent of American adults were morbidly obese, with a BMI over 40.[36]

Limitations of BMI Like other assessments of fatness, the BMI has its limitations. Water, muscle, and bone mass are not included in BMI calculations, and BMI levels don't account for the fact that muscle weighs more than fat. BMI levels can be inaccurate for people who are under 5 feet tall, are highly muscled, or who are older and have little muscle mass. Although a combination of measures might be most reliable in assessing fat levels, BMI continues to be a quick, inexpensive, and useful tool for developing basic health recommendations.[37]

Youth and BMI Today, over 30 percent of youth in America are obese, three times higher than rates in the 1980s.[38] Although the labels *obese* and *morbidly obese* have been used for years for adults, there is growing concern that such labels increase bias and *obesity stigma* against youth.[39] BMI ranges above a normal weight for children and teens are often labeled differently, as

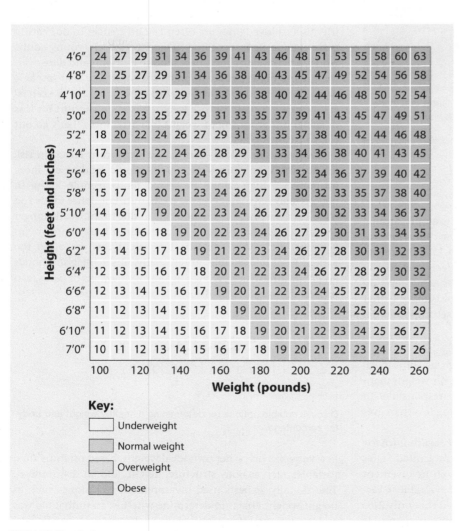

FIGURE 10.3 Body Mass Index (BMI)

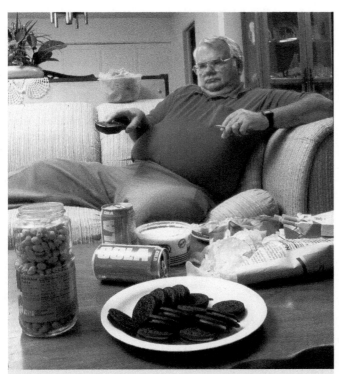

Abdominal obesity puts individuals at increased risk of CVD, stroke, and diabetes, particularly among men.

The waist circumference-to-hip ratio measures regional fat distribution. A waist-to-hip ratio greater than 1 in men and 0.8 in women indicates increased health risks.[42] Newer research has pointed to waist-to-hip ratio being more effective than waist circumference alone or BMI use when measuring body fat in children and adolescents.[43] A waist circumference-to-height ratio is a simple screening tool that says that your waist should be approximately one half of your height; if you were 70 inches tall, your waist shouldn't be more than 35 inches.

Measures of Body Fat

There are numerous ways to assess whether your body fat levels are too high. One low-tech way is simply to look in the mirror or consider how your clothes fit now compared with how they fit last year. For those who wish to take a more precise measurement of their percentage of body fat, more accurate techniques are available, several of which are described and depicted in FIGURE 10.4. These methods usually involve the help of a skilled professional and typically must be done in a lab or clinical setting. Before undergoing any procedure, make sure you understand the expense, potential for accuracy, risks, and training of the tester. Also, consider why you are seeking this assessment and what you plan to do with the results.

Although opinion varies somewhat, most experts agree that men's bodies should contain between 8 and 20 percent total body fat, and women should be within the range of 20 to 30 percent (see TABLE 10.1). Generally, men who exceed 22

"at risk of overweight" and "overweight," to avoid the sense of shame such words may cause. In addition, BMI ranges for children and teens take into account normal differences in body fat between boys and girls and the differences in body fat that occur at various ages. Specific guidelines for calculating youth BMI are available at the Centers for Disease Control and Prevention website, www.cdc.gov.

Waist Circumference and Ratio Measurements

Knowing where your fat is carried may be more important than knowing how much you carry. Men and postmenopausal women tend to store fat in the upper regions of the body, particularly in the abdominal area. Premenopausal women usually store fat in the lower regions of their bodies, particularly the hips, buttocks, and thighs. Waist circumference measurements, including *waist circumference* only, the *waist circumference-to-hip ratio*, and the *waist circumference-to-height ratio*, have all been used to measure abdominal fat as an indicator of obesity and health risk. Where you carry the weight may be of particular importance in determining whether you develop diabetes, cardiovascular disease, hypertension, or stroke.[40]

A waistline greater than 40 inches (102 centimeters) in men and 35 inches (88 centimeters) in women may be particularly indicative of greater health risk.[41] If a person is less than 5 feet tall or has a BMI of 35 or above, waist circumference standards used for the general population might not apply.

TABLE 10.1 | Body Fat Percentage Norms for Men and Women*

Age (Men)	Very Lean	Excellent	Good	Fair	Poor	Very Poor
20–29	<7%	7%–10%	11%–15%	16%–19%	20%–23%	>23%
30–39	<11%	11%–14%	15%–18%	19%–21%	22%–25%	>25%
40–49	<14%	14%–17%	18%–20%	21%–23%	24%–27%	>27%
50–59	<15%	15%–19%	20%–22%	23%–24%	25%–28%	>28%
60–69	<16%	16%–20%	21%–22%	23%–25%	26%–28%	>28%
70–79	<16%	16%–20%	21%–23%	24%–25%	26%–28%	>28%
Age (Women)	Very Lean	Excellent	Good	Fair	Poor	Very Poor
20–29	<14%	14%–16%	17%–19%	20%–23%	24%–27%	>27%
30–39	<15%	15%–17%	18%–21%	22%–25%	26%–29%	>29%
40–49	<17%	17%–20%	21%–24%	25%–28%	29%–32%	>32%
50–59	<18%	18%–22%	23%–27%	28%–30%	31%–34%	>34%
60–69	<18%	18%–23%	24%–28%	29%–31%	32%–35%	>35%
70–79	<18%	18%–24%	25%–29%	30%–32%	33%–36%	>36%

*Assumes nonathletes. For athletes, recommended body fat is 5 to 15 percent for men and 12 to 22 percent for women. Please note that there are no agreed-upon national standards for recommended body fat percentage.

Source: Based on data from The Cooper Institute, Dallas, Texas, www.cooperinstitute.org

Underwater (hydrostatic) weighing:
Measures the amount of water a person displaces when completely submerged. Fat tissue is less dense than muscle or bone, so body fat can be computed within a 2%–3% margin of error by comparing weight underwater and out of water.

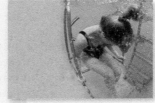

Skinfolds:
Involves "pinching" a person's fold of skin (with its underlying layer of fat) at various locations of the body. The fold is measured using a specially designed caliper. When performed by a skilled technician, it can estimate body fat with an error of 3%–4%.

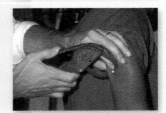

Bioelectrical impedance analysis (BIA):
Involves sending a very low level of electrical current through a person's body. As lean body mass is made up of mostly water, the rate at which the electricity is conducted gives an indication of a person's lean body mass and body fat. Under the best circumstances, BIA can estimate body fat with an error of 3%–4%.

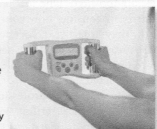

Dual-energy X-ray absorptiometry (DXA):
The technology is based on using very-low-level X ray to differentiate between bone tissue, soft (or lean) tissue, and fat (or adipose) tissue. The margin of error for predicting body fat is 2%–4%.

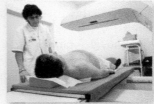

Bod Pod:
Uses air displacement to measure body composition. This machine is a large, egg-shaped chamber made from fiberglass. The person being measured sits in the machine wearing a swimsuit. The door is closed and the machine measures how much air is displaced. That value is used to calculate body fat, with a 2%–3% margin of error.

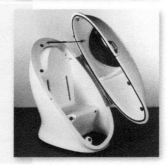

FIGURE 10.4 Overview of Various Body Composition Assessment Methods

Source: Adapted from J. Thompson and M. Manore, *Nutrition: An Applied Approach My Plate Edition*, 3rd edition, © 2012. Printed and electronically reproduced by permission of Pearson Education, Inc., Upper Saddle River, New Jersey.

percent body fat and women who exceed 35 percent are considered overweight, but these ranges vary with age and stages of life. In addition, there are percentages of body fat below which a person is considered underweight, and health is compromised. In men, this lower limit is approximately 3 to 7 percent of total body weight and in women it is approximately 8 to 15 percent.

LO 4 | MANAGING YOUR WEIGHT: INDIVIDUAL ROLES

Explain the effectiveness and potential pros/cons of various weight control strategies, including exercise, diet, lifestyle modification, supplements/diet drugs, surgery, and other options.

At some point in our lives, almost all of us will decide to lose weight. Many will have mixed success. Failure is often related to thinking about losing weight in terms of short-term "dieting" rather than adjusting long-term behaviors. Drugs and intensive counseling can contribute to positive weight loss, but even then, many people regain weight after treatment. Maintaining a healthful body takes constant attention and nurturing. The Student Health Today box looks at characteristics of successful weight losers.

Understanding Calories and Energy Balance

A *calorie* is a unit of measure that indicates the amount of energy gained from food or expended through activity. Each time you consume 3,500 calories more than your body needs to maintain weight, you gain a pound of storage fat. Conversely, each time your body expends an extra 3,500 calories, you lose a pound of fat. If you consume 140 calories (the amount in one can of regular soda) more than you need every single day and make no other changes in diet or activity, you would gain 1 pound in 25 days (3,500 calories ÷ 140 calories per day = 25 days). Conversely, if you walk for 30 minutes each day at a pace of 15 minutes per mile (172 calories burned) in addition to your regular activities, you would lose 1 pound in 20 days (3,500 calories ÷ 172 calories per day = 20.3 days). FIGURE 10.5 illustrates the concept of energy balance.

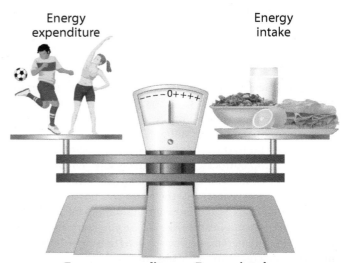

Energy expenditure

Energy intake

Energy expenditure = Energy intake

FIGURE 10.5 The Concept of Energy Balance If you consume more calories than you burn, you gain weight. If you burn more than you consume, you lose weight. If both are equal, your weight will not change.

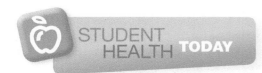

WHO WINS IN LOSING?
Characteristics of Successful Losers

Millions of Americans start their New Year with the most popular resolution: to lose weight and keep it off. Even so, the majority who lose some weight ultimately regain it. But what about those few losers who manage to keep it off?

In general, the literature indicates success rates between 2 and 15 percent, using a variety of weight and BMI parameters, as well as timelines for defining success. From there, success measures look at short-term initial success, 6-month success, and 1-year success, with few studies looking at success rates past 24 months. Based on these studies, characteristics of those likely to be successful include the following:

- High self-esteem, self-efficacy, and realistic body image.
- A strong locus of control—being motivated by internal rather than external factors.
- Having awareness of their current risks and reasonable knowledge of healthy nutrition.
- Having supportive friends and family.
- Utilizing community resources.
- Journaling and tracking calories, nutrients, and/or portion sizes; they also regularly monitor weight.
- Ultimately aiming to follow a healthy, realistic eating and exercise pattern.
- Incorporating some type of incentive into their program
- Praising small successes and avoiding becoming discouraged by setbacks.

A recent meta-analysis of some of the most comprehensive research studies to

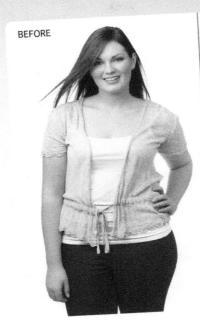

BEFORE

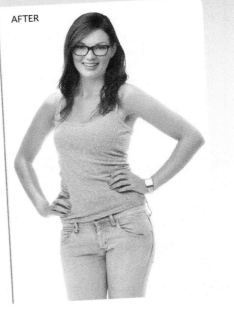

AFTER

date indicated that behavioral interventions that focus on diet and exercise show small but significant weight loss and that long-term maintenance is aided by selected pharmaceutical aids. Those who focus on the above are most likely to win at the losing game.

Sources: J. Kassier and M. Angell, "Losing Weight—An Ill-Fated New Year's Resolution," *New England Journal of Medicine* 338, no. 1 (1998): 52–54; S. Dombrowski et al. "Long Term Maintenance of Weight Loss with Non-surgical Interventions in Obese Adults: Systematic Review and Meta-analyses of Randomized Controlled Trials," *British Medical Journal* 348 (2014): g2646; Look AHEAD Research Group, "Eight Year Weight Losses with an Intensive Lifestyle Intervention: The Look Ahead Study," *Obesity* 22, no 1 (2014): 5–13; M. Butryn et al., "Consistent Self-Monitoring of Weight: A Key Component of Successful Weight Loss Maintenance," *Obesity* 15, no. 12 (2007): 3091–3096; T. Wadden et al., "One Year Weight Losses in the Look Ahead Study: Factors Associated with Success," *Obesity* 17, no. 4 (2009): 713–22; J. Moreno and C. Johnston, "Success Habits of Weight Losers," *American Journal of Lifestyle Medicine* 6, no. 2 (2012): 113–15; Centers for Disease Control and Prevention, "Keeping It Off," September 2011, www.cdc.gov/healthyweight/losing_weight/keepingitoff.html; S. Ramage et al., "Healthy Strategies for Successful Weight Loss and Weight Maintenance: A Systematic Review," *Applied Physiology, Nutrition, and Metabolism* 39, no. 1 (2013): 1–20; S. Simpson et al., "What Is the Most Effective Way to Maintain Weight Loss in Adults?," *British Medical Journal,* 343 (2011):d8042.

Diet and Eating Behaviors

Successful weight loss requires shifting energy balance. The first part of the equation is to reduce calorie intake through modifying eating habits and daily diet.

Improving Your Eating Habits Before you can change an unhealthy eating habit, you must first determine what causes or triggers it. Keeping a detailed daily log of eating triggers—when, what, where, and how much you eat—for at least a week can give clues about what causes you to want unneeded food. Typically, dietary triggers center on patterns and problems in everyday living rather than real hunger pangs. For example, your daily commute might take you past your favorite fast food restaurant. Or maybe there are numerous vending machines on campus. Many people eat compulsively when stressed; however, for other people, the same circumstances diminish their appetite, causing them to lose weight. See the

Skills for Behavior Change box for tips on healthy snacking, and see FIGURE 10.6 for ways to adjust your eating triggers.

Choosing a Diet Plan

Once you have determined your triggers, begin to devise a plan for improved eating by doing the following:

- Seeking assistance from reputable sources such as MyPlate (www.choosemyplate.gov), a registered dietitian (RD), some physicians, health educators, or exercise physiologists with nutritional training.
- Being wary of nutritionists or nutritional life coaches, since there is no formal credential for those titles.

- Avoiding weight-loss programs that promise quick, "miracle" results or that are run by "trainees," often people with short courses on nutrition and exercise that are designed to sell products or services.
- Assessing the nutrient value of any prescribed diet, verifying dietary guidelines are consistent with reliable nutrition research, and analyzing the suitability of the diet to your tastes, budget, and lifestyle.

Any diet that requires radical behavior changes or sets up artificial dietary programs through prepackaged products is likely to fail. The most successful plans allow you to make food choices in real-world settings and do not ask you to

If your trigger is . . .	→ then	try this strategy . . .
A stressful situation		Acknowledge and address feelings of anxiety or stress, and develop stress management techniques to practice daily.
Feeling angry or upset		Analyze your emotions and look for a noneating activity to deal with them, such as taking a quick walk or calling a friend.
A certain time of day		Change your eating schedule to avoid skipping or delaying meals and overeating later; make a plan of what you'll eat ahead of time to avoid impulse or emotional eating.
Pressure from friends and family		Have a response ready to help you refuse food you do not want, or look for healthy alternatives you can eat instead when in social settings.
Being in an environment where food is available		Avoid the environment that causes you to want to eat: Sit far away from the food at meetings, take a different route to class to avoid passing the vending machines, shop from a list and only when you aren't hungry, arrange nonfood outings with your friends.
Feeling bored and tired		Identify the times when you feel low energy and fill them with activities other than eating, such as exercise breaks; cultivate a new interest or hobby that keeps your mind and hands busy.
The sight and smell of food		Stop buying high-calorie foods that tempt you to snack, or store them in an inconvenient place, out of sight; avoid walking past or sitting or standing near the table of tempting treats at a meeting, party, or other gathering.
Eating mindlessly or inattentively		Turn off all distractions, including phones, computers, television, and radio, and eat more slowly, savoring your food and putting your fork down between bites so you can become aware of when your hunger is satisfied.
Spending time alone in the car		Get a book on tape to listen to, or tape your class notes and use the time for studying. Keep your mind off food. Don't bring money into the gas station where snacks are tempting.
Alcohol use		Drink plenty of water and stay hydrated. Seek out healthy snack choices. After a night out, brush your teeth immediately upon getting home and stay out of the kitchen.
Feeling deprived		Allow yourself to eat "indulgences" in moderation, so you won't crave them; focus on balancing your calorie input to calorie output.
Eating out of habit		Establish a new routine to circumvent the old, such as taking a new route to class so you don't feel compelled to stop at your favorite fast-food restaurant on the way.
Watching television		Look for something else to occupy your hands and body while your mind is engaged with the screen: Ride an exercise bike, do stretching exercises, doodle on a pad of paper, or learn to knit.

FIGURE 10.6 Avoid Trigger-Happy Eating

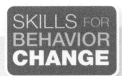
sacrifice everything you enjoy. See **TABLE 10.2** for an analysis of some popular diets marketed today. For information on other plans, check out the regularly updated list of reviews on the website of the Academy of Nutrition and Dietetics (formerly the American Dietetic Association) at www .eatright.org.

Including Exercise

Any increase in the intensity, frequency, and duration of daily exercise can lead to an increase in muscle mass, which can have a significant impact on total calorie expenditure because lean (muscle) tissue is more metabolically active than fat tissue. Exact estimates vary, but experts currently think that 2 to 50 more calories per day are burned per pound of muscle than each pound of fat tissue. Thus, the base level of calories needed to maintain a healthy weight varies greatly from person to person.

The number of calories spent through physical activity depends on three factors:

1. The number and proportion of muscles used
2. The amount of weight moved
3. The length of time the activity takes

An activity involving both the arms and legs burns more calories than one involving only the legs. An activity performed by a heavy person burns more calories than the same activity performed by a lighter person. And, an activity performed for 40 minutes requires twice as much energy as the same activity performed for only 20 minutes.

TABLE 10.2 | Analyzing Popular Diet Programs

Diet Name	Basic Principles	Good for Diabetes and Heart Health?	Weight Loss Effectiveness	Pros, Cons, and Other Things to Consider
DASH (Dietary Approaches to Stop Hypertension)	A balanced plan developed to fight high blood pressure. Eat fruits, veggies, whole grains, lean protein, and low-fat dairy. Avoid sweets, fats, red meat, and sodium.	Yes	Not specifically designed for weight loss.	A balanced, safe and healthy diet, rated the no. 1 best diet overall by 2015 *U.S. News & World Report*. Although not designed for weight reduction per se, it is regarded as very effective in improving cholesterol levels and other biomarkers long term.
TLC (Therapeutic Lifestyle Change)	Developed by NIH. Focus on CVD risk reduction with fruits and veggies, lean protein, low fat, etc. Balanced and effective.	Yes	Weight loss likely; cholesterol key.	Safe, balanced, and healthy diet rated no. 2 diet by 2015 *U.S. News & World Report*. Particularly good for heart health.
Mediterranean	A plan that emphasizes fruits, vegetables, fish, whole grains, beans, nuts, legumes, olive oil, and herbs and spices. Poultry, eggs, cheese, yogurt, and red wine can be enjoyed in moderation, whereas sweets and red meat are saved for special occasions.	Yes	Effective	Widely considered to be one of the more healthy, safe, and balanced diets. Weight loss may not be as dramatic but long-term health benefits have been demonstrated. Tied for third best diet overall—with the Mayo Clinic and Weight Watchers—by 2015 *U.S. News & World Report*. Relatively easy to follow.
Weight Watchers	The program assigns every food a point value based on its nutritional values and how hard your body has to work to burn it off. Total points allowed depend on activity level and personal weight goals. In-person group meetings or online membership are options.	Yes (depending on individual choices)	Effective	Experts consider Weight Watchers effective and easy to follow for both short- and long-term weight loss. Other pluses include an emphasis on group support and room for occasional indulgences. But while not as expensive as some plans, there are membership fees. Tied for third best diet overall in 2015 *U.S. News & World Report*.

continued

TABLE **10.2** | Analyzing Popular Diet Programs (*continued*)

Diet Name	Basic Principles	Good for Diabetes and Heart Health?	Weight Loss Effectiveness	Pros, Cons, and Other Things to Consider
Jenny Craig	Prepackaged meals do the work of restricting calorie intake. Members get personalized meal and exercise plans, plus weekly counseling sessions.	Yes	Effective short term, long-term results dependent on adopting healthful eating later.	Support and premade meals make weight loss easier; however, it may be difficult to maintain for the long run. Cons include cost, which will run hundreds of dollars per month for food alone, plus membership fees. Lactose- and gluten-intolerant individuals cannot join due to available foods.
Biggest Loser	Four servings a day of fruits and vegetables, three of protein foods, two of whole grains, and no more than 200 calories of "extras" like desserts. Exercise, food journals, portion control, and calculating personal calorie allowances are all stressed.	Yes	Effective	This diet is effective at weight loss. Ranked no. 1 by *U.S. News and World Report*, 2015 for those with pre-diabetes or diabetes. Helps reduce blood glucose levels and reduces other biomarkers such as cholesterol, triglycerides, etc.
Nutrisystem	Low-calorie, prepackaged meals are ordered online and delivered to your home.	Not for heart health per se, but may help reduce diabetes risks.	Effective short-term, long-term results dependent on adopting healthful eating later.	Nutrisystem is quite safe, easier to follow than many other diets, and has few nutritional deficiencies if followed as directed, according to experts. It is also expensive (similar to Jenny Craig) due to the cost of ordering food and may not help you learn to eat healthfully after diet is done.
Medifast	Dieters eat six meals a day, five of them 100-calorie Medifast products. After goal weight loss, people wean from Medifast food and gradually add back in starchy veggies, whole grains, fruit, and low-fat dairy products.	Likely yes	Effective in short term; long-term results unproven.	Medifast scored above average in short-term weight loss but gets lower marks for keeping weight off. Because of the extremely low calorie intakes on the program, it is hard to stay on the program for long; doesn't teach healthy eating as part of plan.
Low Carb Diets (Atkins, South Beach, and other variations)	Carbs—sugars and "simple starches" like potatoes, white bread, and rice—are avoided, and some minimize all carb-based foods. Emphasis on proteins and fat from meat and eggs are embraced.	Not likely with so much fat eaten.	Effective in short term, mixed long-term results.	Low carb diets in most forms are often extremely effective at short-term weight loss, but many experts worry that fat intake is up to three times higher than standard daily recommendations and some even omit fruits, vegetables, and healthy grains.
Paleo	Based on the theory that digestive systems have not evolved to deal with many modern foods such as diary, legumes, grains and sugar, this plan emphasizes meats, fish, poultry, fruits, and vegetables.	Unknown (too few studies)	Unknown (too few studies)	Gets low marks by health and nutrition experts due to avoidance of grains, legumes, and dairy and higher fat than the government recommends. Missing essential nutrients, costly to maintain. It can be hard to follow long term and has had only a few very small studies done to document effectiveness.
Fast Diet (also known as the 5:2 diet or Intermittent Fasting Diet)	Based on the theory that by drastically reducing calories on two days (500 cal/day) each week and eating normally the other five, you will lose weight.	Not likely as it doesn't follow guidelines for carbohydrates. Should talk with registered dietician or health care provider.	Effective, but weight loss is relatively slow unless calorie intake is monitored on non-fast days and exercise is part of regimen.	Exceeds dietary guidelines for fat and protein and falls short on carbohydrate recommendation. Does encourage fruits and veggies, but feast and famine regimen is hard to sustain.

Source: Opinions on diet pros and cons are based on *U.S. News & World Report*, "Best Diet Rankings," 2015, http://health.usnews.com/best-diet/best-over-all-diets?int=9c2508; dietary reviews are available online from registered dieticians at the Academy of Nutrition and Dietetics, 2015, http://www.eatrightpro.org/resources/media/trends-and-reviews.

Keeping Weight Control in Perspective

Weight loss is a struggle for many people, and many factors influence success or failure. To reach and maintain a healthy weight, develop a program of exercise and healthy eating behaviors that you can maintain. Remember, you didn't gain your weight in a week or two, and it is both unrealistic and potentially dangerous to take drastic weight loss measures. Instead, try to lose a healthy 1 to 2 pounds during the first week, and stay with this slow and easy regimen. Adding exercise and cutting back on calories to expend about 500 calories more than you consume each day will help you lose weight at a rate of 1 pound per week. You may find tracking your intake and activity easier with one of the apps described in the Tech & Health box on the next page. See the Skills for Behavior Change box for strategies to help your weight management program succeed.

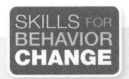

WHY SHOULD I CARE?

It may be easy to grab a fast-food meal, but unless you are very physically active, your body will likely store that "super-sized" meal as fat, which is anything but easy to lose. Eating 500 extra calories a day—less than the average hamburger—can lead to a pound of weight gain in just a week's time. A 150-pound person would need to walk for about 90 minutes at 4 mph to burn that off. if you walk slower, it would take even longer.

One particularly dangerous potential complication of VLCDs is *ketoacidosis,* a condition that occurs when your cells don't have enough of the glucose they need for energy. When this happens, the body begins to burn fat for energy, producing *ketones*—acidic chemicals that can cause major risks to health. As ketones increase initially, you may not feel hungry or thirsty and weight loss may occur. As levels increase, you may begin to develop *ketosis,* which can progress to *ketoacidosis* or acidic blood levels. Early symptoms may include excessive thirst, excessive urination, and high blood sugar, progressing to extreme fatigue, nausea, vomiting, abdominal pain, "fruity breath," fainting, possible coma, and death. Extreme diets that allow very few carbohydrates and/or calories are often the culprits. People with untreated type 1 diabetes and individuals with anorexia or bulimia are also at high risk.

very-low-calorie diets (VLCDs) Diets with a daily caloric value of 400 to 700 calories.

Considering Drastic Weight-Loss Measures?

When nothing seems to work, people become frustrated and pursue high-risk, unproven methods of weight loss or seek medical interventions. Dramatic weight loss may be recommended in cases of extreme health risk. Even in such situations, drastic dietary, pharmacological, or surgical measures should be considered carefully and discussed with several knowledgeable, licensed health professionals working in accredited facilities.

Very-Low-Calorie Diets

In severe cases of obesity that are not responsive to traditional dietary strategies, medically supervised, powdered formulas with daily values of 400 to 700 calories plus vitamin and mineral supplements may be given to patients. Many of these diets emphasize high protein and very low carbohydrates. Such **very-low-calorie diets (VLCDs)** should never be undertaken without strict medical supervision. They do not teach healthy eating, and persons who manage to lose weight on VLCDs may experience significant weight regain. Problems associated with any form of severe caloric restriction include blood sugar imbalance, cold intolerance, constipation, decreased BMR, dehydration, diarrhea, emotional problems, fatigue, headaches, heart irregularities, kidney infections and failure, loss of lean body tissue, weakness, and the potential for coma and death.

SEE IT! VIDEOS

Do you snack like crazy when you're watching an exciting movie? Watch **Fast-Paced Movies, Television Shows May Lead to More Snacking** in the Study Area of MasteringHealth™

SKILLS FOR BEHAVIOR CHANGE

KEYS TO SUCCESSFUL WEIGHT MANAGEMENT

Make a Plan
- ▶ Establish short- and long-term plans. What are the diet and exercise changes you can make this week? Once you do 1 week, plot a course for 2 weeks, and so on.
- ▶ Look for balance. Remember it's calories taken in and burned over time that make the difference.

Change Your Habits
- ▶ Be adventurous. Expand your usual foods to enjoy a wider variety.
- ▶ Eat small portions, less often and savor the flavor.
- ▶ Notice whether you are hungry before starting a meal. Eat slowly, noting when you start to feel full, and *stop* before you are full.
- ▶ Eat breakfast, especially low-fat foods with whole grains and protein. This will prevent you from being too hungry and overeating at lunch.
- ▶ Keep healthful snacks on hand for when you get hungry.

Incorporate Exercise
- ▶ Be active and slowly increase your time, speed, distance, or resistance levels.
- ▶ Vary your physical activity. Find activities that you really love and try things you haven't tried before.
- ▶ Find an exercise partner to help you stay motivated.

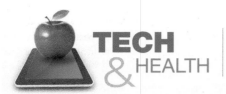

Studies consistently report that people who keep detailed food and exercise journals lose more weight and keep it off longer than those who do not. Want to track what you ate today in terms of total calories and amount of nutrients? There's an app for that. Want to track your walking, running, swimming, lifting, and sleeping activities? There are apps for that, too.

The best programs combine food and physical activity logs, so if you splurge on dessert, you can figure out how many miles you'll need to jog to burn it off. These apps often feature calculators for determining daily calorie intake goals as well as barcode scanners that allow you to quickly add packaged foods to your log. Here are just a few:

- **Lose It!** by FitNow. (Basic Plan Free: Android, iPhone and iPad, Nook tablet, PCs. $39.95 for year subscription to Premium plan), www.loseit.com
- Simple to use, comprehensive database of foods, phone scanning of bar codes, and activities designed to help you log meals and track exercise. Premium model connects to scale for weight-loss monitoring and tracks key health indicators.
- **Restaurant Weight Watcher.** (Modest cost; Android only), http://ellisapps .com Lists nutrition information for the menus of over 200 restaurants and continues to add new ones.

- **MyFitnessPal Calorie Counter & Diet Tracker** (Free: iPhone, Android, Blackberry, PCs) www.myfitnesspal.com A combination of diet and fitness goals as well as a nutritional analysis of what you are eating and your exercise levels. Can scan bar codes on food to help you monitor what you are buying and make healthy choice.
- **Diet Point • Weight Loss** (Free: Android and iPhone) www.dietpointed.com/ Weight loss assistant that offers 55 unique diet plans, from low-carb to vegan to paleo, including grocery lists, instructions, and reminders. Includes BMI and BMR calculator that tracks energy expenditure as well as exercise tracking.

Weight Loss Supplements and Over the Counter Drugs

Thousands of over-the-counter supplements and drugs that claim to make weight loss fast and easy are available for purchase. It's important to note that U.S. Food and Drug Administration (FDA) approval is not required for over-the-counter "diet aids" or supplements. The lack of regular and continuous monitoring of supplements in the United States leaves consumers vulnerable to fraud and potentially toxic "remedies." Most dietary supplements contain stimulants, such as caffeine, or diuretics, and their effectiveness in promoting weight loss has been largely untested and unproved by any scientific studies. In many cases, the only thing that users lose is money. Virtually all persons who used supplements and diet pills in review studies regained their weight once they stopped taking them.[44]

Supplements containing *Hoodia gordonii,* an African, cactus-like plant, have become popular in recent years, and there are many off-market brands produced, including some that contain more unproven ingredients such as bitter orange and other stimulants. Even so, no convincing evidence has been shown for or against *Hoodia gordonii*; to date, it is not FDA approved and has not been tested in clinical trials.[45]

Products containing *ephedra* can cause rapid heart rate, tremors, seizures, insomnia, headaches, and raised blood pressure, all without significant effects on long-term weight control. *St. John's wort* and other alternative medicines reported to enhance serotonin, suppress appetite, and reduce the side effects of depression have not been shown to be effective in weight loss, either.

Historically, FDA-approved diet pills have been available only by prescription and are closely monitored. These lines were blurred in 2007 when the FDA approved the first over-the-counter weight loss pill—a half-strength version of the prescription drug *orlistat* (brand name *Xenical*), marketed as Alli. This drug inhibits the action of lipase, an enzyme that helps the body to digest fats, causing about 30 percent of fats consumed to pass through the digestive system undigested, leading to reduced overall caloric intake. Known side effects of orlistat include gas with watery fecal discharge; oily stools and spotting; frequent, often unexpected, bowel movements; and possible deficiencies of fat-soluble vitamins.

Prescription Weight Loss Drugs

In 2012, the FDA approved the first new weight loss drugs in nearly 13 years. These new drugs, *Belviq* and *Qsymia,* were met with much controversy and carry several warnings and restrictions. Qsymia is an appetite suppressant and antiseizure drug that reduces the desire for food. Belviq affects serotonin levels, helping patients feel full. Newer drugs, such as

39.5%

OF ADULTS AGED 40–59 ARE **OBESE,** FOLLOWED BY 30.3% OBESITY IN THE 20–39 AGE GROUP, AND 35.4% OBESITY IN THE 60+ AGE GROUP.

Contrave combine antidepressants with other approved drugs and carry warnings specific to both. Other weight loss drugs that have been on the market for some time, such as *Meridia*, continue to be marketed. Before taking any weight loss supplements and herbal remedies or prescription drugs, you should always discuss risks, benefits, and options with your doctor and carefully read FDA warnings.

When used as part of a long-term, comprehensive weight-loss program, weight-loss drugs can potentially help those who are severely obese lose up to 10 percent of their weight and maintain the loss. The challenge is to develop an effective drug that can be used over time without adverse effects or abuse, and no such drug currently exists. A classic example of supposedly safe drugs that were later found to have dangerous side effects are Pondimin and Redux, known as *fen-phen* (from their chemical names fenfluramine and phentermine), two of the most widely prescribed diet drugs in U.S. history.[46] When they were found to damage heart valves and contribute to pulmonary hypertension, a massive recall and lawsuit ensued.

Surgery When all else fails, particularly for people who are severely overweight and have weight-related diseases, a person may be a candidate for weight-loss surgery. Generally,

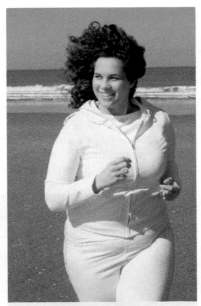

Participating in daily physical activity is key to managing your weight, as well as overall fitness and health.

these surgeries fall into one of two major categories: *restrictive surgeries,* such as gastric banding or lap banding, that limit food intake, and *malabsorption surgeries,* such as gastric bypass, which decrease the absorption of food into the body.

To select the best option, a physician will consider that operation's benefits and risks, the patient's age, BMI, eating behaviors, obesity-related health conditions, mental history, dietary history, and previous operations. Like drugs prescribed for weight loss, surgery for obesity also carries risks for consumers.[47] Some health advocates have proposed that obesity be classified as a disability (see the **Points of View** box on the next page), which could potentially affect a physician's decision on recommending surgery.

In gastric banding and other restrictive surgeries, the surgeon uses an inflatable band to partition off part of the stomach. The band is wrapped around that part of the stomach and is pulled tight, like a belt, leaving only a small opening between the two parts of the stomach. The upper part of the stomach is smaller, so the person feels full more quickly, and food digestion slows so that the person also feels full longer. Although the bands are designed to stay in place, they can be removed surgically. They can also be inflated to different levels to adjust the amount of restriction.

Sleeve gastrectomy is another form of restrictive weight loss that is often done laparoscopically. In this surgery, about 75 percent of the stomach is removed, leaving only a tube (about the size of a banana) or sleeve that is connected directly to the intestines. Usually, this procedure is done on extremely obese or ill patients who need an interim, less invasive procedure before more invasive gastric bypass. However, this procedure isn't reversible and potential risks may be higher.

Gastric bypass is one of the most common types of weight loss surgery and it combines restrictive and malabsorption elements. It can be done laparoscopically or via full open surgery. In this surgery, a major section (as much as 70%) of the stomach is sutured off, restricting the amount of food you can eat and absorb. The remaining pouch is hooked up directly to the small intestine. Results are fast and dramatic, with health issues related to obesity, such as diabetes, high blood pressure, arthritis, sleep apnea, and other problems diminishing or being reduced drastically in a short time.

While weight loss tends to be maintained and health problems decline, there are many risks, including nutritional deficiencies, blood clots in the legs, a leak in a staple line in the stomach, pneumonia, infection, and although rare, even death.

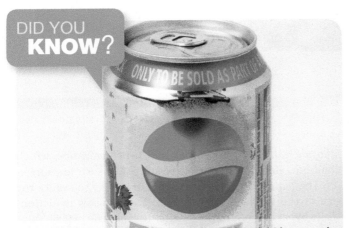

DID YOU KNOW?

Diet soda drinkers may be sabotaging their weight loss—and increasing risks for a variety of health problems! In fact, diet soda drinkers may consume more calories than sugared soda drinkers. Why? Artificial sweeteners may change perceptions of fullness and increase appetite. Others suggest a form of "cognitive distortion" whereby we justify a few more snacks or dessert because our drinks have fewer calories.

Sources: S. N. Bleich, J. A. Wolfson, and S. Vine, "Diet-Beverage Consumption and Caloric Intake among US Adults, Overall and by Body Weight," *American Journal of Public Health* 104, no. 3 (2014): e72–e78

SEE IT! VIDEOS

How can you control your urge to go overboard with meal portions? Watch **Experiment Shows Portion Control Is the Key to Healthy Eating** on **Mastering**Health™

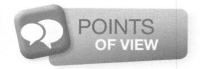
Obesity

Is It a Disability?

A person 150 to 200 pounds over-weight can have difficulty walking, running, standing, and doing other daily tasks. Some believe obesity should be considered a disability legally entitling individuals to certain health benefits and accommodations. Others believe that labeling obesity a disability would add to its stigma and create more problems than it solves.

The federal Americans with Disabilities Act (ADA) defines *disability* as "a physical or mental impairment that substantially limits one or more of the major life activities of [an] individual." Currently, people must have BMIs over 40, or be at least 100 pounds overweight with an underlying disorder before the ADA classifies them as disabled. These strict criteria mean the ADA currently receives few valid claims relating to obesity.

Arguments Favoring Disability Status for Obese People

- Labeling obesity as a disability would provide obese individuals with increased options for health insurance.
- Labeling would protect individuals against weight-based discrimination.
- Labeling would help persons with chronic diseases that require use of walkers, wheelchairs, and other special accommodations at work or home to receive them.

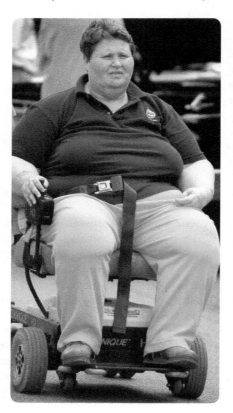

Arguments Opposing Disability Status for Obese People

- Some doctors worry that defining obesity as a disability would make them vulnerable to lawsuits from obese patients who don't want to discuss their weight. Such a threat would prevent doctors from discussing obesity with their overweight patients and recommending specific actions.
- Issues of unfair insurance or job practices could be handled with antidiscrimination laws, not disability status.
- Not all obese people are disabled by their weight, so labeling them all as such would be discriminatory.

WHERE DO YOU STAND?

- What consequences might result from classifying overweight or obese individuals as disabled?
- Do you think labeling obesity as a disability would alter the way our society perceives and behaves toward overweight and obese individuals? If so, how?

Another risk is rapid gastric emptying, commonly referred to as "dumping," in which undigested foods rush through the small intestine, causing cramping and problems with uncontrollable diarrhea.[48] Because the stomach pouch that remains after surgery is only the size of a lime, the person can drink only a few tablespoons of liquid and consume only a very small amount of food at a time. For this reason, other possible side effects include nausea, vitamin and mineral deficiencies, and dehydration. Additional risks include the potential for excess bleeding, ulcers, hernia, and the typical risks from anesthesia.

A technique gaining in popularity because it's even more effective than gastric bypass for rapid weight loss, is the *biliopancreatic diversion* or *duodenal switch procedure*, which combines elements of restrictive and malabsorption surgeries. The patient receives a partial gastrectomy to reduce the size of the stomach (less than gastric bypass's reduction) while bypassing less of the small intestine. The pyloric valve remains intact, which helps prevent dumping syndrome, ulcers, blockages, and other problems that can occur with other techniques. This surgery is one of the most difficult and highest risk surgeries for patients, with the risk of death and other complications higher than those of other options.[49]

Considerable research has demonstrated exciting, unexpected results from gastric surgeries: Even prior to weight

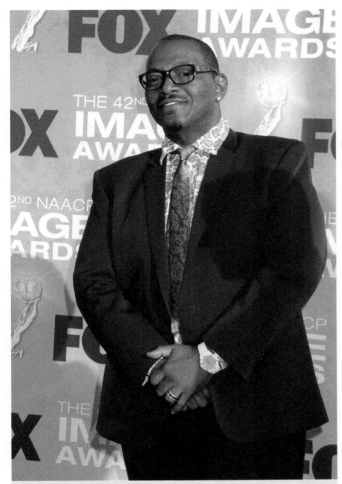

Former *American Idol* judge and record producer Randy Jackson and NBC weatherman Al Roker each have undergone gastric bypass surgery to shed well over 100 pounds and reduce the risks of serious chronic diseases such as type 2 diabetes.

within 5 years after surgery. For those at high risk from these diseases, the choice of undergoing a high-risk surgery may ultimately be similar to the risk of maintaining their current weight.

Unlike surgeries that help make weight loss easier, *liposuction* is a surgical procedure in which fat cells are actually removed from specific areas of the body. Generally, liposuction is considered cosmetic surgery rather than true weight-loss surgery, even though people who have it lose weight and contour their bodies. Liposuction is not risk-free. If you are considering this procedure, check the credentials of the surgeon, the certification of the facility, and the proximity to emergency care if problems arise.

WHAT DO YOU THINK?

If you wanted to lose weight, what strategies would you most likely choose?

■ Which strategies, if any, have worked for you before?

■ What factors might serve to help or hinder your weight-loss efforts?

Trying to Gain Weight

For some people, trying to gain weight is a challenge. If you have trouble, the first priority is to determine why you cannot gain weight. Perhaps you're an athlete and you burn more calories than you eat. Perhaps you're stressed out and skip meals to increase study time. Among older adults, senses of taste and smell may decline, making food less pleasurable to eat. Visual problems and other disabilities may make meals more difficult to prepare, and dental problems may make eating more difficult. People who engage in extreme energy-burning sports and exercise routines may be at risk for caloric and nutritional deficiencies, which can lead not only to weight loss, but also to immune system problems and organ dysfunction; weakness, which leads to falls and fractures; slower recovery from diseases; and a host of other problems. Underweight individuals need to examine diet and exercise behaviors and take steps achieve and maintain a healthy weight.

loss, patients have shown complete remission of type 2 diabetes in the majority of cases, with drastic reductions in blood glucose levels in others.[50] While extremely promising, newer research indicates that about one third of those who have gastric surgery with remission of diabetic symptoms will relapse and begin to show diabetic symptoms

SEE IT! VIDEOS

Could a diet high in protein and fats lead to weight loss? Watch **Low-Carb Diet Trumps Low Fat in Weight-Loss Study** in the Study Area of **MasteringHealth™**

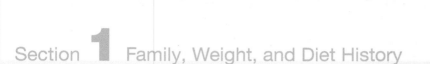

If you are overweight or obese, complete each of the following questions by circling the response(s) that best represents your situation or attitudes, then total your points for each section.

Section 1 Family, Weight, and Diet History

1. How many people in your immediate family (parents or siblings) are overweight or obese?

    a. No one is overweight or obese (0 points)

    b. One person (1 point)

    c. Two people (2 points)

    d. Three or more people (3 points)

2. During which periods of your life were you overweight or obese? (Circle all that apply.)

    a. Birth through age 5 (1 point)

    b. Ages 6 to 11 (1 point)

    c. Ages 12 to 13 (1 point))

    d. Ages 14 to 18 (2 points)

    e. Ages 19 to present (2 points)

3. How many times in the last year have you made a major effort to lose weight but had little or no success?

    a. None. (0 points)

    b. I've thought about it, but never tried. (1 point)

    c. I have tried 2 to 3 times. (1 point)

    d. I have tried at least once a month. (2 points)

    e. I have too many times to count. (3 points)

    Total points: _____

Scoring

A score higher than 4 suggests you may have several challenges ahead as you begin a weight loss program. Your weight is often a product of learned patterns of eating and exercise. If you've tried repeatedly to lose and have not been successful, you may have to reframe your thinking and try something new.

Section 2 Readiness to Change

1. What is/are your main reason(s) for wanting to lose weight? (Circle all that apply.)

    a. I want to please someone I know or attract a new person. (0 points)

    b. I want to look great and/or fit into smaller size clothes for an upcoming event (wedding, vacation, date, etc.). (1 point)

    c. Someone I know has had major health problems because of being overweight/obese. (1 point)

    d. I want to improve my health and/or have more energy. (2 points)

    e. I was diagnosed with a weight-related problem. (2 points)

2. What do you think about your weight and body shape? (Circle all that apply.)

    a. I'm fine with being overweight, and if others don't like it, tough! (0 points)

    b. My weight hurts my energy levels and my performance. (1 points)

    c. I feel good about myself, but think I will be happier if I lose weight. (1 points)

    d. I'm self-conscious about my weight and uncomfortable in my skin. (1 point)

    e. I'm really worried I will have a major health problem if I don't change my behaviors now. (2 points)

3. Which of the following statements describes you? (Circle all that apply.)

    a. I think about food several times a day, even when I'm not hungry. (0 point)

    b. There are some foods or snacks that I can't stay away from, and I eat them even when I'm not hungry. (0 point)

    c. I tend to eat more meat and fatty foods and seldom get enough fruits and veggies. (0 points)

    d. I've thought about the weaknesses in my diet and have some ideas about what I need to do. (1 point)

    e. I haven't really tried to eat a "balanced" diet, but I know that I need to start now. (1 point)

4. When you binge or eat things you shouldn't, what are you likely to do? (Circle all that apply.)

    a. Not care and go off of my diet. (0 points)

    b. Feel guilty for a while, but then do it again the next time I am out. (0 points)

    c. Fast for the next day or two to help balance the high consumption day. (0 points)

    d. Plan ahead for next time and have options in mind so that I do not continue to overeat. (1 point)

    e. Acknowledge that I have made a slip and get back on my program the next day. (1 point)

5. On a typical day, what are your eating patterns? (Circle all that apply.)

    a. I skip breakfast and save my calories for lunch and dinner. (0 point)

    b. I never really sit down for a meal. I am a "grazer" and eat whatever I find that is readily available. (0 point)

    c. I try to eat at least five servings of fruits and veggies and restrict saturated fats in my diet. (1 points)

    d. I eat several small meals, trying to be balanced in my portions and getting foods from different food groups. (1 points)

6. How would you describe your current support system for helping you lose weight? (Circle all that apply.)

    a. I believe I can do this best by doing it on my own. (0 points)

    b. I am not aware of any sources that can help me. (0 points)

    c. I have two to three friends or family members I can count on to help me. (1 point)

    d. There are counselors on campus with whom I can meet to plan a successful approach to weight loss. (1 point)

    e. I have the resources to join Weight Watchers or other community or online weight loss programs. (1 point)

7. How committed are you to exercising? (Circle all that apply.)

    a. Exercise is uncomfortable, embarrassing, and/or I don't enjoy it. (0 points)

    b. I don't have time to exercise. (0 points)

    c. I'd like to exercise, but I'm not sure how to get started. (1 point)

    d. I've visited my campus recreation center or local gym to explore my options. (2 points)

    e. There are specific sports or physical activities I do already, and I can plan to do more of them. (2 points)

8. What statement best describes your motivation to start a weight loss/lifestyle change program?

    a. I don't want to start losing weight. (0 points)

    b. I am thinking about it sometime in the distant future. (0 points)

    c. I am considering starting within the next few weeks; I just need to make a plan. (1 point)

    d. I'd like to start in the next few weeks, and I'm working on a plan. (2 points)

    e. I already have a plan in place, and I'm ready to begin tomorrow. (3 points)

    Total points: _____

Scoring

A score higher than 8 indicates that you may be ready to change; the higher your score above 8, the more successful you may be. Take a close look at areas that you could work on. Your behaviors, resources, readiness to change, and overall plan for change may give you the extra edge necessary to be successful.

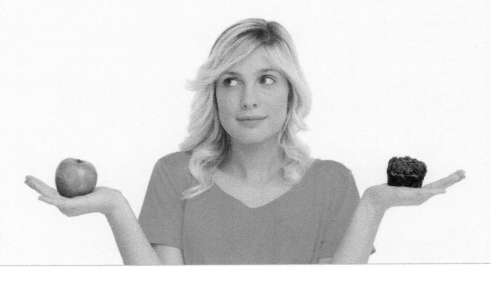

YOUR PLAN FOR CHANGE

The ASSESS YOURSELF identifies six areas of importance in determining your readiness for weight loss. If you wish to lose weight to improve your health, understanding your attitudes about food and exercise will help you succeed.

TODAY, YOU CAN:

☐ Set SMART goals for weight loss and give them a reality check: Are they **s**pecific, **m**easurable, **a**chievable, **r**elevant, and **t**ime oriented? For example, rather than aiming to lose 15 pounds this month (which probably wouldn't be healthy or achievable), set a comfortable goal to lose 1 pound per week by diet and exercise changes.

☐ Keep a food log to identify the triggers that influence your eating habits. Think about what you can do to eliminate or reduce the influence of your two most common food triggers.

WITHIN THE NEXT TWO WEEKS, YOU CAN:

☐ Get in the habit of incorporating more fruits, vegetables, and whole grains in your diet and eating less fat. The next time you make dinner, look at the proportions on your plate. If vegetables and whole grains do not take up most of the space, substitute 1 cup of the meat, non-whole grains, or cheese in your meal with 1 cup of legumes, salad greens, or a favorite vegetable.

☐ Ramp up your exercise in small increments. Visit your campus recreation center or a local gym, and familiarize yourself with the equipment and facilities that are available. Try a new machine or sports activity, and experiment until you find something you really like.

BY THE END OF THE SEMESTER, YOU CAN:

☐ Get in the habit of grocery shopping every week and buying healthy, nutritious foods while avoiding high-fat, high-sugar, or overly processed foods. As you make healthy foods more available and unhealthy foods less available, you'll find it easier to eat better.

☐ Chart your progress and reward yourself as you meet your goals. Do something fun like see a movie, or buy that new pair of skinny jeans you've been wanting for (which will likely fit better than before!).

STUDY PLAN

Customize your study plan—and master your health!—in the Study Area of MasteringHealth™

CHAPTER REVIEW

To hear an MP3 Tutor Session, scan here or visit the Study Area in MasteringHealth.

LO 1 | Overweight and Obesity: A Growing Challenge

- Overweight, obesity, and weight-related health problems have reached epidemic levels. *Globesity,* or global rates of obesity, threatens the health of many countries. Societal costs from obesity include increased health care costs and lowered worker productivity. Individual health risks from overweight and obesity include increased chance of developing cardiovascular diseases, arthritis, stroke, diabetes, gastrointestinal problems, low back pain, and a number of other diseases. Overweight individuals are also at risk of struggling with depression, low self-esteem, and high levels of stress.

LO 2 | Factors Contributing to Overweight and Obesity

- It is important to consider environmental, cultural, and socioeconomic factors when working to prevent obesity. In addition to genetics, metabolism, hormonal influences, excess fat cells, and physical risks, key environmental influences, such as poverty, socioeconomic status, education level, and lack of access to nutritious food, and lifestyle factors, including sedentary lifestyle and high calorie consumption, all make weight loss challenging.

LO 3 | Assessing Body Weight and Body Composition

- Percentage of body fat is a fairly reliable indicator for levels of overweight and obesity. There are many different methods of assessing body fat. Body mass index (BMI) is one of the most commonly accepted measures of weight based on height. *Overweight*

is most commonly defined as a BMI of 25 to 29.9 and *obesity* as a BMI of 30 or greater. Waist circumference, or the amount of fat in the belly region, is believed to be related to the risk for several chronic diseases, particularly type 2 diabetes.

LO 4 | Managing Your Weight

- Increased physical activity, a balanced, healthy diet that controls caloric intake, and other strategies are recommended for controlling your weight. When these options fail and risks increase, doctor-recommended prescription medications, weight loss surgery, and other strategies are used to maintain or lose weight. However, sensible eating behavior and aerobic exercise and exercise that builds muscle mass offer the best options for weight loss and maintenance.

POP QUIZ

Visit MasteringHealth to personalize your study plan with Chapter Review Quizzes and Dynamic Study Modules.

LO 1 | Overweight and Obesity: A Growing Challenge.

1. All of the following statements are true *except* which?
   a. Hispanic and non-Hispanic white men are more likely to be overweight/obese than non-Hispanic Black or Asian men.
   b. Children and adolescents living in higher income homes where parents are more educated have a greatly increased risk of obesity over those living in low income homes where parents are less educated and/or unemployed.
   c. Non-Hispanic black and Hispanic women are more likely to be overweight or obese than non-Hispanic white women.
   d. The United States has the distinction of being one of the fattest developed nations on earth.

LO 2 | Factors Contributing to Overweight and Obesity

2. The rate at which your body consumes food energy to sustain basic functions is your
   a. basal metabolic rate.
   b. resting metabolic rate.
   c. body mass index.
   d. set point.

3. All of the following statements are true *except* which?
   a. A slowing basal metabolic rate may contribute to weight gain after age 30.
   b. Hormones are increasingly implicated in hunger impulses and eating behavior.
   c. The more muscles you have, the fewer calories you will burn.
   d. Yo-yo dieting can make weight loss more difficult.

LO 3 | Assessing Body Weight and Body Composition

4. The proportion of your total weight that is made up of fat is called
   a. body composition.
   b. lean mass.
   c. percentage of body fat.
   d. BMI.

5. All of the following statements about BMI are true *except* which?
   a. BMI is based on height and weight measurements.
   b. BMI is accurate for everyone, including athletes with high amounts of muscle mass.
   c. Very low and very high BMI scores are associated with greater risk of mortality.
   d. BMI stands for "body mass index."

6. Which of the following body circumferences is most strongly associated with risk of heart disease and diabetes?
   a. Hip circumference
   b. Chest circumference
   c. Waist circumference
   d. Thigh circumference

LO 4 | Managing Your Weight

7. One pound of additional body fat is created through consuming how many extra calories?
   a. 1,500 calories
   b. 3,500 calories
   c. 5,000 calories
   d. 7,000 calories

8. To lose weight, you must establish a(n)
   a. negative caloric balance.
   b. isocaloric balance.
   c. positive caloric balance.
   d. set point.

9. Successful weight maintainers are most likely to do which of the following?
   a. Eat two large meals a day before 1 P.M.
   b. Skip meals
   c. Drink diet sodas
   d. Eat high-volume but low-calorie density foods

10. Successful, healthy weight loss is characterized by
    a. a lifelong pattern of healthful eating and exercise.
    b. cutting out all fats and carbohydrates and eating a lean, mean, high-protein diet.
    c. never eating foods that are considered bad for you and rigidly adhering to a plan.
    d. a pattern of repeatedly losing and regaining weight.

Answers to the Pop Quiz can be found on page A-1. If you answered a question incorrectly, review the section tagged by the Learning Outcome. For even more study tools, visit MasteringHealth.

THINK ABOUT IT!

LO 1 Overweight and Obesity: A Growing Challenge

1. Why do you think that obesity rates are rising in both developed and less-developed regions of the world? What strategies can we take collectively and individually to reduce risks of obesity nationally? Internationally?

LO 2 Factors Contributing to Overweight and Obesity

2. List the risk factors for your being overweight or obese right now. Which seem most likely to determine whether you will be obese in middle age?

LO 3 Assessing Body Weight and Body Composition

3. Which measurement would you choose to assess your fat levels? Why?

LO 4 Managing Your Weight

4. Are you satisfied with your body weight? If so, what do you do to maintain a healthy weight? If not, what are some lifestyle changes you could make to improve your weight and overall health?

ACCESS YOUR HEALTH ON THE INTERNET

Visit **MasteringHealth** for links to the websites and RSS feeds. The following websites explore further topics and issues related to personal health. For links to these websites, visit MasteringHealth.

Academy of Nutrition and Dietetics. This site includes recommended dietary guidelines and other current information about weight control. www.eatright.org

Weight Control Information Network. This is an excellent resource for diet and weight control information. http://win.niddk.nih.gov/index.htm

The Rudd Center for Food Policy and Obesity. This website provides excellent information on the latest in obesity research, public policy, and ways we can stop the obesity epidemic at the community level. www.uconnruddcenter.org/

The Obesity Society. Key site for information/education about our national obesity epidemic, including statistics, research, consumer issues, and fact sheets. www.obesity.org

Enhancing Your Body Image

Dissatisfaction with one's appearance and shape is an all-too-common feeling in today's society that can foster unhealthy attitudes and thought patterns, as well as disordered eating and exercising behaviors.

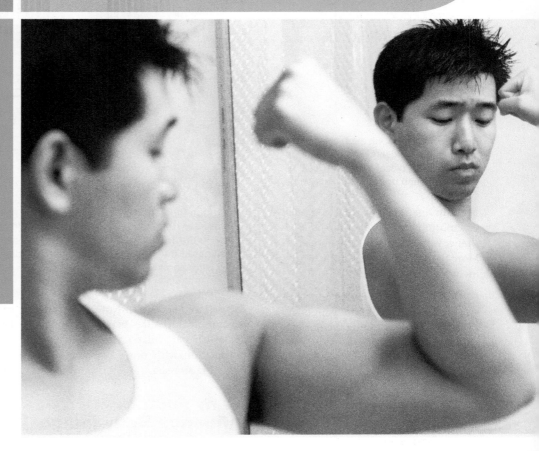

LEARNING OUTCOMES

1 Define body image, list the factors that influence it, and identify the difference between being dissatisfied with your appearance and body image disorders.

2 Describe the signs and symptoms of disordered eating, as well as the physical effects and treatment options for anorexia nervosa, bulimia nervosa, orthorexia nervosa, and binge-eating disorder.

3 List the criteria, symptoms, and treatment for exercise disorders such as muscle dysmorphia and female athlete triad.

When you look in the mirror, do you like what you see? If you feel disappointed, frustrated, or even angry, you're not alone. Preoccupation with appearance and a distorted image of how we look is a major problem for a wide range of people. In a UK study, 93 percent of the women reported negative thoughts about their appearance during the past week and wanted to lose weight, even though the majority were in the underweight or normal weight ranges.[1] Concerns about weight seem to be central to many people's body dissatisfaction. As body mass increases, dissatisfaction increases, particularly during transitional periods in life. Females, in particular, seem to experience peak levels of body dissatisfaction when transitioning from high school to young adulthood.[2] Sadly, dissatisfaction with your body can result in behaviors that disrupt your relationships, affect your mental health, and lead to life-threatening illness. Developing and maintaining a healthy body image can enhance your interactions with others, reduce stress, give you an increased sense of personal empowerment, and bring confidence and joy to your life.

80%

OF ADULT AMERICAN WOMEN REPORT DISSATISFACTION WITH THEIR **APPEARANCE**.

LO 1 | **WHAT** IS BODY IMAGE?

Define body image, list the factors that influence it, and identify the difference between being dissatisfied with your appearance and body image disorders.

Body image refers to what you believe or emotionally feel about your body's shape, weight, and general appearance. More than what you see in the mirror, it includes the following:

- How you see yourself in your mind
- What you believe about your own appearance (including memories, assumptions, and generalizations)
- How you feel about your body, including your height, shape, and weight
- How you sense and control your body as you move

A *negative body image* is defined as either a distorted perception of your shape or feelings of discomfort, shame, or anxiety about your body. It may involve being certain that only people other than you are attractive and that your body is a sign of personal failure. In contrast, a *positive body image* is a true perception of your appearance: You see yourself as you really are. You understand that everyone is different, and you celebrate your uniqueness—including your perceived "flaws," which you know have nothing to do with your value as a person.

Is your body image negative or positive—or somewhere in between? Researchers have developed a body image continuum that may help you

body image How you see yourself in your mind, what you believe about your appearance, and how you feel about your body.

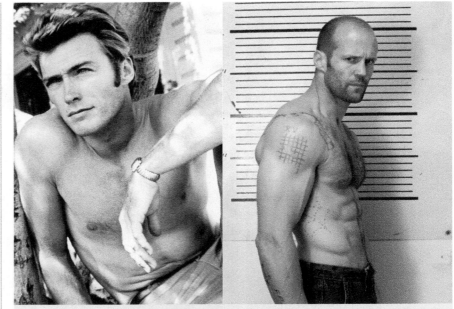

Although the exact nature of the "in" look may change from generation to generation, unrealistic images of both male and female celebrities are nothing new. In the 1960s, images of brawny film stars such as Clint Eastwood dominated the media. The physique of today's male celebrities is even more muscular and still very difficult for most to achieve themselves.

decide (see **FIGURE 1**). Notice that the continuum identifies behaviors associated with particular states, from total dissociation with one's body to body not being an issue.

Many Factors Influence Body Image

You're not born with a body image, but you do begin to develop one at an early age. Let's look more closely at the factors that probably played a role in the development of your body image.

The Media and Popular Culture

Media images tend to set the standard for what we find attractive, leading some people to go to dangerous extremes to have the biggest biceps or fit into size zero jeans. Changing our bodies or body parts to better achieve what current society feels is beautiful has long been part of American culture. During the early twentieth century, while men idolized the strong, hearty outdoorsman President Teddy Roosevelt, women pulled their corsets ever tighter to achieve unrealistically tiny waists. In the 1920s and 1930s, men emulated the burly cops and robbers in

gangster films, while women dieted and bound their breasts to achieve the boyish "flapper" look. By the 1960s, tough guys were the male ideal, whereas rail-thin supermodels embodied the nation's standard of female beauty. Today's societal obsession around appearance—even when many images are airbrushed or Photoshopped—isn't much different.

Social media popularity has also increased concerns regarding negative body images.[3] Many social media sites actively warn against posts promoting or glorifying self-harm, but even messages promoting unhealthy body images can still be hard to avoid. Such messages are often disguised as a type of encouragement—images of unrealistically thin bodies are coupled with catch phrases telling young people to get "thin" or avoid being "fat."[4] See **Student Health Today** on page 320 for more on "thinspiration."

Today, more than 69 percent of American adults 20 years and older are overweight or obese; thus, a significant disconnect exists between the media's idealized images of male and female bodies and the typical American body.[5] We are bombarded with unrealistic images of "beauty." In fact, one study conducted with college women of

Body hate/ disassociation	Distorted body image	Body preoccupied/ obsessed	Body acceptance	Body ownership
I often feel separated and distant from my body—as if it belonged to someone else. I hate my body, and I often isolate myself from others. I don't see anything positive or even neutral about my body shape and size. I don't believe others when they tell me I look okay. I hate the way I look in the mirror.	I spend a significant amount of time exercising and dieting to change my body. My body shape and size keeps me from dating or finding someone who will treat me the way I want to be treated. I have considered changing (or have changed) my body shape and size through surgical means. I wish I could change the way I look in the mirror.	I weigh and measure myself a lot. I spend a significant amount of time viewing myself in the mirror. I compare my body to others. I have days when I feel fat. I accept society's ideal body shape and size as the best body shape and size. I'd be more attractive if I were thinner, more muscular, etc.	I pay attention to my body and my appearance because it is important to me, but it only occupies a small part of my day. I would like to change some things about my body, but I spend most of my time highlighting my positive features. My self-esteem is based on my personality traits, achievements, and relationships—not just my body image.	I feel fine about my body. I don't worry about changing my body shape or weight. I never weigh or measure myself. My feelings about my body are not influenced by society's concept of an ideal body shape. I know that the significant others in my life will always love me for who I am, not for how I look.

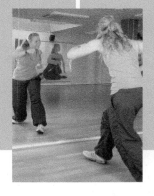

VIDEO TUTOR
Body Image Continuum

FIGURE 1 **Body Image Continuum** This continuum shows a range of attitudes and behaviors toward body image. Functioning at either extreme—not caring at all or being obsessed—leads to problems. When you are functioning in the "body acceptance" area, you are taking care of your body and emotions.

Source: Adapted from Smiley/King/Avery, "Eating Issues and Body Image Continuum," Campus Health Service 1996. Copyright © 1997 Arizona Board of Regents for University of Arizona.

multiple ethnicities found that female body dissatisfaction was attributed to perceptions of celebrity role models and Western culture's thin idealization.[6]

Family, Community, and Cultural Groups

The people with whom we most often interact—our family members, friends, and others—strongly influence the way we see ourselves. Parents are especially influential in body image development. For instance, it's common and natural for fathers of adolescent girls to experience feelings of discomfort related to their daughters' changing bodies. If they are able to navigate these feelings successfully and validate the acceptability of their daughters' appearance throughout puberty, they'll help their daughters maintain a positive body image. In contrast, even subtle judgments about their daughters' changing bodies may prompt girls to question how males view their bodies in general. In addition, mothers who model body acceptance or body ownership may be more likely to foster a positive body image in their daughters, whereas mothers who are frustrated with or ashamed of their own bodies may foster negative attitudes.

Interactions with siblings and other relatives, peers, teachers, coworkers, and other community members can also influence body image development. For instance, peer harassment (teasing and bullying) is widely acknowledged to contribute to a negative body image. Associations within one's cultural group are also a factor. For example, studies have found that European American females experience the highest rates of body dissatisfaction, and as a minority group becomes more acculturated into the mainstream and exposed to media, the body dissatisfaction levels of women in that group increase.[7]

Physiological and Psychological Factors

Recent neurological research suggests that people who have been diagnosed with a body image disorder show differences in the brain's ability to regulate mood-linked

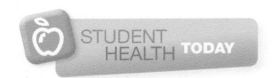
THINSPIRATION AND THE ONLINE WORLD OF ANOREXIA

The pro-anorexia movement has a host of websites, chat rooms, blogs, and discussion boards mostly created and hosted by girls and women struggling with eating disorders. With dangerous and incorrect information about restrictive eating, metabolism, binging, and laxative abuse, many include "thinspiration"—pictures and quotes intended to inspire visitors to thinness—as well as tips and tricks to hide and maintain disordered eating.

Despite the support and understanding that participating women get from each other, they also encourage each other to remain sick. Ambivalent messages about thinness and weight loss coincide with how many visitors feel about their own eating disorder. Many sites claim it is not their intention to recruit new "members"; on the same site, though, you may find tips on "how to become anorexic."

Recently, France voted to punish anyone encouraging people to become dangerously thin with a year in prison and a fine of roughly $11,000. While French authorities have focused on fashion websites, which encourage women to keep their weight as low as possible, pro-anorexia sites are clear violators. Brazil, Italy, and Spain have all taken action against skinny models in fashion shows.

Sources: K. Davis, "Ana & Mia: The Online World of Anorexia and Bulimia," *OHPE Bulletin* 244, no. 1 (2002), www.ohpe.ca/node/160; National Eating Disorder Information Centre, www.nedic.ca; MPA Website, Accessed May 2015, www.myproana.com/index.php/blogs/; P. Allen and I. Sparks, " France Cracks Down on 'Pro-Anorexia" Websites that Encourage Young Women to Keep Their Weight as Low as Possible," *The Daily Mail*, April 2, 2015, www.dailymail.co.uk/news/article-3023026/France-cracks-pro-anorexia-websites-encourage-young-women-weight-low-possible.html

---

chemicals called *neurotransmitters*.[8] Poor regulation of neurotransmitters is also involved in depression, anxiety disorders, and obsessive-compulsive disorder. One study linked distortions in body image, particularly the face, to a malfunction in the brain's visual processing region that was revealed by magnetic resonance imaging (MRI) scanning.[9]

Building a Positive Body Image

To develop a more positive body image, start by challenging some commonly held myths and attitudes in contemporary society.[10]

Myth 1: How you look is more important than who you are. Do you think your weight is important in defining who you are? How much does it matter to you to have thin and attractive friends? How important do you think being thin is for attracting your ideal partner?

Myth 2: Anyone can be slender and attractive if they work at it. When you see someone who is extremely thin, what assumptions do you make about that person? When you see someone who is overweight or obese, what assumptions do you make? Have you ever berated yourself for not having the "willpower" to change some aspect of your body?

Myth 3: Extreme dieting is an effective weight-loss strategy. Do you believe in trying fad diets or "quick-weight-loss" products? How far would you be willing to go to attain the "perfect" body?

Myth 4: Appearance is more important than health. How do you evaluate whether a person is healthy? Is your desire to change some aspect of your body motivated by health reasons or by concerns about appearance?

For ways to bust these toxic myths and attitudes and to build a more positive body image, check out the **Skills for Behavior Change** box.

Body Image Disorders

Although most Americans are dissatisfied with some aspect of their appearance, very few have a true body image

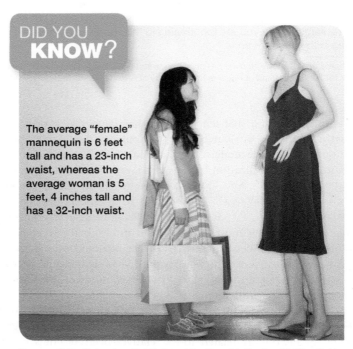

DID YOU KNOW?

The average "female" mannequin is 6 feet tall and has a 23-inch waist, whereas the average woman is 5 feet, 4 inches tall and has a 32-inch waist.

Sources: R. Duyff, *American Dietetic Association Complete Food and Nutrition Guide*, 4th ed. (Hoboken, NJ: John Wiley & Sons, Inc., 2012), 50; C. Fryar, Q. Gu, and C. Ogden, "Anthropometric Reference Data for Children and Adults: United States, 2007–2010," National Center for Health Statistics, *Vital and Health Statistics*, Series 11, no. 252 (2012), www.cdc.gov/nchs/data/series/sr_11/sr11_252.pdf

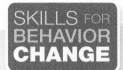

SKILLS FOR BEHAVIOR CHANGE

TEN STEPS TO A POSITIVE BODY IMAGE

One way to turn negative thoughts positive is to think about how to look more healthfully and happily at yourself and your body. The more you try, the better you will feel about who you are and the body you naturally have.

▶ **Step 1.** Appreciate all of the amazing things your body does for you—running, dancing, breathing, laughing, dreaming.

▶ **Step 2.** Make a list of things you like about yourself—things that aren't related to how much you weigh or how you look. Add to it as you notice things.

▶ **Step 3.** Remind yourself that true beauty is not skin deep. When you feel good about yourself and who you are, you carry yourself with a sense of confidence, self-acceptance, and openness that makes you beautiful.

▶ **Step 4.** Look at yourself as a whole person. When you see yourself in a mirror or in your mind, choose not to focus on specific body parts.

▶ **Step 5.** Surround yourself with positive people. It is easier to feel good about yourself when you are around those who are supportive and who recognize the importance of liking yourself as you naturally are.

▶ **Step 6.** Shut down those voices in your head that tell you your body is not "right" or that you are a "bad" person.

▶ **Step 7.** Wear comfortable clothes that make you feel good about your body. Work with your body, not against it.

▶ **Step 8.** Become a critical viewer of social and media messages. Pay attention to images, slogans, and attitudes that make you feel bad about your appearance.

▶ **Step 9.** Show appreciation for your body. Take a bubble bath, make time for a nap, or find a peaceful place outside to relax.

▶ **Step 10.** Use the time and energy you might have spent worrying about food, calories, and your weight to do something to help others. Reaching out to other people can help you feel better about yourself and make a positive change in our world.

Source: "10 Steps to Positive Body Image," from National Eating Disorders Association website, April 22, 2013. Copyright © 2013 National Eating Disorders Association. Reprinted with permission. For more information visit **www.NationalEatingDisorders.org** or call NEDA's helpline 1-800-931-2237.

body dysmorphic disorder (BDD) Psychological disorder characterized by an obsession with one's appearance and a distorted view of one's body or with a minor or imagined flaw in appearance.

social physique anxiety (SPA) A desire to look good that has a destructive effect on a person's ability to function well in social interactions and relationships.

estimated that 10 percent of people seeking dermatology or cosmetic treatments have BDD.[13] Not only do such actions fail to address the underlying problem, but also they are actually considered diagnostic signs of BDD. Psychiatric treatment, including psychotherapy and/or antidepressant medications, can help.

Social Physique Anxiety

An emerging problem for both young men and women is **social physique anxiety (SPA).** The desire to "look good" becomes so strong it has a destructive and sometimes disabling effect on the person's ability to

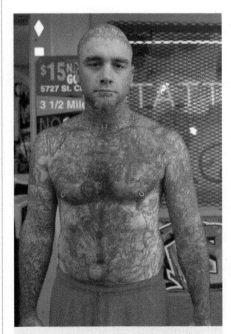

It's not always easy to spot people who are highly dissatisfied with their bodies. People who cover their bodies with tattoos may have a strong sense of self-esteem. On the other hand, extreme tattooing can be an outward sign of a severe body image disturbance known as body dysmorphic disorder.

disorder. However, several diagnosable body image disorders affect a small percentage of the population. Two of the most common are body dysmorphic disorder and social physique anxiety.

Body Dysmorphic Disorder

Approximately 1 percent of people in the United States suffer from **body dysmorphic disorder (BDD).**[11] Persons with BDD are obsessively concerned with their appearance and have a distorted view of their own body shape, size, weight, perceived lack of muscles, facial blemishes, size of body parts, etc. Although the cause of the disorder isn't known, an anxiety disorder or obsessive-compulsive disorder is often present as well. Contributing factors may include genetic susceptibility, childhood teasing, physical or sexual abuse, low self-esteem, and rigid sociocultural expectations of beauty.[12]

People with BDD may try to fix their perceived flaws through abuse of steroids, excessive bodybuilding, cosmetic surgeries, extreme tattooing, or other appearance-altering behaviors. It is

Eating disordered	Disruptive eating patterns	Food preoccupied/ obsessed	Concerned in a healthy way	Food is not an issue
I worry about what I will eat or when I will exercise all the time. I follow a very rigid eating plan and know precisely how many calories, fat grams, or carbohydrates I eat every day. I feel incredible guilt, shame, and anxiety when I break my diet. I regularly stuff myself and then exercise, vomit, or use laxatives to get rid of the food. My friends and family tell me I am too thin, but I feel fat. I am out of control when I eat. I am afraid to eat in front of others. I prefer to eat alone.	My food and exercise concerns are starting to interfere with my school and social life. I use food to comfort myself. I have tried diet pills, laxatives, vomiting, or extra time exercising in order to lose or maintain my weight. I have fasted or avoided eating for long periods of time in order to lose or maintain my weight. If I cannot exercise to burn off calories, I panic. I feel strong when I can restrict how much I eat. I feel out of control when I eat more than I wanted to.	I think about food a lot. I'm obsessed with reading books and magazines about dieting, fitness, and weight control. I sometimes miss school, work, and social events because of my diet or exercise schedule. I divide food into "good" and "bad" categories. I feel guilty when I eat "bad" foods or when I eat more than what I feel I should be eating. I am afraid of getting fat. I wish I could change how much I want to eat and what I am hungry for.	I pay attention to what I eat in order to maintain a healthy body. Food and exercise are important parts of my life, but they only occupy a small part of my time. I enjoy eating, and I balance my pleasure with my concern for a healthy body. I usually eat three balanced meals daily, plus snacks, to fuel my body with adequate energy. I am moderate and flexible in my goals for eating well and being physically active. Sometimes I eat more (or less) than I really need, but most of the time I listen to my body.	I am not concerned about what or how much I eat. I feel no guilt or shame no matter what I eat or how much I eat. Exercise is not really important to me. I choose foods based on cost, taste, and convenience, with little regard to health. My eating is very sporadic and irregular. I don't worry about meals; I just eat whatever I can, whenever I can. I enjoy stuffing myself with lots of tasty food at restaurants, holiday meals, and social events.

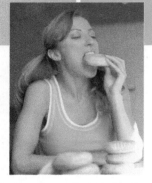 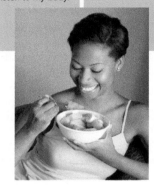

FIGURE 2 Eating Issues Continuum This continuum shows progression from eating disorders to normal eating. Being concerned in a healthy way is the goal, rather than functioning at either extreme.

Source: Adapted from Smiley/King/Avery, "Eating Issues and Body Image Continuum," Campus Health Service 1996. Copyright © 1997 Arizona Board of Regents for University of Arizona.

function effectively in relationships and interactions with others. People suffering from SPA spend a disproportionate amount of time fixating on their bodies, working out, and performing tasks that are ego centered and self-directed, rather than focusing on interpersonal relationships and general tasks.[14] Experts speculate that this anxiety may contribute to disordered eating.

disordered eating A pattern of atypical eating behaviors that is used to achieve or maintain a lower body weight.

LO 2 | DISORDERED EATING AND EATING DISORDERS

Describe the signs and symptoms of disordered eating, as well as the physical effects and treatment options for anorexia nervosa, bulimia nervosa, orthorexia nervosa, and binge-eating disorder.

People with a negative body image can fixate on a wide range of self-perceived "flaws." The so-called flaw that distresses the majority of people with negative body image is feeling overweight.

Some people channel weight-related anxiety into self-defeating thoughts and harmful behaviors. The far left of the eating issues continuum (FIGURE 2) identifies a pattern of thoughts and behaviors associated with **disordered eating**, including chronic dieting, rigid eating patterns, abusing diet pills and laxatives, self-induced vomiting, and many others.

Few people who exhibit disordered eating patterns progress to a clinical **eating disorder.** The eating disorders defined by the American Psychiatric Association (APA) in the *Diagnostic and*

Statistical Manual of Mental Disorders, Fifth Edition (DSM-5) are *anorexia nervosa, bulimia nervosa, binge-eating disorder,* and a cluster of less-distinct conditions collectively referred to as other specified feeding or eating disorder (OSFED).[15]

Twenty million women and 10 million men in the United States will suffer from some sort of eating disorder over their lifetimes.[16] Although anorexia nervosa and bulimia nervosa used to affect people primarily in their teens and twenties, increasing numbers of children as young as 7 have been diagnosed, as have women as old as 80.[17] In 2014, 2.1 percent of college students self-reported as having anorexia or bulimia.[18] Disordered eating and eating disorders are also common among ballet dancers and athletes, particularly athletes in sports with an aesthetic component (e.g., figure skating or gymnastics) or tied to a weight class (e.g., tae kwon do, judo, or wrestling).[19]

Eating disorders are on the rise among men, who make up nearly 25 percent of all anorexia and bulimia patients.[20] Many men suffering from eating disorders fail to seek treatment because these illnesses are traditionally thought of as a woman's problem.

What factors put individuals at risk? Many people with eating disorders feel disenfranchised in other aspects of their lives and try to gain a sense of control through food. Many are clinically depressed, suffer from obsessive-compulsive disorder, or have other psychiatric problems. In addition, individuals with low self-esteem, negative body image, and a high tendency for perfectionism are at risk.[21]

Anorexia Nervosa

Anorexia nervosa is a persistent, chronic eating disorder characterized by deliberate food restriction and severe, life-threatening weight loss. It has the highest death rate (20%) of any psychological illness.[22] It involves self-starvation motivated by an intense fear of gaining weight and an extremely distorted body image. Initially, most people with anorexia nervosa lose weight by reducing total food intake, particularly of high-calorie foods. Eventually, they progress to restricting their intake of almost all foods. The little they do eat, they may purge through vomiting or using laxatives. Although they lose weight, people with anorexia nervosa never feel thin enough. An estimated 0.3 percent of females suffer from anorexia nervosa in their lifetime.[23]

FIGURE 3 illustrates physical symptoms and negative health consequences associated with anorexia nervosa.

Causes of anorexia nervosa are complex and variable. Many people with anorexia have other coexisting psychiatric problems, including low self-esteem, depression, an anxiety disorder such as obsessive-compulsive disorder, and substance abuse. Some people have a history of being physically or sexually abused, and others have troubled interpersonal relationships. Cultural norms that value appearance and glorify thinness as beauty are factors, as are weight-based shame, peer comparisons, and weight bias.[24] Physical factors are thought to include an imbalance of neurotransmitters and genetic susceptibility.[25]

Bulimia Nervosa

Individuals with **bulimia nervosa** often binge on huge amounts of

SEE IT! VIDEOS

How do you treat the most common but least well known eating disorder?

Watch **EDNOS: Most Dangerous, Unheard of Eating Disorder** on MasteringHealth™

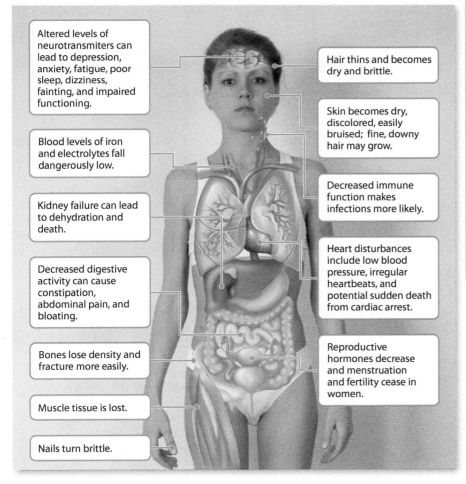

Altered levels of neurotransmiters can lead to depression, anxiety, fatigue, poor sleep, dizziness, fainting, and impaired functioning.

Blood levels of iron and electrolytes fall dangerously low.

Kidney failure can lead to dehydration and death.

Decreased digestive activity can cause constipation, abdominal pain, and bloating.

Bones lose density and fracture more easily.

Muscle tissue is lost.

Nails turn brittle.

Hair thins and becomes dry and brittle.

Skin becomes dry, discolored, easily bruised; fine, downy hair may grow.

Decreased immune function makes infections more likely.

Heart disturbances include low blood pressure, irregular heartbeats, and potential sudden death from cardiac arrest.

Reproductive hormones decrease and menstruation and fertility cease in women.

FIGURE 3 What Anorexia Nervosa Can Do to the Body

eating disorder A psychiatric disorder characterized by severe disturbances in body image and eating behaviors.

anorexia nervosa Eating disorder characterized by deliberate food restriction, self-starvation, or extreme exercising to achieve weight loss, and an extremely distorted body image.

bulimia nervosa Eating disorder characterized by binge eating followed by inappropriate purging measures or compensatory behavior, such as vomiting or excessive exercise, to prevent weight gain.

food—often with a feeling of being out of control—and then engage in some kind of purging or compensatory behavior, such as vomiting, taking laxatives, or exercising excessively, to lose the calories they have just consumed. People with bulimia are obsessed with their bodies, weight gain, and appearance, but unlike those with anorexia, their problem is often hidden from the public eye because their weight may fall within a normal range or they may be overweight. Up to 3 percent of adolescents and young women are bulimic; rates among men are about 10 percent of the rate among women.[26]

FIGURE 4 illustrates the physical symptoms and negative health consequences associated with bulimia nervosa.

A combination of genetic and environmental factors is thought to cause bulimia nervosa.[27] A family history of obesity, an underlying anxiety disorder, and an imbalance in neurotransmitters are all possible contributing factors. In support of the role of neurotransmitters, a study showed that brain circuitry involved in regulating impulsive behavior seems to be less active in women with bulimia than in healthy women.[28] However, it is unknown whether such differences exist before bulimia develops or arise as a consequence of the disorder.

Binge-Eating Disorder

Individuals with **binge-eating disorder** gorge themselves, but do not take excessive measures to lose the weight gained. Thus, they are often clinically obese. Binge-eating episodes are typically characterized by eating large amounts of food rapidly, even when not feeling

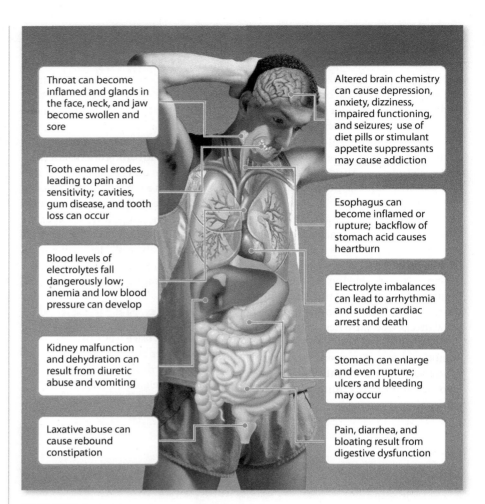

Throat can become inflamed and glands in the face, neck, and jaw become swollen and sore

Tooth enamel erodes, leading to pain and sensitivity; cavities, gum disease, and tooth loss can occur

Blood levels of electrolytes fall dangerously low; anemia and low blood pressure can develop

Kidney malfunction and dehydration can result from diuretic abuse and vomiting

Laxative abuse can cause rebound constipation

Altered brain chemistry can cause depression, anxiety, dizziness, impaired functioning, and seizures; use of diet pills or stimulant appetite suppressants may cause addiction

Esophagus can become inflamed or rupture; backflow of stomach acid causes heartburn

Electrolyte imbalances can lead to arrhythmia and sudden cardiac arrest and death

Stomach can enlarge and even rupture; ulcers and bleeding may occur

Pain, diarrhea, and bloating result from digestive dysfunction

FIGURE 4 What Bulimia Nervosa Can Do to the Body

hungry, and feeling guilty or depressed after overeating.[29]

A national survey reported a lifetime prevalence of binge-eating disorder in the study participants of 1.4 percent.[30]

Other Specified Feeding or Eating Disorder

The APA recognizes that some patterns of disordered eating qualify as a legitimate psychiatric illness but don't fit into the strict diagnostic criteria for anorexia, bulimia, or binge-eating disorder. Called **other specified feeding or eating disorders (OSFED),** this group of disorders includes five specific subtypes: *night eating syndrome, purging disorder, binge-eating disorder of low frequency/limited duration, bulimia*

nervosa of low frequency/duration, and atypical anorexia nervosa. Atypical anorexia nervosa is defined in this category as displaying anorexic features without low weight.[31] All of these subtypes can cause remarkable distress or impairment but don't exhibit the full criteria of another feeding or eating disorder.

binge-eating disorder A type of eating disorder characterized by gorging on food once a week or more, but not typically followed by a purge.

other specified feeding or eating disorder (OSFED) Eating disorders that are a true psychiatric illness but that do not fit the strict diagnostic criteria for anorexia nervosa, bulimia nervosa, or binge-eating disorder.

orthorexia nervosa An eating disorder characterized by fixation on food quality and purity.

Orthorexia Nervosa

Literally meaning "fixation on righteous eating," **orthorexia nervosa** is an unhealthy obsession with what would otherwise be healthy eating. What typically begins as a simple attempt to eat more healthfully can become a fixation with food quality and purity. Those with orthorexia nervosa become consumed with what and how much to eat and how to deal with eating mistakes. Eventually, food choices become so restrictive that health suffers.

Treatment for Eating Disorders

Because eating disorders are caused by a combination of factors, there are no simple solutions. Without treatment, approximately 20 percent of people with a serious eating disorder will die as a result; with treatment, long-term full recovery rates range from 44 to 76 percent for anorexia nervosa and from 50 to 70 percent for bulimia nervosa.[32]

Treatment often focuses first on reducing the threat to life. Once the patient is stabilized, long-term therapy focuses on the psychological, social, environmental, and physiological factors that have led to the problem. Through therapy, the patient works on adopting new eating behaviors, building self-confidence, and finding healthy ways to deal with life's problems. Support groups can help the family and the individual learn positive actions and interactions. Treatment of an underlying anxiety disorder or depression may also be a focus.

Helping Someone with Disordered Eating

Although every situation is different, there are several things you can do if you suspect someone you know is struggling with disordered eating:[33]

- **Learn** as much as you can about disordered eating.
- **Know the facts** about weight, nutrition, and exercise. Accurate

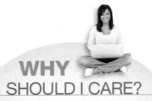

WHY SHOULD I CARE?

Although exercising is generally beneficial to your health, doing it compulsively can lead to broken bones, joint injuries, and even depression—all of which can put you out of commission for the other things you enjoy. Remember that moderation is essential and taking rest days is important to your health.

information can help you reason against excuses used to maintain a disordered eating pattern.

- **Be honest** and talk openly about your concerns.
- **Be caring, but be firm** because caring about your friend does not mean allowing him or her to manipulate you. Your friend must be responsible for his or her actions and the

consequences of those actions. Avoid making statements that you cannot or will not uphold.

- **Compliment** your friend's personality, successes, and accomplishments.
- **Be a good role model** for healthy eating, exercise, and self-acceptance.
- **Tell someone,** and don't wait until your friend's life is in danger. Addressing disordered eating patterns in their beginning stages offers your friend the best chance for working through these issues and becoming healthy again.

There are many resources for people who are considering seeking help or finding out if they are at risk for developing an eating disorder. The National Eating Disorders Association has a general online screening tool allowing individuals to assess their own patterns to determine if they should seek professional help (www .nationaleatingdisorders.org/online-eating-disorder-screening). They also have additional information and a helpline (1-800-931-2237) for guidance, treatment referrals, and support.[34]

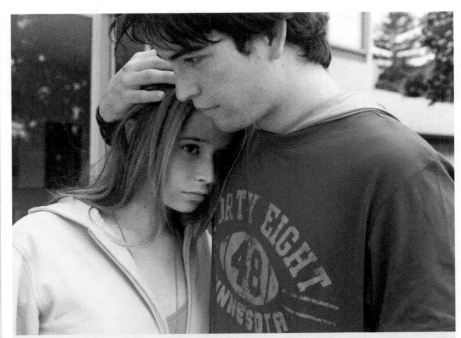

When talking to a friend about an eating disorder or disordered eating patterns, avoid casting blame, preaching, or offering unsolicited advice. Instead, be a good listener, let the person know that you care, and offer your support.

List the criteria, symptoms, and treatment for exercise disorders such as muscle dysmorphia and female athlete triad.

Although exercise is generally beneficial, in excess it can be a problem. In addition to being a common compensatory behavior used by people with anorexia or bulimia, exercise can become a compulsion or contribute to more complex disorders such as muscle dysmorphia or the female athlete triad.

Compulsive Exercise

In a recent study, researchers showed that participants used excessive exercise or **compulsive exercise** as a way to regulate their emotions.[35] Also called *anorexia athletica,* compulsive exercise is characterized not by a *desire* to exercise but a *compulsion*; that is, the person struggles with guilt and anxiety if he or she doesn't work out. Compulsive exercisers, like people with eating disorders, often define their self-worth externally. They overexercise in order to feel more in control of their lives. Disordered eating or an eating disorder is often part of the picture.

Compulsive exercise can contribute to a variety of injuries. It can also put significant stress on the heart, especially if combined with disordered eating. Psychologically, people who engage in compulsive exercise are often plagued by anxiety and/or depression. Their social life and academic success can suffer as they fixate more and more on exercise.

Muscle Dysmorphia

Muscle dysmorphia is a form of body image disturbance and exercise disorder in which a person (usually male) believes his body is insufficiently lean or muscular.[36] Men who have muscle dysmorphia believe, despite looking normal or even unusually brawny, that they look "puny." Because of their adherence to a meticulous diet and time-consuming workout schedule, and their shame over their perceived appearance flaws, important social or occupational activities may fall by the wayside. Other behaviors characteristic of muscle dysmorphia include comparing oneself unfavorably to others, checking one's appearance in the mirror, and camouflaging one's appearance. Men with muscle dysmorphia also are likely to abuse anabolic steroids and dietary supplements.[37]

The Female Athlete Triad

In an effort to be the best, some women may put themselves at risk for developing a syndrome called the **female athlete triad.** *Triad* means "three," and the three interrelated problems are low energy (food) intake, typically prompted by disordered eating behaviors; menstrual dysfunction such as amenorrhea; and poor bone density (FIGURE 5).[38]

How does the female athlete triad develop, and what makes it so dangerous? First, a chronic pattern of low energy intake and intensive exercise alters normal body functions. For example, when an athlete restricts her

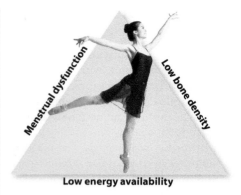

FIGURE 5 The Female Athlete Triad

eating, she can deplete her body stores of nutrients essential to health. At the same time, her body begins to burn its stores of fat tissue for energy. Adequate body fat is essential to maintaining healthy levels of the female reproductive hormone *estrogen*; when an athlete isn't getting enough food, estrogen levels decline. This can manifest as amenorrhea: The body is using all calories to keep the athlete alive, and nonessential body functions such as menstruation cease. In addition, fat-soluble vitamins, calcium, and estrogen are all essential for dense, healthy bones, so their depletion weakens the athlete's bones, leaving her at high risk for fracture.

The female athlete triad is particularly prevalent in women who participate in highly competitive individual sports or activities that emphasize leanness and require body-contouring clothing. Gymnasts, figure skaters, cross-country runners, and ballet dancers are among those at highest risk for the female athlete triad.

SEE IT! VIDEOS

Can you go too far with extreme exercise? Watch **Young Boys Exercising to Extremes,** available on MasteringHealth™

---

compulsive exercise Disorder characterized by a compulsion to engage in excessive amounts of exercise and feelings of guilt and anxiety if the level of exercise is perceived as inadequate.

muscle dysmorphia Body image disorder in which men believe that their bodies are insufficiently lean or muscular.

female athlete triad A syndrome of three interrelated health problems seen in some female athletes: disordered eating, amenorrhea, and poor bone density.

ASSESS | YOURSELF

Are Your Efforts to Be Thin Sensible—Or Are You Spinning Out of Control?

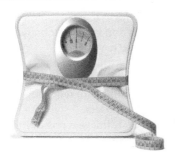

Just because you weigh yourself, count calories, or work out every day doesn't necessarily mean you have any of the health concerns discussed in this chapter. On the other hand, efforts to lose a few pounds can spiral out of control. To assess whether your efforts to be thin are harmful to you, take the following quiz from the National Eating Disorders Association (NEDA).

			T	F
1.	I constantly calculate numbers of fat grams and calories.		T	F
2.	I weigh myself often and find myself obsessed with the number on the scale.		T	F
3.	I exercise to burn calories and not for health or enjoyment.		T	F
4.	I sometimes feel out of control while eating.		T	F
5.	I often go on extreme diets.		T	F
6.	I engage in rituals to get me through mealtimes and/or secretively binge.		T	F
7.	Weight loss, dieting, and controlling my food intake have become my major concerns.		T	F
8.	I feel ashamed, disgusted, or guilty after eating.		T	F
9.	I constantly worry about the weight, shape, and/or size of my body.		T	F
10.	I feel my identity and value are based on how I look or how much I weigh.		T	F

If any of these statements is true for you, you could be dealing with disordered eating. If so, talk about it! Tell a friend, parent, teacher, coach, youth group leader, doctor, counselor, or nutritionist what you're going through. Check out the NEDA's Sharing with EEEase handout at www.nationaleatingdisorders .org/sharing-eeease for help planning what to say the first time you talk to someone about your eating and exercise habits.

Source: Adapted from "NEDA Screening for Eating Disorders" by the National Eating Disorders Association (NEDA) and Screening for Mental Health, Inc. (SMH), from NEDA website. Copyright © 2013 NEDA and SMH. Reprinted with permission.

YOUR PLAN FOR **CHANGE**

The **ASSESS YOURSELF** activity gives you a chance to evaluate your feelings about your body. Below are some steps you can take to improve your body image.

TODAY, YOU CAN:

☐ Talk back to the media. Write letters to advertisers and magazines that depict unhealthy and unrealistic body types. Boycott their products or start a blog commenting on harmful body image messages in the media.

☐ Just for today, eat the recommended number of servings from every food group at every meal. And don't count calories!

WITHIN THE NEXT TWO WEEKS, YOU CAN:

☐ Find a photograph of a person you admire for his or her contributions to humanity. Put it up next to your mirror to remind yourself that true beauty comes from within and benefits others.

☐ Start a journal. Each day, record one thing you are grateful for that has nothing to do with your appearance. At the end of each day, record one small thing you did to make someone's world a little brighter.

BY THE END OF THE SEMESTER, YOU CAN:

☐ Establish a group of friends who support you for who you are, not what you look like and who get the same support from you. Form a group on a favorite social-networking site, and keep in touch, especially when you feel troubled by self-defeating thoughts or have the urge to engage in unhealthy behaviors.

☐ Borrow from the library or purchase one of the many books on body image now available, and read it!

Customize your study plan—and master your health!—in the Study Area of MasteringHealth™

CHAPTER **REVIEW**

To head an MP3 Tutor Session, scan here or visit the Study Area in **MasteringHealth**.

LO **1** | **What Is Body Image?**

- Body image refers to what you believe or emotionally feel about your body's shape, weight, and general appearance.

LO **2** | **Disordered Eating and Eating Disorders**

- Millions of Americans will struggle with an eating disorder at some point in their lives. Media, family, community, cultural groups, and psychological and physiological factors all influence body image.
- Anorexia nervosa is a persistent, chronic eating disorder characterized by deliberate food restriction and severe, life-threatening weight loss.
- Individuals with bulimia nervosa rapidly consume large amounts of food and purge either with vomiting or laxative abuse or by using non-purging techniques such as excessive exercise and/or fasting.
- Individuals with binge-eating disorder gorge themselves but do not take excessive measures to lose weight.
- Orthorexia nervosa is an unhealthy obsession with a rigid diet focused on food quality and purity.
- Eating disorders are caused by a combination of many factors, and there are no simple solutions. Without treatment, approximately 20 percent of people with a serious eating disorder will die from it. Long-term treatment focuses on the psychological, social, environmental, and physiological factors that have led to the problem.

LO **3** | **Exercise Disorders**

- Compulsive exercise is used as a way to regulate emotions. Also called *anorexia athletica,* compulsive exercise is characterized by a compulsion to exercise, resulting in guilt and anxiety if the person doesn't work out.
- Muscle dysmorphia, typically found in men, is characterized by a distorted belief that their body is insufficiently muscular or lean. As a result, they spend an inordinate amount of time working out.
- The female triad syndrome occurs when female athletes restrict their food intake and train intensively, altering their normal body functions. Three interrelated problems occur: low energy intake; menstrual dysfunction, and poor bone density.
- Treatment requires a multidisciplinary approach involving the coach, psychologist, and family members.

POP **QUIZ**

Visit **MasteringHealth** to personalize your study plan with Chapter Review Quizzes and Dynamic Study Modules.

LO **1** | **What Is Body Image?**

1. All of the statements about body image are true *except* which?
   a. The obsession with having big biceps or being able to wear size zero skinny jeans began in the late 1990s.
   b. Concerns about weight seems to be central to many people's dissatisfaction with their body.
   c. People who have been diagnosed with a body image disorder show differences in the brain's ability to regulate neurotransmitters.
   d. Positive body image is possessing a true perception of your appearance.

LO **2** | **Disordered Eating and Eating Disorders**

2. Orthorexia nervosa is
   a. an excessive focus on eating foods high in calcium and vitamin D.
   b. characterized by a fixation on the quality and purity of food.
   c. an obsession with bone health.
   d. a condition that results from binging and purging.

LO **3** | **Exercise Disorders**

3. Muscle dysmorphia
   a. is a muscular disease that results from an autoimmune disorder.
   b. occurs only in women.
   c. results in menstrual dysfunction.
   d. occurs most often in men.

Answers to the Pop Quiz questions can be found on page A-1. If you answered a question incorrectly, review the section identified by the Learning Outcome. For even more study tools, visit MasteringHealth.

11 Improving Your Personal Fitness

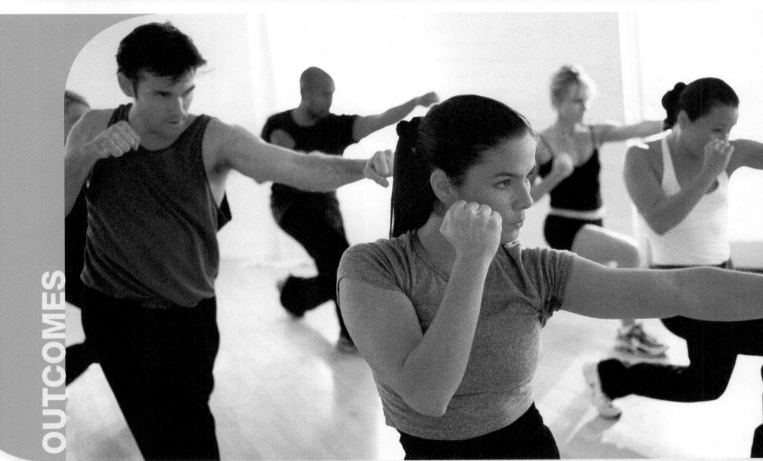

LEARNING OUTCOMES

1 Describe the health benefits of being physically active.

2 Distinguish between the physical activity required for health, physical fitness, and performance.

3 Identify lifestyle obstacles to physical activity, describe ways to surmount them, and make a commitment to getting physically fit.

4 Understand and be able to use the FITT (frequency, intensity, time, and type) principles for the health-related components of physical fitness.

5 Devise a plan to implement your safe and effective fitness program.

6 Describe optimal foods and fluids consumption recommendations for exercise and recovery.

7 Explain how to prevent and treat common exercise injuries.

Most Americans are aware of the wide range of physical, social, and mental health benefits of physical activity and know that they should be more physically active. The physiological changes in the body that result from regular physical activity reduce the likelihood of coronary artery disease, high blood pressure, type 2 diabetes, obesity, and other chronic diseases. Furthermore, engaging in physical activity regularly helps to control stress, increases self-esteem, and contributes to that "feel-good" feeling.

physical activity Refers to all body movements produced by skeletal muscles, resulting in substantial increases in energy expenditure.

exercise Planned, structured, and repetitive bodily movement done to improve or maintain one or more components of physical fitness.

Despite knowledge of the importance of physical activity for health and wellness, most people are not sufficiently active to obtain these optimal health benefits. Recent statistics indicate that 50.2 percent of American adults met the 2008 guidelines for aerobic exercise, and 29.6 percent met the guidelines for strengthening exercise.[1] However, only 20.2 percent reported meeting the guidelines for both aerobic and strengthening exercise, and 26.3 percent reported no leisure activities.[2] These statistics are based on activity reported during one's "down" time in the previous month.[3] The growing percentage of Americans who live physically inactive lives has been linked to the current high incidences of obesity, type 2 diabetes, and other chronic and mental health diseases.[4]

In general, college students are more physically active than older adults, but a recent survey indicated that 51.0 percent of college women and 47.0 percent of college men do not meet recommended guidelines for engaging in moderate or vigorous physical activities.[5]

LO 1 | PHYSICAL ACTIVITY FOR HEALTH

Describe the health benefits of being physically active.

Physical activity refers to all body movements produced by skeletal muscles that result in substantial increases in energy expenditure. Physical activities can vary by intensity: light, moderate, or vigorous. For example, walking on a flat surface at a casual pace requires little effort (light), whereas

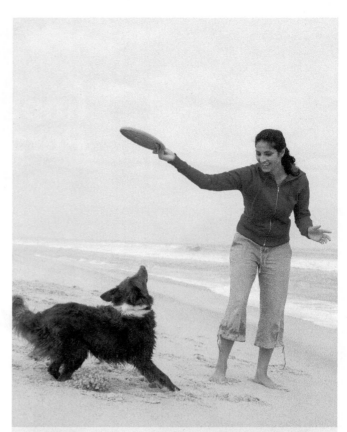

Activities such as walking and playing with your dog count toward your recommended daily physical activity.

walking uphill is more intense and harder to do (moderate). Jogging and running are examples of vigorous intensity physical activities. There are three general categories of physical activity defined by the purpose for which they are done: leisure-time physical activity, occupational physical activity, and lifestyle physical activity.

Exercise is defined as planned, repetitive, and structured bodily movement undertaken to maintain or better any number of physical fitness components—for example, cardiorespiratory fitness, muscular strength or endurance, or flexibility. Although all exercise is physical activity, not all physical activity would be considered exercise. For example, walking from your car to class is physical activity, whereas going for a brisk 30-minute walk to maintain a healthy body weight is considered exercise.

150 MINUTES

OF MODERATE PHYSICAL ACTIVITY A WEEK—ALONG WITH STRENGTH EXERCISES TWO DAYS A WEEK—PROVIDES SUBSTANTIAL **HEALTH BENEFITS**. MORE IS EVEN BETTER!

Adding more physical activity to your day, like walking or cycling to school, can benefit your health. In fact, it is estimated that if the number of adults meeting the 2008 Physical Activity Guidelines (see TABLE 11.1) increased by 25 percent, there would be 1.3 million fewer deaths per year and the life expectancy would increase. In the United Stated, it is estimated that physical inactivity is responsible for 6.7 percent of the cases of coronary heart disease, 8.3 percent cases of type 2 diabetes, 12.4 percent cases of breast cancer, and 12.0 percent cases of colon cancer. Furthermore, physical inactivity accounts for approximately 10.8 percent of deaths in the United States.[6]

Regular participation in physical activity improves more than 50 different physiological, metabolic, and psychological aspects of human life. FIGURE 11.1 summarizes some of these major health-related benefits.

Reduced Risk of Cardiovascular Diseases

Aerobic exercise is good for the heart and lungs and reduces the risk for heart-related diseases. It improves blood flow and eases

WHY SHOULD I CARE?

Being physically active reduces your risk for many chronic diseases. That may not seem like an immediate concern, but there are a lot more immediate benefits: Becoming physically fit can help improve your physical appearance and sense of self-esteem, boost your resistance to diseases like colds and flus, reduce your stress level, improve your sleep, and help you concentrate. All that, and it's fun, too!

the performance of everyday tasks. Regular exercise makes the cardiovascular and respiratory systems more efficient by strengthening the heart muscle, enabling more blood to be pumped with each stroke, and increasing the number of *capillaries* (small blood vessels that allow gas exchange between blood and surrounding tissues) in trained skeletal muscles, which supply more blood to working muscles. Exercise also improves the respiratory system by increasing the amount of oxygen that is inhaled with each breath and distributed to body tissues.[7]

Regular physical activity can reduce hypertension, or chronic high blood pressure, a cardiovascular disease itself, and a significant risk factor for other coronary heart diseases and stroke (see Chapter 12).[8] Regular aerobic exercise also improves the blood lipid profile. It typically increases high-density lipoproteins (HDLs, or "good" cholesterol), which are associated with lower risk for coronary artery disease because of their role in removing plaque built up in the arteries.[9] Triglycerides (a blood fat) typically decrease with aerobic exercise. Low-density lipoproteins (LDLs, or "bad" cholesterol) and total cholesterol are often improved with exercise due to weight loss and the improvements in HDL and triglycerides.

TABLE 11.1 | 2008 Physical Activity Guidelines for Americans

	Key Guidelines for Health*	For Additional Fitness or Weight Loss Benefits*	Additional Exercises
Adults	150 min/week moderate-intensity physical activity OR 75 min/week of vigorous-intensity physical activity OR Equivalent combination of moderate- and vigorous-intensity physical activity (e.g., 100 min moderate intensity + 25 min vigorous intensity)	300 min/week moderate-intensity physical activity OR 150 min/week of vigorous-intensity physical activity OR Equivalent combination of moderate- and vigorous-intensity physical activity (e.g., 200 min moderate intensity + 50 min vigorous intensity) OR More than the previously described amounts	Muscle-strengthening activities for all the major muscle groups at least 2 days/week
Older Adults	If unable to follow above guidelines, then as much physical activity as their condition allows	If unable to follow above guidelines, then as much physical activity as their condition allows	In addition to muscle-strengthening activities, those with limited mobility should add exercises to improve balance and reduce risk of falling.
Children and Youth	60 min or more of moderate- or vigorous-intensity physical activity daily; should include at least 3 days/week or vigorous activity	At least 60 min of moderate- or vigorous-intensity physical activity on every day of the week	Include muscle-strengthening activities at least 3 days/week. Include bone-strengthening activities at least 3 days/week.

*Avoid inactivity (some activity is better than none), accumulate physical activity in sessions of 10 minutes or more at one time, and spread activity throughout the week.
Source: Office of Disease Prevention and Health Promotion, U.S. Department of Health and Human Services, *2008 Physical Activity Guidelines for Americans: Be Active, Healthy, and Happy!* (Washington, DC: U.S. Department of Health and Human Services, 2008), ODPHP Publication no. U0036, www.health.gov

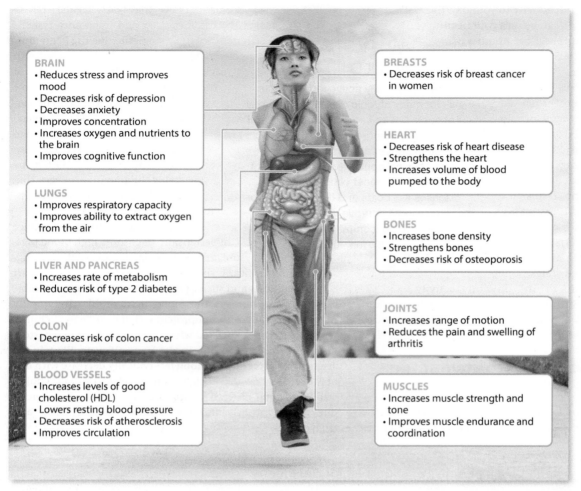

FIGURE 11.1 Some Health Benefits of Regular Exercise

→ VIDEO TUTOR
Health Benefits of Regular Exercise

Reduced Risk of Metabolic Syndrome and Type 2 Diabetes

Regular physical activity reduces the risk of metabolic syndrome, a combination of heart disease and diabetes risk factors that produces a synergistic increase in risk.[10] Specifically, metabolic syndrome includes high blood pressure, abdominal obesity, low levels of HDLs, high levels of triglycerides, and impaired glucose tolerance.[11] Regular participation in moderate-intensity physical activities reduces risk for each factor individually and collectively.[12]

Research indicates that a healthy dietary intake combined with sufficient physical activity could prevent many of the current cases of type 2 diabetes.[13] In a major national clinical trial, researchers found that exercising 150 minutes per week and eating fewer calories and less fat could prevent or delay the onset of type 2 diabetes.[14] (For more on diabetes prevention and management, see **Focus On: Minimizing Your Risk for Diabetes** on page 386.)

Reduced Cancer Risk

After decades of research, most cancer epidemiologists believe that 25 percent to 37 percent of cancers can be avoided by healthier lifestyle and environmental choices.[15] In fact, a report released by the World Cancer Research Fund, in conjunction with the American Institute for Cancer Research, stated that one third of cancers could be prevented by being physically active and eating well.[16] Regular physical activity appears to lower the risk for some specific cancers, particularly colon, rectal, and breast cancer.[17] Research on exercise and breast cancer survivors has shown that physical activity helps patients more effectively deal with treatment for the disease and improves survival rates.[18]

Improved Bone Mass and Reduced Risk of Osteoporosis

A common affliction for older people is *osteoporosis,* a disease characterized by low bone mass and deterioration of bone tissue, which increases fracture risk. Regular weight-bearing and strength-building physical activities are recommended to maintain bone health and prevent osteoporotic fractures. Although men and women are both negatively affected by osteoporosis, it is more common in women. Bone mass levels are significantly higher among active individuals than among sedentary persons.[19] However, it appears that the full bone-related benefits of physical activity can only be achieved with sufficient hormone levels (estrogen in women, testosterone in men) and adequate calcium, vitamin D, and total caloric intakes.[20]

Improved Weight Management

For many people, the desire to lose weight or maintain a healthy weight is the main reason for physical activity. On the most basic level, physical activity requires your body to generate energy through calorie expenditure; if calories expended exceed calories consumed over a span of time, the net result will be weight loss. Some activities are more intense or vigorous than others and result in more calories used. FIGURE 11.2 shows the caloric cost of various activities when done for 30 minutes.

In addition to the calories expended during activity, physical activity has a direct positive effect on metabolic rate, keeping it elevated for several hours following vigorous physical activities. This increase in metabolic rate can lead to body composition changes that favor weight management. After weight loss, increased physical activity also improves your chances of maintaining

If you want to lose weight, you need to move more and often!

the weight loss. If you are currently at a healthy body weight, regular physical activity can prevent significant weight gain.[21]

Improved Immunity

Research shows that regular moderate-intensity physical activity reduces individual susceptibility to disease.[22] Just how regular physical activity positively influences immunity is not well understood. We know that moderate-intensity physical activity temporarily increases the number of white blood cells, which are responsible for fighting infection.[23] Often, the relationship of physical activity to immunity, or more specifically to disease susceptibility, is described as a J-shaped curve. Susceptibility to disease decreases with moderate activity, but then increases as you move to extreme levels of physical activity or exercise or if you continue to exercise without adequate recovery time and/or dietary intake.[24] Athletes engaging in marathon-type events or very intense physical training programs have been shown to be at greater risk for upper respiratory tract infections in the first 8 hours after an intense exercise session.[25]

Improved Mental Health and Stress Management

Most people who engage in regular physical activity are likely to notice the psychological benefits, such as feeling better about oneself and an overall sense of well-being. Although these mental health benefits are difficult to quantify, they are frequently mentioned as reasons for continuing to be physically active. Learning new skills, developing increased ability and capacity in recreational activities, and sticking with a physical activity plan also improve self-esteem. In addition, regular physical activity can improve a person's physical appearance, further increasing self-esteem.

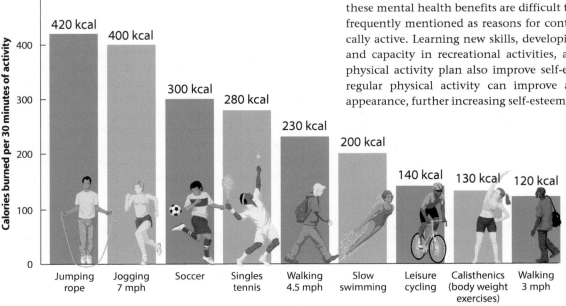

FIGURE 11.2 **Calories Burned by Different Activities** The harder your physical activity, the more energy you expend. Estimated calories burned for various moderate and vigorous activities are listed for 30 minutes of activity. Note that the number of calories burned depends on body weight (generally, the higher your body weight, the greater the number of calories you'll burn).

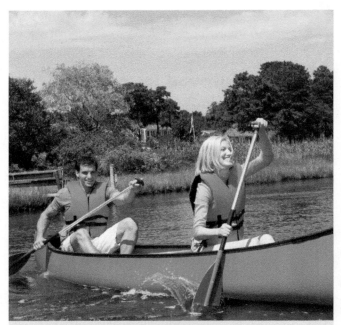

Although physical activity actually stimulates the stress response, a physically fit body adapts efficiently to the eustress of it, and as a result is better able to tolerate and effectively manage stress of all kinds.

particularly among those who have several risk factors and who use physical activity as a means of risk reduction.[31] Results from a study of nearly a million subjects showed that the largest benefits from physical activity occur in sedentary individuals who add a little physical activity to their lives, with additional benefits as physical activity levels increase.[32] Additionally, data from a national sample show that a sedentary lifestyle as associated with a reduced ability to perform activities of daily living.[33] The more sedentary time adults report, the greater reduction in the ability to perform activities of daily living. It is not just structured exercise that is important, but moving as much as possible and sitting as little as possible.

LO 2 | PHYSICAL ACTIVITY FOR FITNESS AND PERFORMANCE

Distinguish between the physical activity required for health, physical fitness, and performance.

Physical fitness refers to a set of attributes that are either health or skill related.

Health-Related Components of Physical Fitness

The health-related attributes—cardiorespiratory fitness, muscular strength and endurance, flexibility, and body composition—allow you to perform moderate- to vigorous-intensity physical activities on a regular basis without getting too tired and with energy left over to handle physical or mental emergencies. FIGURE 11.3 identifies the major health-related components of physical fitness.

Cardiorespiratory Fitness Cardiorespiratory fitness is the ability of the heart, lungs, and blood vessels to supply the body with oxygen efficiently. The primary category of physical activity known to improve cardiorespiratory fitness is aerobic exercise. The word *aerobic* means "with oxygen" and describes any type of exercise that requires oxygen to make energy for prolonged activity. Aerobic activities, such as swimming, cycling, and jogging, are among the best exercises for improving or maintaining cardiorespiratory fitness.

Cardiorespiratory fitness is measured by determining aerobic capacity (power), the volume of oxygen the muscles consume during exercise. Maximal aerobic power (commonly written as VO_{2max}) is defined as the volume of oxygen that the muscles consume per minute during maximal exercise. The

physical fitness A balance of health-related attributes that allows you to perform moderate to vigorous physical activities on a regular basis and complete daily physical tasks without undue fatigue.

cardiorespiratory fitness The ability of the heart, lungs, and blood vessels to supply oxygen to skeletal muscles during sustained physical activity.

aerobic exercise Prolonged exercise that requires oxygen to make energy for activity.

aerobic capacity (power) The functional status of the cardiorespiratory system; refers specifically to the volume of oxygen the muscles consume during exercise.

Regular aerobic physical activity can provide a break from stressors. It can improve the way the body handles stress by its effect on neurotransmitters associated with mood enhancement. Physical activity might also help the body recover from the stress response more quickly as fitness increases.[26]

There is increasing evidence that regular physical activity improves cognitive function across the lifespan. Research has associated regular activity with academic and standardized test performance in school.[27] Recent research indicates that the relationship between physical activity and executive cognitive function is reciprocal.[28] Those with poor executive function experienced greater reductions in physical activity over time compared to those with higher function. Promoting physical activity as we age is important to prevent the decline in cognitive function, which in turn can help maintain regular activity.[29] Regular aerobic activity has also been associated with the prevention and improvement of dementia and Alzheimer's disease in adults.[30]

Longer Life Span

Experts have long debated the relationship between physical activity and longevity. Several studies indicate significant decreases in long-term health risk and increases in years lived,

ONLY 20.2%

OF AMERICAN ADULTS MEET GUIDELINES FOR BOTH CARDIORESPIRATORY AND MUSCULAR FITNESS.

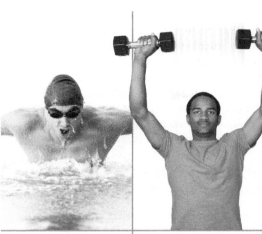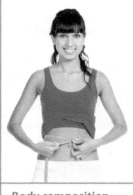

Cardiorespiratory fitness	Muscular strength	Muscular endurance	Flexibility	Body composition
Ability to sustain aerobic whole-body activity for a prolonged period of time	Maximum force able to be exerted by single contraction of a muscle or muscle group	Ability to perform muscle contractions repeatedly without fatiguing	Ability to move joints freely through their full range of motion	The relative proportions of fat mass and fat-free mass in the body

FIGURE 11.3 Health-Related Components of Physical Fitness

most common measure of maximal aerobic capacity is a walk or run test on a treadmill. For greatest accuracy, this is done in a lab with specialized equipment and technicians to measure the precise amount of oxygen entering and exiting the body during the exercise session. To get a more general sense of cardiorespiratory fitness, submaximal tests performed in the classroom or field can predict maximal aerobic capacity.

Muscular Strength **Muscular strength** refers to the amount of force a muscle or group of muscles can generate in one contraction. The most common way to assess the strength of a particular muscle or muscle group is to measure the maximum amount of weight you can move one time (and no more) or your one repetition maximum (1 RM).

Muscular Endurance **Muscular endurance** is the ability of a muscle or group of muscles to exert force repeatedly without fatigue or the ability to sustain a muscular contraction. The more repetitions you can perform successfully (e.g., push-ups) or the longer you can hold a certain position (e.g., flexed arm hang), the greater your muscular endurance.

Flexibility **Flexibility** refers to the range of motion, or the amount of movement possible, at a particular joint or series of joints: the greater the range of motion, the greater the flexibility. Various tests measure the flexibility of the body's joints, including range-of-motion tests for specific joints.

Body Composition **Body composition** is the fifth and final health-related component of physical fitness. Body composition describes the relative proportions and distribution of fat and fat-free (muscle, bone, water, organs) tissues in the body. (For more details on body composition, including its measurement, see Chapter 10.)

Skill-Related Components of Physical Fitness

In addition to the five health-related components of physical fitness, physical fitness for athletes involves attributes that improve their ability to perform athletic tasks. These attributes, called the *skill-related components* of physical fitness, also help recreational athletes and general exercisers increase fitness levels and their ability to perform daily tasks. The skill-related components of physical fitness (also

muscular strength The amount of force that a muscle is capable of exerting in one contraction.

muscular endurance A muscle's ability to exert force repeatedly without fatiguing or the ability to sustain a muscular contraction for a length of time.

flexibility The range of motion, or the amount of movement possible, at a particular joint or series of joints.

body composition The relative proportions of fat and fat-free (muscle, bone, water, organs) tissues in the body.

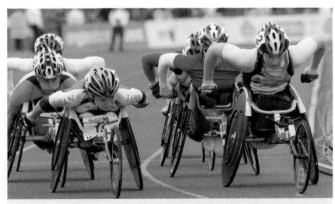

It is important for all people, including those with disabilities, to develop optimal levels of physical fitness and participate in physical activities they enjoy—including competitive sports.

called sport skills) are *agility, balance, coordination, power, speed,* and *reaction time.* Note that some of the skill-related fitness components can impact health. For example, consider the importance of balance and coordination for older adults who are at increased risk for falls.

LO 3 | COMMITTING
TO PHYSICAL FITNESS

Identify lifestyle obstacles to physical activity, describe ways to surmount them, and make a commitment to getting physically fit.

To succeed at incorporating physical fitness into your life, you need to design a fitness program that takes obstacles into account and that is founded on the activities you enjoy most.

What If I Have Been Inactive for a While?

If you have been physically inactive for the past few months or longer, first make sure that your physician clears you for exercise. Consider consulting a personal trainer or fitness instructor to help you get started. In this phase of a fitness program, known as *the initial conditioning stage,* you may begin at levels lower than those recommended for physical fitness. For example, you might start your cardiorespiratory program by simply getting moving each day. Take the stairs instead of the elevator, walk farther from your car to the store, and plan for organized movement each day, such as a 10- to 15-minute walk. In addition, you can start your muscle fitness program with simple body weight exercises, emphasizing proper technique and body alignment before adding any resistance.

Overcoming Common Obstacles to Physical Activity

People have real and perceived barriers that prevent regular physical activity, ranging from personal ("I do not have time") to environmental ("I do not have a safe place to be active"). Some people may be reluctant to exercise if they are overweight, feel embarrassed to work out with their more "fit" friends, or feel they lack the knowledge and skills required.

Think about your obstacles to physical activity and write them down. Consider anything that gets in your way of exercising, however minor. Once you honestly evaluate why you are not as physically active as you want to be, review TABLE 11.2 for suggestions on overcoming your hurdles.

TABLE 11.2 | Overcoming Obstacles to Physical Activity

Obstacle	Possible Solution
Lack of time	■ Look at your schedule. Where can you find 30-minute time slots? Perhaps you need to focus on shorter times (10 minutes or more) throughout the day.
	■ Multitask. Read while riding an exercise bike or listen to lectures or podcasts while walking.
	■ Be physically active during your lunch and study breaks as well as between classes. Skip rope or throw a Frisbee with a friend.
	■ Select activities that require less time, such as brisk walking or jogging.
	■ Ride your bike to class, or park (or get off the bus) farther from your destination.
Social influence	■ Invite family and friends to be active with you.
	■ Join an exercise class to meet new people.
	■ Explain the importance of exercise and your commitment to physical activity to people who may not support your efforts.
	■ Find a role model to support your efforts.
	■ Plan for physically active dates—go for a walk, dancing, or bowling.
Lack of motivation, willpower, or energy	■ Schedule your workout time just as you would any other important commitment.
	■ Enlist the help of an exercise partner to make you accountable for working out.
	■ Give yourself an incentive.
	■ Schedule your workouts when you feel most energetic.
	■ Remind yourself that exercise gives you more energy.
	■ Get things ready; for example, if you choose to walk in the morning, set out your clothes and shoes the night before.
Lack of resources	■ Select an activity that requires minimal equipment, such as walking, jogging, jumping rope, or calisthenics.
	■ Identify inexpensive resources on campus or in the community.
	■ Use active forms of transportation.
	■ Take advantage of no-cost opportunities, such as playing catch in the park or green space on campus.

Source: Adapted from National Center for Chronic Disease Prevention and Health Promotion, "How Can I Overcome Barriers to Physical Activity?," Updated May 2011, www.cdc.gov

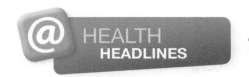
TRANSPORT YOURSELF!

Before we became a car culture, much of our transportation was human powered. Historically, bicycling and walking were important means of transportation and recreation in the United States. Since World War II, however, the development of automobile-oriented communities has led to a steady decline of bicycling and walking. Currently, less than 12 percent of trips are made by foot or bike, but the number varies according to region of the country and size of the city.

Many people are now embracing a movement toward more active transportation. *Active transportation* means using your own power to get from place to place—whether walking, riding a bike, skateboarding, or roller skating. You can cycle to work or to do errands even if you do not own a bike. Check to see whether your city has a bike share program at http://bikeshare.com. Here are just a few of the many reasons to make active transportation a bigger part of your life:

- **You will be adding more exercise into your daily routine.** People who use active forms of transportation to complete errands are more likely to meet physical activity guidelines.
- **Walking or biking can save you money.** It is significantly less expensive to own a bike than a car when

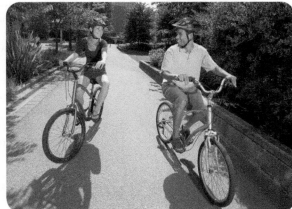

Hop on that bike and join the green revolution! Active transportation is an excellent want to add physical activity to your day, especially on nonexercise days.

you consider gas and maintenance. It is estimated that it is costs 30 times more to maintain a care than a bike! Additionally, those who cycle to work are eligible for up to $20 per month in a tax-free reimbursement!

- **Walking or biking may save you time!** Short commutes of three to five files are usually as fast or faster via bicycle rather than via car.
- **You will enjoy being outdoors.** Research is emerging on the physical and mental health benefits of nature and being outdoors. So much of what we do is inside, with recirculated air and artificial lighting, that our bodies are deficient in fresh air and sunlight.

- **You will make a significant contribution to reducing air pollution.** Choosing to walk or bike instead of driving only 2 days a week can reduce greenhouse gas emissions by an average of 4,000 pounds a year.
- **You will help reduce traffic.** More active commuters means fewer cars on the roads and less traffic congestion.
- **You will contribute to global environmental health.** Reducing vehicle trips will help reduce overall greenhouse gas emissions and the need to source more fossil fuel. Swapping waking or cycling for the car when taking short trips is estimated to save over 10 billion gallons of fuel per year.

Sources: Rails-to-Trails Conservancy, "Investing in Trails: Cost-Effective Improvements—for Everyone," 2013, www.railstotrails.org /resourcehandler.ashx?id=3629; M. Woodruff, "13 Reasons You Should Start Biking to Work," *Business Insider,* October 2012, www .businessinsider.com/13-reasons-you-should -bike-to-work-2012-10#ixzz3fFS2Ovre; U.S. Environmental Protection Agency, "Climate Change: What You Can Do: On the Road," Updated April 2014, www.epa.gov/climatechange /wycd/road.html; B. McKenzie, "Modes Less Traveled—Bicycling and Walking to Work in the United States: 2008–2012," U.S. Department of Commerce, May 2014, www.census .gov/prod/2014pubs/acs-25.pdf

Incorporating Physical Activity in Your Life

When designing your fitness program, there are several factors to consider. First, choose activities that are appropriate for you, convenient, and that you genuinely enjoy. For example, choose jogging because you like to run and there are beautiful trails nearby versus swimming when you do not really like the water and the pool is difficult to get to. Likewise, choose activities that are suitable for your current fitness level. If you are overweight or have not exercised in months, start slowly, plan fun activities, and progress to more challenging physical activities as your physical fitness improves. You may choose to simply walk more in an attempt to achieve the recommended goal

of 10,000 steps per day; keep track with a pedometer. Try to make physical activity a part of your routine by incorporating it into something you already have to do—such as getting to class or work. See the Health Headlines box for more on using your transportation for fitness.

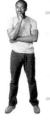

WHICH **PATH** WOULD YOU TAKE **?**

Scan the QR code to see how different physical fitness choices YOU make today can affect your overall health tomorrow.

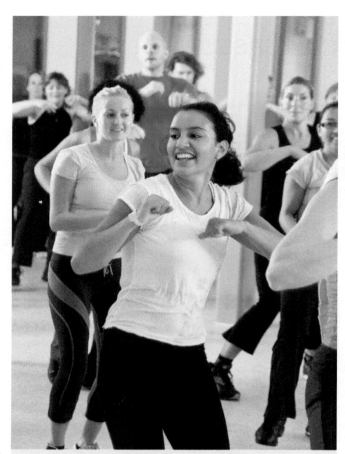

One great way to motivate yourself is to sign up for an exercise class. The structure, schedule, social interaction, and challenge of learning a new skill can be the motivation you need to get moving!

LO 4 | CREATING YOUR OWN FITNESS PROGRAM

Understand and be able to use the FITT (frequency, intensity, time, and type) principles for the health-related components of physical fitness.

FITT Acronym for frequency, intensity, time, and type; the terms that describe the essential components of a program or plan to improve a health-related component of physical fitness.

frequency As part of the FITT prescription, refers to how many days per week a person should exercise.

intensity As part of the FITT prescription, refers to how hard or how much effort is needed when a person exercises.

time As part of the FITT prescription, refers to the duration of an exercise session.

type As part of the FITT prescription, refers to what kind of exercises a person needs to do.

The first step in creating a personal physical fitness program is identifying your goals. Do you want to be better at sports or feel better about your body? Is your goal to manage stress or reduce your risk of chronic diseases? Perhaps your most vital goal will be to establish a realistic schedule of diverse physical activities that you can maintain and enjoy throughout your life. Your physical fitness goals and objectives should be both achievable for you and in line with what you truly want.

Set SMART Goals

To set successful goals, try using the *SMART* system. SMART goals are **s**pecific, **m**easurable, **a**ction-oriented, **r**ealistic, and **t**ime-oriented.

A vague goal would be "Improve fitness by exercising more." A SMART goal would be as follows:

- *Specific*—"I'll participate in a resistance-training program that targets all of the major muscle groups 3–5 days per week."
- *Measurable*—"I'll improve my fitness classification from average to good."
- *Action-oriented*—"I'll meet with a personal trainer to learn how to safely do resistance exercises and to plan a workout for the gym and home."
- *Realistic*—"I'll increase the weight I can lift by 20 percent."
- *Time-oriented*—"I'll try my new weight program for 8 weeks, then reassess."

Use the FITT Principle

To improve your health-related physical fitness (or performance-related physical fitness), use the **FITT** (Frequency, Intensity, Time, and Type)[34] principle to define your exercise program. The FITT prescription (**FIGURE 11.4**) uses the following criteria:

- **Frequency** refers to the number of times per week you need to engage in particular exercises to achieve the desired level of physical fitness in a particular component.
- **Intensity** refers to how hard your workout must be to achieve the desired level of physical fitness.
- **Time**, or the *duration,* refers to how many minutes or repetitions of an exercise are required at a specified intensity during any one session to attain the desired level of physical fitness for each component.
- **Type** refers to what kind of exercises should be performed to improve the specific component of physical fitness.

The FITT Principle for Cardiorespiratory Fitness

The most effective aerobic exercises for building cardiorespiratory fitness are total body activities involving the large muscle groups of your body. The FITT prescription for cardiorespiratory fitness includes 3 to 5 days per week of vigorous, rhythmic, continuous activity at 64 to 96 percent of your estimated maximal heart rate for 20 to 60 minutes.[35]

Frequency The frequency of your program is related to your intensity. If you choose to do moderate-intensity exercises, you should aim for a frequency of at least 5 days (frequency drops to at least 3 days per week with vigorous-intensity activities). Newcomers to exercise can still improve by doing less-intense exercise (light to moderate level), but doing it more days during a week. In this case, follow the recommendations from the Centers for Disease Control and Prevention (CDC) for moderate physical activity (refer to Table 11.1 on page 331).

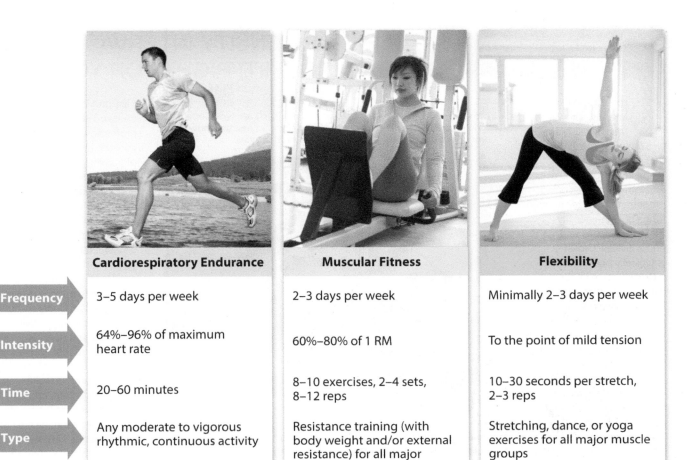

	Cardiorespiratory Endurance	**Muscular Fitness**	**Flexibility**
Frequency	3–5 days per week	2–3 days per week	Minimally 2–3 days per week
Intensity	64%–96% of maximum heart rate	60%–80% of 1 RM	To the point of mild tension
Time	20–60 minutes	8–10 exercises, 2–4 sets, 8–12 reps	10–30 seconds per stretch, 2–3 reps
Type	Any moderate to vigorous rhythmic, continuous activity	Resistance training (with body weight and/or external resistance) for all major muscle groups	Stretching, dance, or yoga exercises for all major muscle groups

FIGURE 11.4 The FITT Principle Applied to Cardiorespiratory Fitness, Muscular Strength and Endurance, and Flexibility

Intensity The most common methods used to determine the intensity of cardiorespiratory endurance exercises are target heart rate, rating of perceived exertion, and the talk test. The exercise intensity required to improve cardiorespiratory endurance is a heart rate between 64 and 96 percent of your maximum heart rate (moderate to vigorous intensity). Before calculating your **target heart rate**, you must first estimate your maximal heart rate with the formula [207 – 0.7(age)]. The example below is based on a 20-year-old. Substitute your age to determine your own maximal heart rate, then multiply by 0.64 and 0.94 to determine the lower and upper limits of your target range.

1. 207 – 0.7(20) = maximal heart rate for a 20-year old
2. 207 – 14 = 193 (maximal heart rate)
3. 193(0.64) = 123.52 (lower target limit)
4. 193.5(0.94) = 185.28 (upper target limit)
5. Target range = 124–186 beats per minute

To determine how close you are to your target heart rate, take your pulse. Lightly place your index and middle fingers (not your thumb) over the carotid artery in your neck or on the radial artery on the inside of your wrist (**FIGURE 11.5**). Count your pulse while exercising, if possible, or start counting your pulse immediately after you stop exercising, as your heart rate decreases rapidly when you stop. Using a watch or a clock, take your pulse for 10 seconds (the first pulse is "0" if you are starting a stopwatch, but 1 if you are using a watch that is already running) and multiply this number by 6 to get the number of beats per minute.

> **target heart rate** The heart rate range of aerobic exercise that leads to improved cardiorespiratory fitness (i.e., 64% to 96% of maximal heart rate).

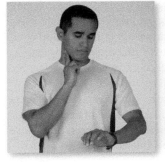

ⓐ Carotid pulse

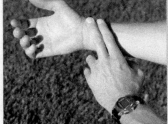

ⓑ Radial pulse

FIGURE 11.5 **Taking a Pulse** Palpation of the carotid (neck) or radial (wrist) artery is a simple way of determining heart rate.

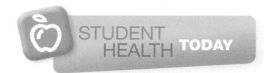
IS HIGH INTENSITY INTERVAL TRAINING (HIIT) RIGHT FOR YOU?

CrossFit and high-intensity interval training (HIIT) are two methods of training that are increasing in popularity. CrossFit is a strength and conditioning program that utilizes a broad range of high-intensity functional movements and activities. CrossFit is typically performed in a CrossFit gym or "Box" within a group or class. It is an intense specialized training program, so there are special requirements and certifications to become a CrossFit trainer or coach.

HIIT is a type of training that combines alternating high-intensity bouts and active rest bouts within your exercise session. For example, after the warm-up phase, you might do 2 minutes of a near-maximal-paced run, and then jog for 2 minutes to rest. This type of training can provide a very efficient workout. The volume of exercise is generally less than a continuous bout at a constant pace, but similar fitness gains can be seen with the lower volume of exercise as with the

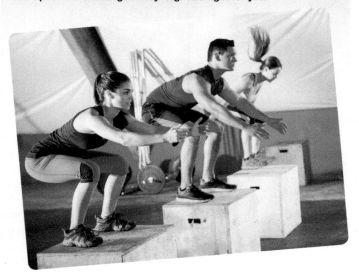

CrossFit and high-intensity interval training (HIIT) are two methods of training that are increasing in popularity. If you're healthy enough—and up for the challenge—they might be right for you.

tradition exercise bout. The intervals can be varied depending on your fitness level and goals.

How do you know whether either type of training is right for you? If you are a beginner, have risk factors for cardiovascular disease or musculoskeletal disorders, are obese, or have been sedentary, make sure you get clearance from your health

care provider. After getting checked out, find a fitness professional who can help you get started. Both types of training can be modified to accommodate varying levels of fitness.

If you like a challenge, a variety of exercises, and the motivation of the gym, CrossFit might be right for you. HIIT might be a good option if time is barrier or you are trying to improve your performance. Because both are high-intensity activities, it is important to allow your body time to rest and recover to reduce the risk of injury. Using different activities on consecutive days and not doing more than 3 consecutive days of exercise are recommendations for CrossFit. HIIT should be alternated with other activities throughout the week. If you are up for the challenge, give one of these nontraditional training programs a try.

Sources: CrossFit, /www.crossfit.com/; L. Kravitz, "High-Intensity Interval Training," ACSM, www.acsm.org/docs/brochures/high-intensity-interval-training.pdf

---

Another way to determine the intensity of cardiorespiratory exercise intensity is to use Borg's rating of perceived exertion (RPE) scale. **Perceived exertion** refers to how hard you feel you are working, which you might base on your heart rate, breathing rate, sweating, and level of fatigue. This scale uses a rating from 6 (no exertion at all) to 20 (maximal exertion). An RPE of 12 to 16 is generally recommended for training the cardiorespiratory system.

perceived exertion The subjective perception of effort during exercise that can be used to monitor exercise intensity

The easiest method of measuring cardiorespiratory exercise intensity is the "talk test." A "moderate" level of exercise (heart rate at 64 to 76 percent of maximum) is a conversational level of exercise. At this level you are able to talk with a partner while exercising. If you can talk, but only in short fragments and not sentences, you may be at a "vigorous" level of exercise (heart rate at 76 to 96 percent of maximum). If you are breathing so hard that speaking at all is difficult, the intensity of your exercise may be too high. Conversely, if you are able to sing or

laugh heartily while exercising, the intensity of your exercise is light and may be insufficient for maintaining or improving cardiorespiratory fitness.

Time For cardiorespiratory fitness benefits, the American College of Sports Medicine (ACSM) recommends that vigorous activities be performed for at least 20 minutes at a time, and moderate activities for at least 30 minutes.[36] See also the **Student Health Today** box for information on a few exercise programs that can really give you a lot of bang for your buck. Free time for exercise can vary from day to day, so you can also set a time goal for the entire week as long as you keep your sessions to at least 10 minutes (150 minutes per week for moderate intensity, and 75 minutes per week for vigorous intensity).

Type Any sort of rhythmic, continuous, and physical activity that can be done for 20 or more minutes will improve cardiorespiratory fitness. Examples include walking briskly, cycling, jogging, fitness classes, and swimming.

The FITT Principle for Muscular Strength and Endurance

The FITT prescription for muscular strength and endurance includes 2 to 3 days per week of exercises that train the major muscle groups, using enough sets, repetitions, and resistance to maintain or improve muscular strength and endurance.[37]

Frequency For frequency, training the major muscle groups 2 to 3 days a week is recommended. It is believed that overloading the muscles, a normal part of resistance training described below, causes microscopic tears in muscle fibers, and the rebuilding process that increases the muscle's size and capacity takes about 24 to 48 hours. Thus, resistance training exercise programs should include at least 1 day of rest between workouts before the same muscles are overloaded again. But don't wait too long between workouts: One of the important principles of strength training is the idea of *reversibility*. Reversibility means that if you stop exercising, the body responds by deconditioning. Within 2 weeks, muscles begin to revert to their untrained state.[38] The saying "use it or lose it" applies!

Intensity To determine the intensity of exercise needed to improve muscular strength and endurance, you need to know the maximum amount of weight you can lift (or move) in one contraction. This value is called your **one repetition maximum (1 RM)**. Once your 1 RM is determined, it is used as the basis for intensity recommendations for improving muscular strength and endurance. Muscular strength is improved when resistance loads are greater than 60 percent of your 1 RM, whereas muscular endurance is improved using loads less than 50 percent of your 1 RM.

Everyone begins a resistance-training program at an initial level of strength. To become stronger, you must *overload* your muscles, that is, regularly create a degree of tension in your muscles that is greater than what they are accustomed to. Overloading them forces your muscles to adapt by getting larger, stronger, and capable of producing more tension. If you "underload" your muscles, you will not increase strength. If you create too great an overload, you may experience muscle injury, muscle fatigue, and potentially a loss in strength.

> **one repetition maximum (1 RM)** The amount of weight or resistance that can be lifted or moved only once.

Time The time recommended for muscular strength and endurance exercises is measured, not in minutes of exercise, but rather in repetitions and sets.

- **Repetitions and sets.** To increase muscular strength, you need higher intensity and fewer repetitions and sets: Use a resistance of at least 60 percent of your 1 RM, performing 8 to 12 repetitions per set, with two to four sets performed overall. If improving muscular endurance is your goal, use less resistance and more repetitions: Perform one to two sets of 15 to 25 repetitions using a resistance that is less than 50 percent of your 1 RM.
- **Rest periods.** Resting between exercises is crucial to reduce fatigue and help with performance and safety in subsequent sets. A rest period of 2 to 3 minutes is recommended when using the guidelines for general health benefits. However, the rest period when working to develop strength or endurance will vary. Note that the rest period refers specifically to the muscle group being exercised. For example, you can alternate a set of push-ups with curl-ups, as the muscle groups worked in one set can rest while you are working the other muscle groups.

Type To improve muscular strength or endurance, it is recommended that resistance training use either the body's weight or devices that provide a fixed or variable resistance (see **TABLE 11.3**). When selecting strength-training exercises,

TABLE 11.3 | Methods of Providing Muscular Resistance

Body Weight Resistance (Calisthenics)	Fixed Resistance	Variable Resistance
- Uses your own body weight to develop muscular strength and endurance - Improves overall muscular fitness and, in particular, core body strength and overall muscle tone **Examples:** Push-ups, pull-ups, curl-ups, dips, leg raises, chair sits, etc.	- Provides a constant resistance throughout the full range of movement - Requires balance and coordination; promotes development of core body strength **Examples:** Free weights, such as barbells, dumbbells, medicine balls, and kettlebells	- Resistance altered so that the muscle's effort is consistent throughout the full range of motion - Provides more controlled motion and isolates certain muscle groups **Examples:** Weight machines in gyms and homes

there are three important principles to bear in mind: specificity, exercise selection, and exercise order. According to the *specificity principle,* the effects of resistance exercise training are specific to the muscles exercised; thus, to improve total body strength, include exercises for all the major muscle groups.

The second important concept is *exercise selection.* It is important to select exercises that will meet your goals. Selecting eight to ten exercises targeting all major muscle groups is generally recommended and will ensure that exercises are balanced for opposing muscle groups.

Finally, for optimal training effects, pay attention to *exercise order.* When training all major muscle groups in a single workout, complete large muscle group exercises (e.g., the bench press or leg press) before small muscle group exercises, multiple-joint exercises before single-joint exercises (e.g., biceps curls, triceps extension), and high-intensity exercises before lower-intensity exercises.

The FITT Principle for Flexibility

Although often overshadowed by cardiorespiratory and muscular fitness training, flexibility is important. Inflexible muscles are susceptible to injury, and flexibility training reduces the incidence and severity of lower back problems and muscle or tendon injuries.[39] Improved flexibility also means less tension and pressure on joints, resulting in less joint pain and joint deterioration.[40] This means that remaining flexible can help prevent the decreased physical function that often occurs with aging.[41]

Frequency The FITT principle calls for a minimum of 2 to 3 days per week for flexibility training.

Intensity Intensity recommendations for flexibility are that you perform or hold stretching positions at an individually determined "point of mild tension." You should be able to feel tension or mild discomfort in the muscle(s) you are stretching, but the stretch should not hurt.[42]

Time The time recommended to improve flexibility is based upon time per stretch. Once you are in a stretching position, you should hold at the "point of tension" for 10 to 30 seconds for each stretch and repeat two to four times in close succession.[43]

Type The most effective exercises for increasing flexibility involve stretching the major muscle groups of your body when the body is already warm, such as after your cardiorespiratory workout. The safest exercises for improving flexibility involve **static stretching.** The primary strategy is to decrease the resistance to stretch (tension) within a tight muscle targeted for increased range of motion.[44] To do this, you repeatedly stretch the muscle and its tendons of attachment to elongate them. With each repetition of a static stretch, your range of motion improves temporarily due to the slightly lessened sensitivity of tension receptors in the stretched muscles; when done regularly, range of motion increases.[45] FIGURE 11.6 illustrates some basic stretching exercises to increase flexibility.

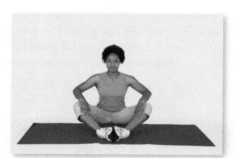
a Stretching the inside of the thighs

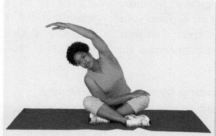
b Stretching the upper arm and the side of the trunk

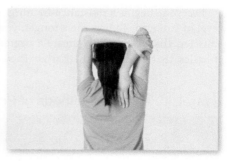
c Stretching the triceps

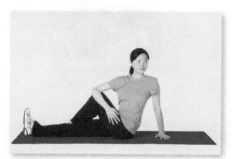
d Stretching the trunk and the hip

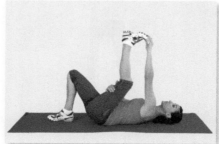
e Stretching the hip, back of the thigh, and the calf

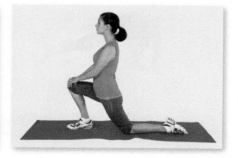
f Stretching the front of the thigh and the hip flexor

FIGURE 11.6 **Stretching Exercises to Improve Flexibility** Use these stretches as part of your cool-down. Hold each stretch for 10 to 30 seconds, and repeat two to four times for each limb.

LO 5 | IMPLEMENTING YOUR FITNESS PROGRAM

Devise a plan to implement your safe and effective fitness program.

As your physical fitness improves, you need to adjust the frequency, intensity, time, and type of your exercise to maintain or continue to improve your level of physical fitness. Below are a few suggestions to get started and stay on track. (If you're looking for a little more direction, the Money & Health box on page 344 offers suggestions on choosing a personal trainer or fitness coach.)

Develop a Progressive Plan

Experts recommend beginning an exercise regimen by picking an exercise and gradually increasing the frequency or time of your workouts. For example, in week 1, you might exercise 3 days for 20 minutes per day, and then move to 4 days in week 3 or 4. Then, consider increasing your duration to 30 minutes per session over the next couple of weeks. Gradual increases in intensity are typically made once the duration and frequency goals are met.

Finding a variety of exercises can reduce the risk of overuse injuries. Choosing different exercises for your workouts will also provide for a more complete training program by targeting more muscle groups. Reevaluate your physical fitness goals and action plan monthly to ensure that they are still working for you. A mistake many people make when they decide to become more physically active (or to make any other behavior

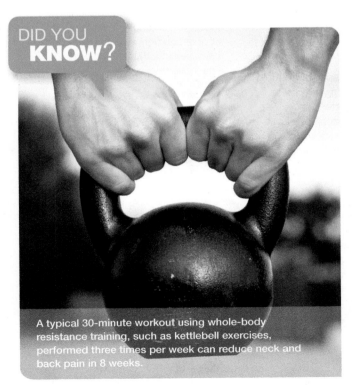

DID YOU KNOW?

A typical 30-minute workout using whole-body resistance training, such as kettlebell exercises, performed three times per week can reduce neck and back pain in 8 weeks.

Source: K. Jay et al., "Kettlebell Training for Musculoskeletal and Cardiovascular Health: A Randomized Controlled Trial," *Scandinavian Journal of Work, Environment, and Health* 37, no. 3 (2011): 196–203.

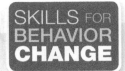

SKILLS FOR BEHAVIOR CHANGE — PLAN IT, START IT, STICK WITH IT!

The most successful physical activity program is one that you enjoy, is realistic, and is appropriate for your skill level and needs.

▶ **Make it enjoyable.** Pick activities you like to do so you will make the effort and find the time to do it.

▶ **Start slowly.** If you have been physically inactive for a while, any type and amount of physical activity is a step in the right direction. Start slowly, letting your body adapt so there is not too much pain the next day.

▶ **Make only one lifestyle change at a time.** It is not realistic to change everything at once. Furthermore, success with one behavioral change will increase your confidence and encourage you to make other positive changes.

▶ **Set reasonable expectations for yourself and your physical fitness program.** You will not become "fit" overnight. Focus on the changes you do see immediately (e.g., improved sleep, feeling relaxed, stress management, feeling good about yourself). These things will help you stay motivated while working to meet long-term goals. Be patient and enjoy!

▶ **Choose a time to be physically active and stick with it.** Learn to establish priorities and keep to a schedule. Try different times of the day to learn what works best for you. Yet, be flexible, so if something comes up that you cannot work around, you will still find time to do some physical activity.

▶ **Record your progress.** Include the intensity, time, and type of physical activities; your emotions; and your personal achievements.

▶ **Take lapses in stride.** Sometimes life gets in the way. Start again and do not despair; your commitment to physical fitness has ebbs and flows like most everything else in life.

▶ **Reward yourself.** Find meaningful and healthy ways to reward yourself when you reach your goals.

change) is putting so much effort into getting started that they allow their efforts to dwindle once in the action phase. The Skills for Behavior Change box offers more tips on starting and sticking with an exercise plan.

Design Your Exercise Session

A comprehensive workout should include a warm-up, cardiorespiratory and/or resistance training, and then a cool-down to finish the session.

Warm-Up The warm-up prepares the body physically and mentally for cardiorespiratory and/or resistance training.

static stretching Stretching techniques that slowly and gradually lengthen a muscle or group of muscles and their tendons.

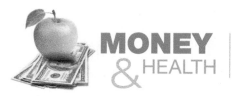

MONEY & HEALTH | ALL CERTIFICATIONS ARE NOT CREATED EQUAL

Using a personal trainer or fitness trainer is a great way to get on track with a new exercise program. So, how do you select the best fit for you and your goals?

First, make sure your trainer is certified and carries personal liability insurance, but be careful! There are a lot of certifications available, and not all are reputable. You can use the Internet to review the organizations that award certifications. Consider the following characteristics when reviewing certifications:

- **Quality of Certification.** Avoid using a trainer with a certification that is very easily obtainable. The reputable certifications have workshops, test review materials, online study materials, and minimal standards to qualify (e.g., a high school diploma). The National Commission for Certifying Agencies, an accrediting agency for health professions (www.credential-ingexcellence.org/p/cm/ld/fid=121), lists accredited fitness certifications.
- **Continuing Education Credits.** Review the continuing education requirements to maintain the certification. Workshops, professional conferences, tests in scientific journals, and online courses should be options for maintaining the certification. It's a good sign when other certifying bodies use an organization's conferences and classes for continuing education.

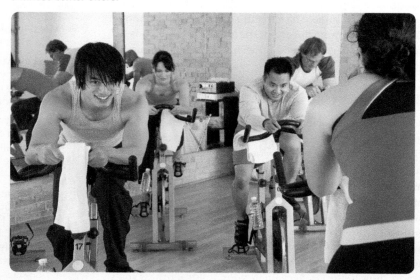

Before you sign on the dotted line, check out the classes, equipment, and personnel a fitness center offers.

- **Readily Available Information.** You should be able to readily find information about the certification or organization that provides the certification.

In addition to certification, also consider characteristics of the trainer and get recommendations from whose you trust.

- The trainer's area of specialty should fit with your goals (e.g., weight loss, improved athletic performance).
- The trainer should teach you about fitness, and not just give you a workout plan. And, the trainer should

explain things to you at a level you understand. Consider the trainer's education level.

- You should not feel judged by the trainer.
- The trainer's style should match your needs. For example, if you need a lot of encouragement and reinforcement, select a trainer who will provide those things.

Sources: ACE, "How to Choose the Right Personal Trainer," 2015, www.acefitness.org/acefit/healthy_living_fit_facts_content.aspx?itemid=19; ACSM, "Using a Personal Trainer," www.acsm.org/docs/default-source/brochures/using-a-personal-trainer.pdf?sfvrsn=4.

A warm-up should involve large body movements, generally using light cardiorespiratory activities, followed by range-of-motion exercises of the muscle groups to be used during the exercise session. Usually 5 to 15 minutes long, a warm-up is shorter when you are geared up and ready to go and longer when you are struggling to get moving or your muscles are cold or tight. The warm-up provides a transition from rest to physical activity by slowly increasing heart rate, blood pressure, breathing rate, and body temperature. These gradual changes improve joint lubrication, increase muscle and tendon elasticity, and enhance blood flow throughout the body, facilitating performance during the next stage of the workout.

Cardiorespiratory and/or Resistance Training
The next stage of your workout may involve cardiorespiratory training, resistance training, or a little of both. If completing aerobic and resistance exercise in the same session, it is often recommended to perform your aerobic

SEE IT! VIDEOS

Get moving to benefit your brain in a variety of ways! Watch **New Study Shows Exercise May Build Brain Power** in the Study Area of MasteringHealth™

exercise first. This order will provide additional warm-up for the resistance session, and your muscles will not be fatigued for the aerobic workout.

Cool-down and Stretching A cool-down is an essential component of a fitness program; it involves another 10 to 15 minutes of activity time. Start your cool-down with 5 to 10 minutes of moderate- to low-intensity activity, and follow it with approximately 5 to 10 minutes of stretching. Because of the body's increased temperature, the cool-down is an excellent time to stretch to improve flexibility. The purpose of the cool-down is to gradually reduce your heart rate, blood pressure, and body temperature to pre-exercise levels. In addition, the cool-down reduces the risk of blood pooling in the extremities and facilitates quicker recovery between exercise sessions.

Explore Activities That Develop Multiple Components of Fitness

Some forms of activity have the potential to improve several components of physical fitness and thus improve your everyday functioning ("functional" exercises). For example, core strength training improves posture and can prevent back pain. In addition, yoga, tai chi, and Pilates improve flexibility, muscular strength and endurance, balance, coordination, and agility. They also develop the mind-body connection through concentration on breathing and body position.

Core Strength Training The body's core muscles are the foundation for all movement.[46] These muscles include the deep back, abdominal, and hip muscles that attach to the spine and pelvis. The contraction of these muscles provides the basis of support for movements of the upper and lower body and powerful movements of the extremities. A weak core generally results in poor posture, low back pain, and muscle injuries. A strong core provides a more stable center of gravity, and as a result, a more stable platform for movements, thus reducing the chance of injury.

You can develop core strength by doing various exercises, including calisthenics, yoga, or Pilates. Holding yourself in a front or reverse plank (an upward-facing version of a push-up position) or doing abdominal curl-ups are examples of exercises that increase core strength. Increased core strength does not happen from one single exercise,

but rather from a structured regime of postures and exercises.[47] The use of instability devices (stability ball, wobble boards, etc.) and exercises to train the core have become popular.[48]

Yoga Yoga, based on ancient Indian practices, blends the mental and physical aspects of exercise—a union of mind and body that participants often find relaxing and satisfying. The practice of yoga focuses attention on controlled breathing as well as physical exercise and incorporates a complex array of static stretching and strengthening exercises expressed as postures (*asanas*). Done regularly, yoga improves flexibility, vitality, posture, agility, balance, coordination, and core muscular strength and endurance. Many people report an improved sense of general well-being, too.

Tai Chi Tai chi is an ancient Chinese form of exercise that combines stretching, balance, muscular endurance, coordination, and meditation. It increases range of motion and flexibility while reducing muscular tension. It involves continuously performing a series of positions called *forms*. Tai chi is often described as "meditation in motion" because it promotes serenity through gentle movements that connect the mind and body.

Pilates Pilates was developed by Joseph Pilates in 1926 as an exercise style that combines stretching with movement against resistance, frequently aided by devices such as tension springs or heavy rubber bands. It differs from yoga and tai chi in that it includes a component specifically designed to increase strength. Some movements are carried out on specially designed equipment, whereas others can be performed on mats. It teaches body awareness, good posture, and easy, graceful body movements while improving flexibility, coordination, core strength, muscle tone, and economy of motion.

SEE IT! VIDEOS

Can you use some tips on stretching before and after exercise? Watch **The Do's and Don'ts of Stretching** in the Study Area of MasteringHealth™

Resistance training to improve muscular strength and endurance can be done with free weights, machines, or even your own body weight.

LO **6** | TAKING IN PROPER NUTRITION FOR EXERCISE

Describe optimal foods and fluids consumption recommendations for exercise and recovery.

It's important to evaluate your eating habits in light of your exercise habits. Whether you're a seasoned fitness buff or a beginner, the importance of proper nutrition for exercise can't be overstated.

Foods for Exercise and Recovery

To make the most of your workouts, follow the recommendations from the MyPlate plan and make sure that you eat sufficient carbohydrates, the body's main source of fuel. Your body stores carbohydrates as glycogen primarily in the muscles and liver and then uses this stored glycogen for energy when you are physically active. Fats are also an important source of energy, packing more than double the energy per gram compared to carbohydrates. Protein plays a role in muscle repair and growth, but is not normally a source of energy.

When you eat is almost as important as what you eat. Eating a large meal before exercising can cause upset stomach, cramping, and diarrhea, because your muscles have to compete with your digestive system for energy. After a large meal, wait 3 to 4 hours before you begin exercising. Smaller meals (snacks) can be eaten about an hour before activity. Not eating at all before a workout can cause low blood sugar levels that in turn cause weakness and slower reaction times.

hyponatremia or water intoxication Overconsumption of water, which leads to a dilution of sodium concentration in the blood, with potentially fatal results.

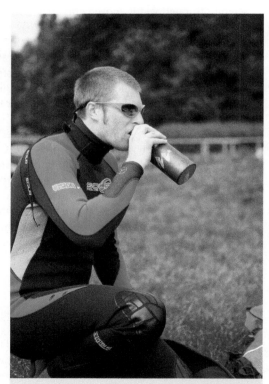

The American College of Sports Medicine and the National Athletic Trainers' Association recommend consuming 14 to 22 ounces of fluid several hours prior to exercise and about 6 to 12 ounces per 15 to 20 minutes during—assuming you are sweating.

After your workout, help your muscles recover by eating a snack or meal that contains plenty of carbohydrates and a little protein, too. Today, there is a burgeoning market for dietary supplements that claim to deliver the nutrients needed for muscle recovery, as well as additional "performance-enhancing" ingredients; one thing to keep in mind, especially if you consider these products, is that there are few standards and virtually no Food and Drug Administration (FDA) approval needed for many to grace store shelves. (See Chapter 9 on nutrition for more on supplements).

Fluids for Exercise and Recovery

In addition to eating well, staying hydrated is also crucial. How much fluid do you need? Keep in mind that the goal of fluid replacement is to prevent excessive dehydration (greater than 2% loss of body weight). The ACSM and the National Athletic Trainers Association recommend consuming 5 to 7 milliliters per kilogram of body weight (approximately 0.7 to 1.07 ounces per 10 pounds body weight) 4 hours prior to exercise.[49] Drinking fluids during exercise is also important, but it is difficult to provide guidelines for how much or when because intake should be based on time, intensity, and type of activity performed. A good way to monitor how much fluid you need to replace is to weigh yourself before and after your workout. The difference in weight is how much you should drink. So, for example, if you lost 2 pounds during a training session, you should drink 32 ounces of fluid.[50]

For exercise sessions lasting less than 1 hour, plain water is sufficient for rehydration. If your exercise session exceeds 1 hour—and you sweat profusely—consider a sports drink containing electrolytes. The electrolytes in these products are minerals and ions such as sodium and potassium that are needed for proper functioning of your nervous and muscular systems. Replacing electrolytes is particularly important for endurance athletes. In endurance events lasting more than 4 hours, an athlete's overconsumption of plain water can dilute the sodium concentration in the blood with potentially fatal results, an effect called **hyponatremia** or **water intoxication**.

Although water is the best choice in most cases, there are situations in which you might need to choose something different. Some people are likely to consume more when their drink is flavored, a point that may be significant in ensuring proper hydration. Recently, research has considered low-fat chocolate milk as a recovery drink.[51] Chocolate milk is a liquid that not only hydrates, but also is a source of sodium, potassium, carbohydrates, and protein. Consuming carbohydrates and protein immediately after exercise will help replenish muscle and liver glycogen stores and stimulate muscle protein synthesis for better recovery from exercise. The protein in milk, whey protein, is ideal because it contains all of the essential amino acids and is rapidly absorbed by the body. Low-fat chocolate milk is a good choice to hydrate and recover after exercise.

LO 7 | PREVENTING AND TREATING FITNESS-RELATED INJURIES

Explain how to prevent and treat common exercise injuries.

Two basic types of injuries stem from fitness-related activities: traumatic injuries and overuse injuries. **Traumatic injuries** occur suddenly and usually by accident. Typical traumatic injuries are broken bones, torn ligaments and muscles, contusions, and lacerations. If a traumatic injury causes a noticeable loss of function and immediate pain or pain that does not go away after 30 minutes, consult a physician.

Overuse injuries result from the cumulative effects of day-after-day stresses. These injuries occur most often in repetitive activities such as swimming, running, bicycling, and step aerobics. The forces that occur normally during physical activity are not enough to cause a ligament sprain or muscle strain as in a traumatic injury, but when these forces are applied daily for weeks or months, they can result in an overuse injury. Factors such as overweight or obesity, running mechanics, and poor choice of shoe can also contribute to overuse injury.

The three most common overuse injuries are *runner's knee, shin splints,* and *plantar fasciitis.* Runner's knee is a general term describing a series of problems involving the muscles, tendons, and ligaments around the knee. *Shin splints* is a general term used for any pain that occurs below the knee and above the ankle in the shin. Plantar fasciitis is an inflammation of the plantar fascia, a broad band of dense, inelastic tissue in the foot. Rest, variation of routine, and stretching are the first lines of treatment for any of these overuse injuries. If pain continues, visit a physician. Orthotics, physical therapy, or steroid shots are possible treatment options.

WHAT DO YOU THINK?

How do your physical activities put you at risk of injury?

- What changes can you make to your approach to training, your training program, equipment, or footwear to reduce these risks?

Preventing Injuries

To reduce your risk of overuse or traumatic injuries, use common sense and the proper gear and equipment. Vary your physical activities throughout the week, setting appropriate and realistic short- and long-term goals. Listen to your body when working out. Warning signs include muscle stiffness and soreness, bone and joint pains, and whole-body fatigue that simply does not go away.

Appropriate Footwear Proper footwear, replaced in a timely manner, can decrease the likelihood of foot, knee, hip, or back injuries. Biomechanics research has revealed that running is a collision sport—with each stride, the runner's foot collides with the ground with a force three to five times the runner's body weight.[52] Consider the impact for a beginner runner who might have poor mechanics or an overweight individual who participates in weight-bearing activities. The force not absorbed by the running shoe is transmitted upward into the foot, leg, thigh, and back. Our bodies can absorb forces such as these but may be injured by the cumulative effect of repetitive impacts (such as running 40 miles per week). Thus, the shoes' ability to absorb shock is critical—not just for those who run, but for anyone engaged in weight-bearing activities.

> **traumatic injuries** Injuries that are accidental and occur suddenly.
>
> **overuse injuries** Injuries that result from the cumulative effects of day-after-day stresses placed on tendons, muscles, and joints.

In addition to absorbing shock, an athletic shoe should provide a good fit for maximal comfort and performance—see FIGURE 11.7. To get the best fit, shop at a sports or fitness specialty store where there is a large selection and the salespeople are trained in properly fitting athletic shoes. Try on shoes later in the day when your feet are largest, and check to make sure there is a little extra room in the toe and that the width is appropriate. Because different activities place different stresses on your feet and joints, you should choose shoes specifically designed for your sport or activity. Shoes of any type should be replaced once they lose their cushioning. A common rule of thumb is that running shoes ought to be replaced after 300 to 500 miles of use, which is typically between 3 and 9 months, depending on your activity level.

Appropriate Protective Equipment It is essential to use well-fitted, appropriate protective equipment for your physical activities. For example, using the correct racquet with the proper tension helps prevent the general inflammatory condition known as tennis elbow. As another example, eye injuries can occur in virtually all physical activities, although some activities (such as baseball, basketball, and racquet sports) are more risky than others.[53] As many as 90 percent of eye injuries could be prevented by wearing appropriate eye protection, such as goggles with polycarbonate lenses.[54]

Wearing a helmet while bicycle riding is an important safety precaution. An estimated 66 to 88 percent of head injuries among cyclists can be prevented by wearing a helmet.[55] In a

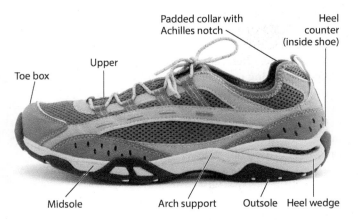

FIGURE 11.7 **Anatomy of a Running Shoe** A good running shoe should fit comfortably; allow room for your toes to move; have a firm, but flexible midsole; and have a firm grip on your heel to prevent slipping.

Toe box · Upper · Padded collar with Achilles notch · Heel counter (inside shoe) · Midsole · Arch support · Outsole · Heel wedge

heat cramps Involuntary and forcible muscle contractions that occur during or following exercise in hot and/or humid weather.

heat exhaustion A heat stress illness caused by significant dehydration resulting from exercise in hot and/or humid conditions.

heatstroke A deadly heat stress illness resulting from dehydration and overexertion in hot and/or humid conditions.

hypothermia Potentially fatal condition caused by abnormally low body core temperature.

recent study of college students, 45.8 percent of students who rode a bike in the past 12 months reported never wearing a helmet, and 24.69 percent said they wore one only sometimes or rarely.[56] The direct medical costs from cyclists' failure to wear helmets is an estimated $81 million a year.[57] Cyclists aren't the only ones who should be wearing helmets. People who skateboard, ski, in-line skate, snowboard, play contact sports, or use kick-scooters should also wear helmets. Look for helmets that meet the standards established by the American National Standards Institute or the Snell Memorial Foundation.

Exercising in the Heat

Exercising in hot or humid weather increases your risk of a heat-related illness. In these conditions, your body's rate of heat production can exceed its ability to cool itself. The three different heat stress illnesses, progressive in their level of severity, are heat cramps, heat exhaustion, and heatstroke.

Heat cramps (heat-related involuntary and forcible muscle contractions that cannot be relaxed), the least serious problem, can usually be prevented by adequate fluid replacement and a dietary intake that includes the electrolytes lost during sweating.

Heat exhaustion is actually a mild form of shock, in which the blood pools in the arms and legs away from the brain and major organs of the body. It is caused by excessive water loss because of intense or prolonged exercise or work in a hot and/or humid environment. Symptoms of heat exhaustion include nausea, headache, fatigue, dizziness and faintness, and, paradoxically, goose bumps and chills. When you are suffering from heat exhaustion, your skin will be cool and moist.

Heatstroke, often called *sunstroke,* is a life-threatening emergency condition with a high morbidity and mortality rate.[58] Heatstroke occurs during vigorous exercise when the body's heat production significantly exceeds its cooling capacities. Core body temperature can rise from normal (98.6°F) to 105°F to 110°F within minutes after the body's cooling mechanism shuts down. A rapid increase in core body temperature can cause brain damage, permanent disability, and death. Common signs of heatstroke are dry, hot, and usually red skin;

very high body temperature; and rapid heart rate. If you experience any of the symptoms mentioned here, stop exercising immediately. Move to the shade or a cool spot to rest and drink plenty of cool fluids for heat cramps and exhaustion. If heatstroke is suspected, seek medical attention immediately.

You can prevent heat stress by following certain precautions. First, acclimatize yourself to hot or humid climates. The process of heat acclimatization, which increases your body's cooling efficiency, requires about 10 to 14 days of gradually increased physical activity in the hot environment. Second, reduce your risk of dehydration by replacing fluids before, during, and after exercise. Third, wear clothing appropriate for the activity and the environment—for example, light-colored nylon shorts and a mesh tank top. Finally, use common sense. For example, on a day when the temperature is 85°F and the humidity is around 80 percent, postpone lunchtime physical activity until the evening when it is cooler or exercise indoors where the conditions are controlled.

Exercising in the Cold

When you exercise in cool weather, especially in windy and damp conditions, your body's rate of heat loss is frequently greater than its rate of heat production. These conditions may lead to **hypothermia**—a condition in which the body's core temperature drops below 95°F.[59] Temperatures need not be frigid for hypothermia to occur; it can also result from prolonged, vigorous exercise in 40°F to 50°F temperatures, particularly if there is rain, snow, or a strong wind.

As body core temperature drops from the normal 98.6°F to about 93.2°F, shivering begins. Shivering—the involuntary contraction of nearly every muscle in the body—increases body temperature by using the heat given off by muscle activity. You may also experience cold hands and feet, poor judgment, apathy, and amnesia. Shivering ceases in most hypothermia victims as body core temperatures drop to between 87°F and 90°F, a sign that the body has lost its ability to generate heat. Death usually occurs at body core temperatures between 75°F and 80°F.[60]

To prevent hypothermia, analyze weather conditions before engaging in outdoor physical activity. Remember that wind and humidity are as significant as temperature. Have a friend join you for safety when exercising outdoors in cold weather, and wear layers of appropriate clothing to prevent excessive heat loss and frostbite (polypropylene or woolen undergarments, a windproof outer garment, and a wool hat and gloves). Keep your head, hands, and feet warm. Finally, do not allow yourself to become dehydrated.[61]

Reducing risk for exercise injuries requires common sense and preventative measures, including wearing protective gear (helmets, knee pads, elbow pads, eyewear).

Treating Injuries

First-aid treatment for virtually all fitness training–related injuries involves **RICE:** **r**est, **i**ce, **c**ompression, and **e**levation.

- *Rest*—is required to avoid further irritation of the injured body part.
- *Ice*—is applied to relieve pain and constrict the blood vessels to reduce internal or external bleeding. To prevent frostbite, wrap the ice or cold pack in a layer of wet toweling or elastic bandage before applying it to your skin. A new injury should be iced for approximately 20 minutes every hour for the first 24 to 72 hours.
- *Compression*—of the injured body part can be accomplished with a 4- or 6-inch-wide elastic bandage; this applies indirect pressure to damaged blood vessels to help stop bleeding. Be careful, though, that the compression wrap does not interfere with normal blood flow. Throbbing or pain indicates that the compression wrap should be loosened.
- *Elevation*—of an injured extremity above the level of your heart also helps control internal or external bleeding by making the blood flow upward to reach the injured area.

Applying ice to an injury such as a sprain can help relieve pain and reduce swelling, but never apply the ice directly to the skin, as that could lead to frostbite.

RICE Acronym for the standard first-aid treatment for virtually all traumatic and overuse injuries: rest, ice, compression, and elevation.

1 Evaluating Your Cardiorespiratory Endurance (The 1.5-Mile Run Test)

This test assesses your cardiorespiratory endurance level.

Procedure

Find a local track, typically .25 mile per lap, to perform your test. Run 1.5 miles; use a stopwatch to measure how long it takes to reach that distance. If you become extremely fatigued during the test, slow your pace or walk—do not overstress yourself! If you feel faint or nauseated or experience any unusual pains in your upper body, stop and notify your instructor. Use the chart below to estimate your cardiorespiratory fitness level based on your age and sex. Note that women have lower standards for each fitness category because they have higher levels of essential fat than men do.

Fitness Categories for 1.5-Mile Run Test

Men, years	Excellent	Good	Fair	Poor
20–29	< 10:10	10:10–11:29	11:30–12:38	> 12:38
30–39	< 10:47	10:47–11:54	11:55–12:58	> 12:58
40–49	< 11:16	11:16–12:24	12:25–13:50	> 13:50
50–59	< 12:09	12:09–13:35	13:36–15:06	> 15:06
60–69	< 13:24	13:24–15:04	15:05–16:46	> 16:46

Women, years	Excellent	Good	Fair	Poor
20–29	< 11:59	11:59–13:24	13:25–14:50	> 14:50
30–39	< 12:25	12:25–14:08	14:09–15:43	> 15:43
40–49	< 13:24	13:24–14:53	14:54–16:31	> 16:31
50–59	< 14:35	14:35–16:35	16:36–18:18	> 18:18
60–69	< 16:34	16:34–18:27	18:28–20:16	> 20:16

Source: The Cooper Institute, *Physical Fitness Assessments and Norms for Adults and Law Enforcement,* Dallas, Texas. Copyright © 2007 by The Cooper Institute. Reprinted with permission.

2 Evaluating Your Muscular Strength and Endurance (Partial Curl-Up Test)

Your abdominal muscles are important for core stability and back support; this test will assess their muscular endurance.

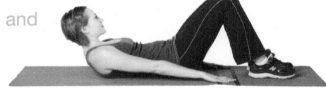

Procedure

Lie on a mat with your arms by your sides, palms flat on the mat, elbows straight, and fingers extended. Bend your knees at a 90-degree angle. Your instructor or partner will mark your starting finger position with a piece of masking tape aligned with the tip of each middle finger. He or she will also mark with tape your ending position, 10 cm (4 inches) away from the first piece of tape—one ending position tape for each hand.

Set a metronome to 50 beats per minute and curl up at this slow, controlled pace: one curl-up every two beats (25 curl-ups per minute). Curl your head and upper back upward, lifting your shoulder blades off the mat (your trunk should make a 30-degree angle with the mat) and reaching your arms forward along the mat to touch the ending tape. Then curl back down so that your upper back and shoulders touch the floor. During the entire curl-up, your fingers, feet, and buttocks should stay on the mat. Your partner will count the number of correct repetitions you complete. Perform as many curl-ups as you can in 1 minute without pausing, to a maximum of 25.

Healthy Musculoskeletal Fitness: Norms and Health Benefit Zones: Curl-Ups

Men, years	Excellent	Good	Fair	Needs Improvement	Women, years	Excellent	Good	Fair	Needs Improvement
20–29	25	21–24	11–20	≤ 10	20–29	25	18–24	5–17	≤ 4
30–39	25	18–24	11–17	≤ 10	30–39	25	19–24	6–18	≤ 5
40–49	25	18–24	6–17	≤ 5	40–49	25	19–24	4–18	≤ 3
50–59	25	17–24	8–16	≤ 7	50–59	25	19–24	6–18	≤ 5
60–69	25	16–24	6–15	≤ 5	60–69	25	17–24	3–16	≤ 2

Source: From *Canadian Physical Activity, Fitness & Lifestyle Approach: CSEP-Health & Fitness Program's Appraisal and Counselling Strategy,* 3rd edition, © 2003. Reprinted with permission from the Canadian Society for Exercise Physiology

3 Evaluating Your Flexibility (The Sit-and-Reach Test)

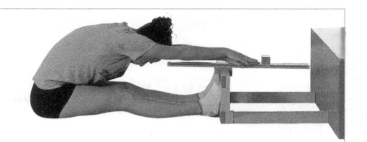

This test measures the general flexibility of your lower back, hips, and hamstring muscles.

Procedure

Warm up with some light activity that involves the total body, range-of-motion exercises, and stretches for the lower back and hamstrings. For the test, start by sitting upright, straight-legged on a mat with your shoes removed and soles of the feet flat against a flexometer (sit-and-reach box) at the 10.25-in mark. Inner edges of the soles are placed within 0.75 in of the measuring scale.

Have a partner on hand to record your measurements. Stretch your arms out in front of you and, keeping the hands parallel to each other, slowly reach forward with both hands as far as possible, holding the position for approximately

2 seconds. Your fingertips should be in contact with the measuring portion of the sit-and-reach box. To facilitate a longer reach, exhale and drop your head between your arms while reaching forward. Keep your knees extended the whole time and breathe normally.

Your score is the most distant point (in inches) reached with the fingertips; have your partner make note of this number for you. Perform the test twice, record your best score, and compare it with the norms presented in the following tables.

Healthy Musculoskeletal Fitness: Norms and Health Benefit Zones: Sit-and-Reach Test*

Men, years	Excellent (in)	Very Good (in)	Good (in)	Fair (in)	Needs Improvement (in)	Women, years	Excellent (in)	Very Good (in)	Good (in)	Fair (in)	Needs Improvement (in)
20–29	≥ 15.5	13.5–15.5	12–13	10–11.5	≤ 10	20–29	≥ 16	14.5–15.5	13–14	11–12.5	≤ 10.5
30–39	≥ 15	13–14.5	11–12.5	9–10.5	≤ 9	30–39	≥ 16	14–15.5	12.5–13.5	10.5–12	≤ 10
40–49	≥ 13.5	11.5–13.5	9.5–11	7–9	≤ 6.5	40–49	≥ 15	13.5–14.5	12–13	10–11.5	≤ 9.5
50–59	≥ 13.5	11–13.5	9.5–10.5	6–9	≤ 6	50–59	≥ 15.5	13–15	12–12.5	10–11.5	≤ 9.5
60–69	≥ 13	10–12.5	8–9.5	6–7.5	≤ 5.5	60–69	≥ 13.5	12–13.5	10.5–12	9–10	≤ 8.5

*Note: These norms are based on a sit-and-reach box in which the zero point is set at 10.25 in. When using a box in which the zero point is set at 9 in, subtract 1.2 in from each value in this table.
Source: From *Canadian Physical Activity, Fitness & Lifestyle Approach: CSEP-Health & Fitness Program's Appraisal and Counselling Strategy*, 3rd edition, © 2003. Reprinted with permission from the Canadian Society for Exercise Physiology.

YOUR PLAN FOR **CHANGE**

The **ASSESS YOURSELF** activity helped you determine your current level of physical fitness. Based on your results, you may decide that you should take steps to improve one or more components of your physical fitness.

TODAY, YOU CAN:

☐ Visit your campus fitness facility (or its website) and familiarize yourself with the equipment and resources. Find out what classes it offers, and take home (or print out) a copy of the schedule.

☐ Walk between your classes; make an extra effort to take the long way to get from building to building. Use the stairs instead of the elevator or escalator.

☐ Take an activity break. Spend 5 to 10 minutes between homework projects or just before bed doing some type of activity, such as abdominal crunches, push-ups, or yoga poses.

WITHIN THE NEXT TWO WEEKS, YOU CAN:

☐ Shop for comfortable workout clothes and appropriate athletic footwear.

☐ Look into group activities on your campus or in your community that you might enjoy.

☐ Ask a friend to join you in your workout once a week. Agree on a date and time in advance so you both will be committed to following through.

☐ Plan for a physically active outing with a friend or date; perhaps you can go dancing, bowling, or shoot hoops. Use active transportation (i.e., walk or cycle) to get to a movie or go out for dinner.

BY THE END OF THE SEMESTER, YOU CAN:

☐ Establish a regular routine of engaging in physical activity or exercise at least three times a week. Mark your exercise times on your calendar and keep a log to track your progress.

☐ Take your workouts to the next level. If you have been working out at home, try going to a gym or participating in an exercise class. If you are walking, try walking up hills, intermittent jogging, or sign up for a fitness event such as a charity 5K.

Customize your study plan—and master your health!—in the Study Area of MasteringHealth™

CHAPTER REVIEW

To hear an MP3 Tutor Session, scan here or visit the Study Area in MasteringHealth.

LO 1 Physical Activity for Health

- Benefits of regular physical activity include reduced risk of cardiovascular diseases, metabolic syndrome and type 2 diabetes, and cancer, as well as improved blood lipoproteins, bone mass, weight control, immunity to disease, mental health, stress management, and life span.

LO 2 Physical Activity for Fitness and Performance

- Physical fitness involves achieving minimal levels in the health-related components of fitness: cardiorespiratory, muscular strength, muscular endurance, flexibility, and body composition. Skill-related components of fitness, such as agility, balance, reaction time, speed, coordination, and power, are essential for elite and recreational athletes to increase their performance in and enjoyment of sport.

LO 3 Committing to Physical Fitness

- Commit to your new lifestyle of physical activity and increased fitness levels by incorporating fitness activities into your life. If you are new to exercise, start slowly, keep your fitness program simple, and consider consulting your physician and/or a fitness instructor for recommendations. Overcome your barriers or obstacles to exercise by identifying them and then planning specific strategies to address them. Choose activities that are fun and convenient to increase your likelihood of sticking with them.

LO 4 Creating Your Own Fitness Program

- The FITT principle can be used to develop a progressive program of physical fitness. For general health

benefits, every adult should participate in moderate-intensity activities for 30 minutes at least 5 days a week. To improve cardiorespiratory fitness, you should engage in vigorous, continuous, and rhythmic activities 3 to 5 days per week at an exercise intensity of 64 to 96 percent of your maximum heart rate for 20 to 30 minutes.

- Three key principles for developing muscular strength and endurance are overload, specificity of training, and reversibility. Muscular strength is improved by engaging in resistance-training exercises two to three times per week, using an intensity of greater than 60 percent of 1 RM, and completing two to four sets of 8 to 12 repetitions. Muscular endurance is improved by engaging in resistance-training exercises two to three times per week, using an intensity of less than 50 percent of 1 RM, and completing one to two sets of 15 to 25 repetitions.

- Flexibility is improved by engaging in two to four repetitions of static stretching exercises at least 2 to 3 days a week, where each stretch is held for 10 to 30 seconds.

LO 5 Implementing Your Fitness Program

- Planning to improve your physical fitness involves setting goals and designing a program to achieve these goals. A comprehensive workout should include a warm-up with some light stretching, strength-development exercises, aerobic activities, and a cool-down period with a heavier emphasis on stretching exercises. Core strength training is important for mobility, stability, and preventing back injury. The popular exercise forms of yoga, tai chi, and Pilates all develop core strength as well as flexibility, strength, and endurance.

LO 6 Taking in Proper Nutrition for Exercise

- Fueling properly for exercise involves eating a balance of healthy foods 3 to 4 hours before exercise. In exercise sessions lasting an hour or more, performance can benefit from some

additional calories ingested during the exercise session. Hydrating properly for exercise is important for performance and injury prevention. Chocolate milk is a good source of carbohydrates and protein for postexercise recovery.

LO 7 Preventing and Treating Common Exercise Injuries

- Physical activity–related injuries are generally caused by overuse or trauma. The most common overuse injuries are plantar fasciitis, shin splints, and runner's knee. Proper footwear and protective equipment help to prevent injuries. Exercising in the heat or cold requires taking special precautions. Minor exercise injuries should be treated with RICE (rest, ice, compression, and elevation).

POP QUIZ

Visit MasteringHealth to personalize your study plan with Chapter Review Quizzes and Dynamic Study Modules.

LO 1 Physical Activity for Health

1. What is physical fitness?
   a. The ability to respond to routine physical demands
   b. Having enough physical reserves to cope with a sudden challenge
   c. A balance of cardiorespiratory, muscle, and flexibility fitness
   d. All of the above

2. Which of the following is not a health benefit associated with regular exercise?
   a. Reduced risk for some cancers
   b. Reduced risk for cardiovascular diseases
   c. Elimination of chronic diseases
   d. Improved mental health

LO 2 Physical Activity for Fitness and Performance

3. The maximum volume of oxygen consumed by the muscles during exercise defines

a. target heart rate.
b. muscular strength.
c. aerobic capacity.
d. muscular endurance.

4. Flexibility is the range of motion around
   a. specific bones.
   b. a joint or series of joints.
   c. the tendons.
   d. the muscles.

LO 3 | Committing to Physical Fitness

5. Miguel is thinking about becoming more active. Which of the following is *not* a good piece of advice to offer him?
   a. Incorporate physical activity into your daily life.
   b. Make multiple changes to diet and exercise routines simultaneously.
   c. Identify obstacles to being active.
   d. Set SMART goals.

LO 4 | Creating Your Own Fitness Program

6. Janice has been lifting 95 pounds while doing three sets of six leg curls. To become stronger, she began lifting 105 pounds while doing leg curls. What principle of strength development does this represent?
   a. Reversibility
   b. Overload
   c. Flexibility
   d. Specificity of training

7. The "talk test" measures
   a. exercise intensity.
   b. exercise time.
   c. exercise frequency.
   d. exercise type.

LO 5 | Implementing Your Fitness Program

8. At the start of an exercise session, you should always
   a. stretch before doing any activity.
   b. do 50 crunches to activate your core muscles.
   c. warm up with light cardiorespiratory activities.
   d. eat a meal to ensure that you are fueled for the activity.

LO 6 | Taking in Proper Nutrition for Exercise

9. Chocolate milk is good for
   a. preworkout energy boost.
   b. postworkout recovery.
   c. slimming down.
   d. staying hydrated during exercise.

LO 7 | Preventing and Treating Common Exercise Injuries

10. Overuse injuries can be prevented by
    a. monitoring the quantity and quality of your workouts.
    b. engaging in only one type of aerobic training.
    c. working out daily.
    d. working out with a friend.

Answers to the Pop Quiz can be found on page A-1. If you answered a question incorrectly, review the section identified by the Learning Outcome. For even more study tools, visit MasteringHealth.

THINK ABOUT IT!

LO 1 | Physical Activity for Health

1. How do you define *physical fitness*? Identify at least four physiological and psychological benefits of physical activity. How would you promote these benefits to nonexercisers?

LO 2 | Physical Activity for Fitness and Performance

2. How are muscle strength and muscle endurance different? What are some ways you might work to increase muscle strength and muscle endurance?

LO 3 | Committing to Physical Fitness

3. What do you do to motivate yourself to engage in physical activity on a regular basis? What and who helps you to be physically active?

LO 4 | Creating Your Own Fitness Program

4. Describe the FITT prescription for cardiorespiratory fitness, muscular strength and endurance, and flexibility training.

LO 5 | Implementing Your Fitness Program

5. Why is core strength important? What are some ways to increase your core strength every day?

LO 6 | Taking in Proper Nutrition for Exercise

6. Why is when you eat as important as what you eat? How might your exercise preparation and routine differ in hot and cold climates?

LO 7 | Preventing and Treating Common Exercise Injuries

7. What precautions do you need to take when exercising outdoors in the heat and in the cold?

ACCESS YOUR HEALTH ON THE INTERNET

Visit **MasteringHealth** for links to the websites and RSS feeds.

The following websites explore further topics and issues related to personal health. For links to the websites below, visit the Study Area in MasteringHealth.

American College of Sports Medicine. This site is the link to the American College of Sports Medicine and all its resources. www.acsm.org

American Council on Exercise. Information is found here on exercise and disease prevention. www.acefitness.org

Centers for Disease Control and Prevention, National Center for Chronic Disease Prevention and Health Promotion, Division of Nutrition, Physical Activity, and Obesity. This site is a great resource for current information on exercise and health. www.cdc.gov/nccdphp/dnpao

National Strength and Conditioning Association. This site is a resource for personal trainers and others interested in conditioning and fitness. www.nsca-lift.org

12 Reducing Your Risk of Cardiovascular Disease and Cancer

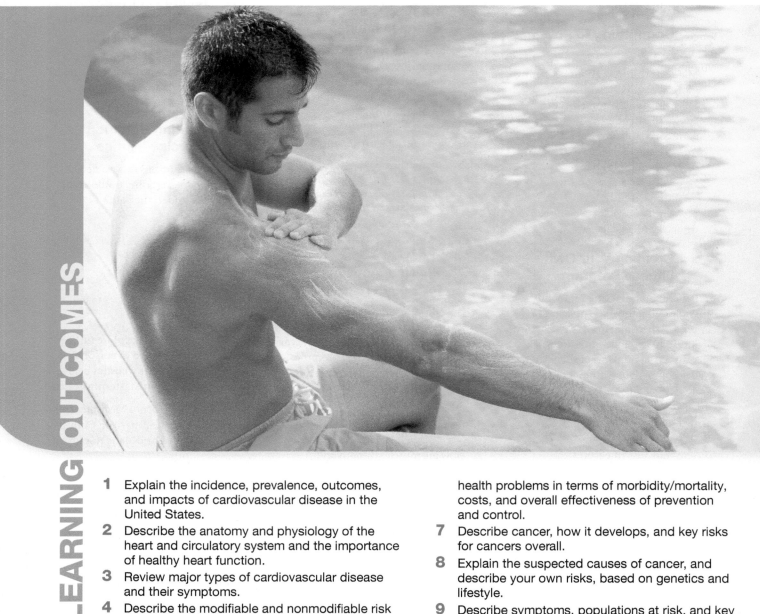

LEARNING OUTCOMES

1 Explain the incidence, prevalence, outcomes, and impacts of cardiovascular disease in the United States.

2 Describe the anatomy and physiology of the heart and circulatory system and the importance of healthy heart function.

3 Review major types of cardiovascular disease and their symptoms.

4 Describe the modifiable and nonmodifiable risk factors for cardiovascular disease and methods of prevention.

5 Examine current strategies for diagnosis and treatment of cardiovascular disease.

6 Describe the impact of cancer on people in the United States and compare it to other major

health problems in terms of morbidity/mortality, costs, and overall effectiveness of prevention and control.

7 Describe cancer, how it develops, and key risks for cancers overall.

8 Explain the suspected causes of cancer, and describe your own risks, based on genetics and lifestyle.

9 Describe symptoms, populations at risk, and key methods of prevention for the most common types of cancer.

10 Discuss cancer diagnosis and treatment, including radiotherapy and chemotherapy, and describe more recent developments in detection and treatment.

When we think of the major disease killers, images of older individuals dying after a long battle with *cancer* or succumbing to a fast and painful death from *cardiovascular disease* (CVD) like heart attack or stroke often come to mind. In reality, more often than not, cancer and CVD are long-term illnesses that exact a huge toll on individuals young and old, their loved ones, and society. In fact, these two categories of disease are among the greatest contributors to the **global burden of disease (GBD)**, a method of quantifying the burden of premature morbidity, disability, and death for a given disease or disease group.[1] GBD is measured in **disability adjusted years (DALYs)** or years lived in ill health or disability.[2] Today, people in many higher income regions of the world often live longer with diseases such as cancer and CVD due to earlier diagnosis, better treatments, and improved medicines, all of which increase disease costs. Diabetes, another major cause of global disease is discussed in **Focus On: Minimizing Your Risk for Diabetes** beginning on page 386.)

Even though death rates have declined and people may live longer, CVD continues to be the leading cause of death in the world, killing more than 17 million each year. If current trends continue, numbers are projected to grow to nearly 24 million by 2030.[3]

Like CVD, cancer is no slouch when it comes to exacting a heavy global burden. In 2012, over 14 million new cases of cancer were diagnosed and slightly over 8.2 million people died from cancer-related causes.[4] These rates are projected to soar to 21.7 million new cases and 13 million deaths by 2030.[5] Cancers of the lungs, stomach, liver, colon, and female breasts account for the largest percentage of cancer death.[6] Those living in poverty are hit hardest and have the worst prognosis once cancer or CVD are diagnosed, as resources necessary for early and comprehensive diagnosis and treatment are often lacking.[7]

Both CVD and cancer are **chronic diseases**, meaning they are prolonged, do not resolve spontaneously, and are rarely cured completely. As such, they are responsible for significant rates of disability, lost productivity, pain, and suffering, not to mention soaring health care costs. Cardiovascular diseases in particular are closely related to lifestyle factors such as obesity, sedentary behavior, poor nutrition, stress, lack of sleep, tobacco use, and excessive alcohol use. The good news is that in many cases, these lifestyle factors can be changed or modified to decrease disease risks for both CVD and cancer.

LO 1 | CARDIOVASCULAR DISEASE IN THE UNITED STATES

Explain the incidence, prevalence, outcomes, and impacts of cardiovascular disease in the United States.

Early in 2015, the American Heart Association (AHA) reported that death rates from **cardiovascular disease (CVD)**—diseases associated with the heart and blood vessels, such as high blood pressure, coronary heart disease (CHD), heart failure, stroke, and congenital cardiovascular defects—had declined by nearly 33 percent in the last decade.[8] Sounds great, doesn't it? In spite of the promising decline, nearly 86 million Americans, more than 1 out of every 3 adults, suffer from one or more types of CVD.[9]

Much of the improvement in death rates is due to better diagnosis, early intervention and treatment, and a multi-billion-dollar market in drugs designed to keep the heart and circulatory system ticking along. We've also improved our understanding about diet, activity, and other behaviors that impact risk of CVD. Yet, CVD continues to be a threat (**FIGURE 12.1**).[10] Nearly *one third* of all deaths in the United States have CVD as an underlying cause—more than cancer, chronic lower respiratory diseases, and accidental deaths combined.[11] Some populations are disproportionately affected; 48 percent of African American women and 46 percent of African American men have a variety of cardiovascular disease.[12]

global burden of disease (GBD) A method of quantifying the burden of premature morbidity, disability, and death for a given disease or disease groups.

disability adjusted life years (DALYs) A measure of overall disease burden expressed as the number of years lost due to ill-health.

chronic disease An illness that is prolonged, does not resolve spontaneously, and is rarely cured.

cardiovascular disease (CVD) Disease of the heart and blood vessels.

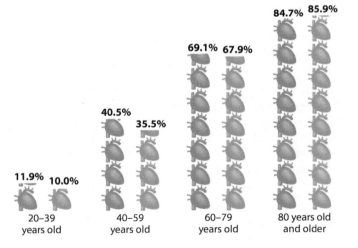

 Men with CVD; each heart = 10% of the population

Women with CVD; each heart = 10% of the population

FIGURE 12.1 **Prevalence of Cardiovascular Diseases (CVDs) in Adults Aged 20 and Older by Age and Sex**

Source: Data from D. Mozaffarian, et al. "Heart Disease and Stroke Statistics, 2015 Update," *Circulation* 131 (2015): e29–2322).

2,150

IS THE NUMBER OF AMERICANS WHO DIE EVERY DAY OF **CVD**. MILLIONS MORE ARE DISABLED OR TAKING MEDICATIONS TO KEEP THEIR CVD UNDER CONTROL.

Although these statistics are grim, the reality is that CVD has been the leading killer of both men and women in the United States every year since 1918, when a pandemic flu killed more people.[13] Recognizing that selected risk factors are key to changing the future course of CVD, the American Heart Association is aiming to improve Americans' cardiovascular health by 20 percent and to reduce death from CVDs and stroke by 20 percent—all by the year 2020.[14] As part of this strategy, the AHA is focusing on **ideal cardiovascular health (ICH)** rather than mortality rates and the disease process. ICH is defined as the absence of clinical indicators of CVD and the simultaneous presence of the following seven behavioral and health factor metrics.[15]

ideal cardiovascular health (ICH) The absence of clinical indicators of CVD and the presence of certain behavioral and health factor metrics.

cardiovascular system Organ system, consisting of the heart and blood vessels, that transports nutrients, oxygen, hormones, metabolic wastes, and enzymes throughout the body.

atria (singular: atrium) The heart's two upper chambers, which receive blood.

ventricles The heart's two lower chambers, which pump blood through the blood vessels.

Behaviors:
1. Not smoking
2. Recommended physical activity
3. A healthy diet pattern
4. A healthy weight

Health Factors:
5. Having optimal total cholesterol without medication
6. Having optimal blood pressure without medication
7. Having optimal fasting blood glucose without medication

How are we doing with respect to these ideal healthy heart measures today? Not so hot. Only 18 percent of U.S. adults meet five or more metrics with ideal levels, whereas 50 percent of children meet five or more metrics.[16] Clearly, we have a long way to go.

The best defense against CVD is to reduce your risks and prevent it from developing in the first place. Considerable research points to the fact that the sooner you start, the better![17]

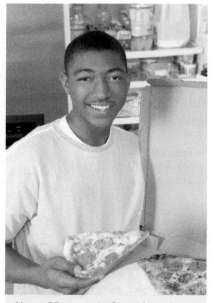

About 25 percent of your blood cholesterol level comes from foods you eat, and this is where you can make real improvements.

LO 2 | UNDERSTANDING THE CARDIOVASCULAR SYSTEM

Describe the anatomy and physiology of the heart and circulatory system and the importance of healthy heart function.

The **cardiovascular system** is the network of organs and vessels through which blood flows as it carries oxygen and nutrients to all parts of the body. It includes the *heart, arteries, arterioles* (small arteries), *veins, venules* (small veins), and *capillaries* (minute blood vessels). Understanding how your cardiovascular system works and the factors that can impair its functioning will help you understand your risk and how to reduce it.

The Heart: A Mighty Machine

The heart is a muscular, four-chambered pump, roughly the size of your fist. It is a highly efficient, extremely flexible organ that contracts 100,000 times each day and pumps the equivalent of 2,000 gallons of blood through the body. In a 70-year lifetime, an average human heart beats 2.5 billion times.

Under normal circumstances, the human body contains approximately 6 quarts of blood, which transports nutrients, oxygen, waste products, hormones, and enzymes throughout the body. Blood also aids in regulating body temperature, cellular water levels, and acidity levels of body components, and it helps defend the body against toxins and harmful microorganisms. An adequate blood supply is essential to health and well-being.

The heart has four chambers that work together to circulate blood constantly throughout the body. The two upper chambers of the heart, called **atria,** are large collecting chambers that receive blood from the rest of the body. The two lower chambers, known as **ventricles,** pump the blood out again. Small valves regulate the steady, rhythmic flow of blood between chambers and prevent leakage or backflow between them.

Heart Function Heart activity depends on a complex interaction of biochemical, physical, and neurological signals. Here are the four basic steps involved in heart function (see **FIGURE 12.2**):

1. Deoxygenated blood enters the right atrium after having been circulated through the body.
2. From the right atrium, blood moves to the right ventricle and is pumped through the pulmonary artery to the lungs, where it receives oxygen.

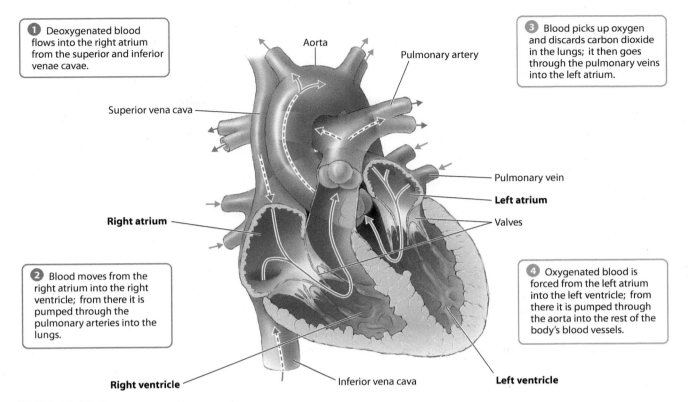

1. Deoxygenated blood flows into the right atrium from the superior and inferior venae cavae.

2. Blood moves from the right atrium into the right ventricle; from there it is pumped through the pulmonary arteries into the lungs.

3. Blood picks up oxygen and discards carbon dioxide in the lungs; it then goes through the pulmonary veins into the left atrium.

4. Oxygenated blood is forced from the left atrium into the left ventricle; from there it is pumped through the aorta into the rest of the body's blood vessels.

Aorta
Pulmonary artery
Superior vena cava
Pulmonary vein
Left atrium
Right atrium
Valves
Right ventricle
Inferior vena cava
Left ventricle

FIGURE 12.2 Blood Flow within the Heart

3. Oxygenated blood from the lungs then returns to the left atrium of the heart.
4. Blood from the left atrium moves into the left ventricle. The left ventricle pumps blood through the aorta to all body parts.

Various blood vessels perform different parts of this process. **Arteries** carry blood away from the heart; all arteries carry oxygenated blood, *except* for pulmonary arteries, which carry deoxygenated blood to the lungs, where the blood picks up oxygen and gives off carbon dioxide. As the arteries branch off from the heart, they branch into smaller blood vessels called **arterioles,** and then into even smaller blood vessels known as **capillaries.** Capillaries have thin walls that permit the exchange of oxygen, carbon dioxide, nutrients, and waste products with body cells. Carbon dioxide and other waste products are transported to the lungs and kidneys through **veins** and **venules** (small veins).

For the heart to function properly, the four chambers must beat in an organized manner. Your heartbeat is governed by an electrical impulse that directs the heart muscle to move when the impulse travels across it, resulting in a sequential contraction of the four chambers. This signal starts in a small bundle of highly specialized cells, the **sinoatrial node (SA node),** located in the right atrium. The SA node serves as a natural pacemaker for the heart. People with a damaged SA node must often have a mechanical pacemaker implanted to ensure the smooth passage of blood

through the heartbeat's sequential phases.

At rest, the average adult heart beats 70 to 80 times per minute; a well-conditioned heart may beat only 50 to 60 times per minute to achieve the same results. If your resting heart rate is routinely in the high 80s or 90s, it may indicate that you are out of shape or suffering from some underlying illness. When overly stressed, a heart may beat more than 200 times per minute. A healthy heart functions more efficiently and is less likely to suffer damage from overwork.

arteries Vessels that carry blood away from the heart to other regions of the body.

arterioles Branches of the arteries.

capillaries Minute blood vessels that branch out from the arterioles and venules; their thin walls permit exchange of oxygen, carbon dioxide, nutrients, and waste products among body cells.

veins Vessels that carry blood back to the heart from other regions of the body.

venules Branches of the veins.

sinoatrial node (SA node) Cluster of electric pulse–generating cells that serves as a natural pacemaker for the heart.

LO 3 | KEY CARDIOVASCULAR DISEASES

Review major types of cardiovascular disease and their symptoms.

Although there are several types of CVD and derivatives thereof, the key ones we will consider are hypertension, atherosclerosis, peripheral arterial disease (PAD), coronary heart disease (CHD), angina pectoris, arrhythmia, congestive heart

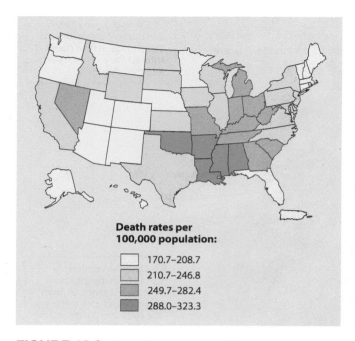

Death rates per 100,000 population:

- 170.7–208.7
- 210.7–246.8
- 249.7–282.4
- 288.0–323.3

FIGURE 12.3 Major Cardiovascular Disease Age-Adjusted Death Rates by State

Source: A. S. Go et al., "Heart Disease and Stroke Statistics—2014 Update: A Report from the American Heart Association," *Circulation* 129 (2014): e28–e292.

failure, and stroke. Many forms of CVD are potentially fatal, and FIGURE 12.3 presents the prevalence CVD-related deaths among adults in the United States.

Hypertension

Blood pressure measures how hard blood pushes against the walls of vessels as your heart pumps. Sustained high blood pressure is called **hypertension**. Known as the "silent killer," it has few overt symptoms. Untreated hypertension damages blood vessels and increases your chance of angina, heart failure, peripheral artery disease, stroke, and heart attack. Hypertension can also cause kidney damage and contribute to vision loss, erectile dysfunction, and memory problems.[18]

Today, nearly 1 in 3 adults in the United States have high blood pressure; based on current trends, rates may reach 41.4 percent by 2030.[19] There are large disparities in self-reported hypertension by race/ethnicity, age, sex, level of education, and state. At approximately 45 percent, African Americans have the highest rates of high blood pressure in the United States and globally.[20] Rates are also much higher among the elderly, men, and those who don't have a high school education.[21]

hypertension Sustained elevated blood pressure.

systolic blood pressure The upper number in the fraction that measures blood pressure, indicating pressure on the walls of the arteries when the heart contracts.

diastolic blood pressure The lower number in the fraction that measures blood pressure, indicating pressure on the walls of the arteries during the relaxation phase of heart activity.

prehypertensive Blood pressure is above normal, but not yet in the hypertensive range.

Although awareness of hypertension has increased and most diagnosed individuals are using hypertension medications, only 53 percent of those on meds have their hypertension under control.[22] Blood pressure is measured by two numbers, for example, 110/80 mm Hg, stated as "110 over 80 millimeters of mercury." The top number, **systolic blood pressure**, refers to the pressure of blood in the arteries when the heart muscle contracts, sending blood to the rest of the body. The bottom number, **diastolic blood pressure**, refers to the pressure of blood on the arteries when the heart muscle relaxes, as blood is reentering the heart chambers. Normal blood pressure varies depending on age, weight, and physical condition, and high blood pressure is usually diagnosed when systolic pressure is 140 or above (see TABLE 12.1). When only systolic pressure is high, the condition is known as *isolated systolic hypertension (ISH)*, the most common form of high blood pressure in older Americans.

Systolic blood pressure tends to increase with age, whereas diastolic blood pressure typically increases until age 55 and then declines. Men under the age of 45 are at nearly twice the risk of becoming hypertensive as their female counterparts and have an increased risk of dying of vascular disease within 10 years of a stroke.[23] Women tend to have higher rates of hypertension after age 65.[24] More and more people (over 30 percent of the population) are considered to be **prehypertensive**, meaning that their blood pressure is above normal, but not yet in the hypertensive range. These individuals have a significantly greater risk of becoming hypertensive.[25]

New guidelines for the management/treatment of high blood pressure among those with a history of diabetes, heart disease, or stroke are available. In general, guidelines for treating and managing high blood pressure provide information about maintaining lower blood pressure levels, recommending certain types of meds, as well as optimal times to begin medicating. People 65 and over are usually put on meds when their blood pressure is 150/90 or higher; those under 60 years of age are recommended to take medications at 140/90 or higher,

TABLE 12.1 | Blood Pressure Classifications

Classification	Systolic Reading (mm Hg)		Diastolic Reading (mm Hg)
Normal	Less than 120	and	Less than 80
Prehypertension	120–139	or	80–89
Hypertension			
Stage 1	140–159	or	90–99
Stage 2	Greater than or equal to 160	or	Greater than or equal to 100
Hypertensive crisis	Greater than or equal to 180	or	Greater than or equal to 110

Source: The American Heart Association, "Understanding Blood Pressure Readings," 2015, http://www.heart.org/HEARTORG/Conditions/HighBloodPressure/HighBloodPressure/Understanding-Blood-Pressure-Readings_UCM_301764_Article.jsp

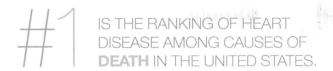

#1

IS THE RANKING OF HEART
DISEASE AMONG CAUSES OF
DEATH IN THE UNITED STATES.

especially if they have kidney disease or diabetes. At current rates, more and more people will begin heart meds at younger and younger ages.[26]

Atherosclerosis

Arteriosclerosis, thickening and hardening of arteries, is a condition that underlies many cardiovascular health problems. **Atherosclerosis** is a type of arteriosclerosis, where fatty substances, cholesterol, cellular waste products, calcium, and fibrin (a clotting material in the blood) accumulate in the inner lining of an artery. *Hyperlipidemia* (abnormally high blood levels of *lipids,* which are non-water-soluble molecules, such as fats and cholesterol) is a key factor in this process, and the resulting buildup is referred to as **plaque.**

As plaque accumulates, it adheres to the inner lining of the blood vessels. Vessel walls become narrow and may eventually block blood flow or rupture. This is similar to putting your thumb over the end of a hose while water is running through it. Pressure builds within arteries just as pressure builds in the hose. If vessels are weakened and pressure persists, the artery may become weak and eventually burst. Fluctuation in the blood pressure levels within arteries may actually damage their internal walls, making it even more likely that plaque will accumulate.

Atherosclerosis is the most common form of *coronary artery disease (CAD).* It occurs as plaques are deposited in vessel walls and restrict blood flow and oxygen to the body's main coronary arteries on the outer surface of the heart, often eventually resulting in a heart attack (see **FIGURE 12.4**). When circulation is impaired and blood flow to the heart is limited, the heart may become starved for oxygen—a condition commonly referred to as **ischemia.** Sometimes coronary artery disease is referred to as ischemic heart disease.

Peripheral Artery Disease

When atherosclerosis occurs in the upper or lower extremities, such as in the arms, feet, calves, or legs, and causes narrowing or complete blockage of arteries, it is often called **peripheral artery disease (PAD).** In the United States, over 8.5 million

> **arteriosclerosis** A general term for thickening and hardening of the arteries.
>
> **atherosclerosis** Condition characterized by deposits of fatty substances (plaque) on the inner lining of an artery.
>
> **plaque** Buildup of deposits in the arteries.
>
> **ischemia** Reduced oxygen supply to a body part or organ.
>
> **peripheral artery disease (PAD)** Atherosclerosis occurring in the lower extremities, such as in the feet, calves, or legs, or in the arms.

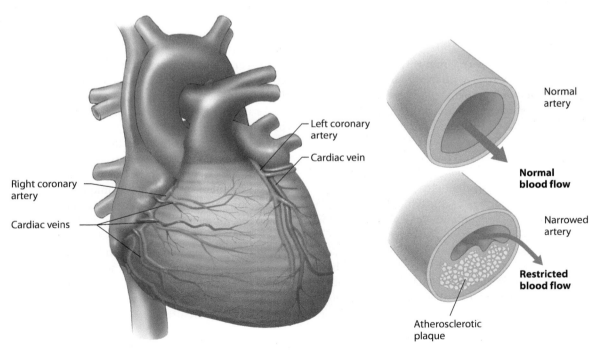

Left coronary artery

Cardiac vein

Right coronary artery

Cardiac veins

Normal artery

Normal blood flow

Narrowed artery

Restricted blood flow

Atherosclerotic plaque

FIGURE 12.4 Atherosclerosis and Coronary Heart Disease The coronary arteries are located on the exterior of the heart and supply blood and oxygen to the heart muscle itself. In atherosclerosis, arteries become clogged by a buildup of plaque. When atherosclerosis occurs in coronary arteries, blood flow to the heart muscle is restricted and a heart attack may occur.

Sources: Adapted from Joan Salge Blake, *Nutrition & You*, and Michael D. Johnson, *Human: Biology: Concepts and Current Issues*, 7th ed. Both copyright © 2014 Pearson Education, Inc. Reprinted by permission.

▶ **VIDEO TUTOR**
Atherosclerosis and
Coronary Artery Disease

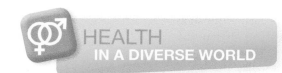
WOMEN AND HEART ATTACKS

"Having a heart attack" usually brings to mind an older man gasping for breath, clutching his chest, toppling over in the middle of a workout. So, the story of comedian and former talk show host Rosie O'Donnell's heart attack doesn't seem to fit the mold: O'Donnell, 50, didn't immediately know she'd had one. At first, she wondered if she might have strained a muscle. Later she felt hot, clammy, and vomited. Fortunately, she took an aspirin and eventually went to the doctor, despite initially doubting a serious problem. It turned out O'Donnell had an almost complete blockage of a heart artery that required a stent.

Unfortunately, Rosie isn't alone. In fact, heart disease is the number one killer of women, affecting 1 out of every 3 in the United States. Like many chronic diseases, certain populations are disproportionately affected, in part because of late access to diagnosis and treatment—largely the result of being uninsured or underinsured, and

lack of nearby information/resources about symptoms and risks. Nearly half of African American women have heart disease.

In addition to the above, women's heart attack symptoms often don't "look" like what people have come to expect. Women who suffer heart attacks under the age of 55 are not only less likely to have classic chest pain or pressure, but they also tend to delay going to the doctor. When they do seek medical attention, they often report atypical symptoms, such as shortness of breath, or pain in the neck, shoulder, arms, and stomach. Many women chalk up heart symptoms to stress, flu, or lack of exercise. Because of treatment delays, women are more likely to have heart damage and to die from a heart attack than are men of the same age.

So how can a woman tell if she is having a heart attack? In addition to the symptoms already mentioned, women may experience chest pressure or pain; radiating pains in the arms, shoulder, neck, jaw,

or back; dizziness; abdominal pain; and unexplained feelings of fatigue, anxiety, or weakness—especially during exertion. But the real answer to the question of how to tell if a woman is having a heart attack is this: *Let a doctor* determine that. If you or someone you know has even a few of these symptoms, don't delay. Crush or chew a full strength aspirin and swallow it with water. In addition to being a pain killer, aspirin has blood-thinning properties; taking one can prevent fatal blood clots from forming. Then, have someone drive you to a health care facility for evaluation, or call 9-1-1 to get an ambulance.

Sources: J. Cant, W. J. Rogers, R. J. Goldberg, et al., "Association of Age and Sex with Myocardial Infarction Symptom Presentation and In-Hospital Mortality," *Journal of the American Medical Association* 307, no. 8 (2012,): 813–22; National Coalition for Women with Heart Disease, "Women Heart, Are You Having a Heart Attack?," 2014, www.heart.org/HEARTORG/Conditions/HeartAttack/WarningSignsofaHeartAttack/Angina-in-Women-Can-Be-Different-Than-Men. 2015_UCM_448902_Article.jsp

---

people—particularly people over 65, non-Hispanic blacks, and women—have PAD; many receive no treatment because they are asymptomatic or don't recognize symptoms until they have a heart attack or stroke.[27] Others have pain and aching in the legs, calves, or feet upon walking/exercising, relieved by rest (known as *intermittent claudication*). PAD is a leading cause of disability in people over the age of 50. While it strikes both men and women, men develop it more frequently. Risk factors include inflammation, smoking, high blood pressure, high cholesterol, and diabetes.[28] Sometimes PAD in the arms can be caused by trauma, certain diseases, radiation therapy, or repetitive motion syndrome, or the combined risks of these factors and atherosclerosis.

> **coronary heart disease (CHD)** A narrowing of the small blood vessels that supply blood to the heart.
>
> **myocardial infarction (MI; heart attack)** A blockage of normal blood supply to an area in the heart.
>
> **angina pectoris** Chest pain occurring as a result of reduced oxygen flow to the heart.

Coronary Heart Disease

Of all the major cardiovascular diseases, **coronary heart disease (CHD)** is the greatest killer, accounting for nearly 1 in 7 deaths in the United States. Nearly 1 million new and recurrent heart attacks occur in the United States each year.[29] A **myocardial infarction (MI)**, or **heart attack**, involves an area

of the heart that suffers permanent damage because its normal blood supply has been blocked—often brought on by a blood clot in a coronary artery or an atherosclerotic narrowing that blocks an artery. When blood does not flow readily, there is a corresponding decrease in oxygen flow. If the blockage is extremely minor, an otherwise healthy heart will adapt over time by enlarging existing blood vessels and growing new ones to reroute blood through other areas. Some populations, particularly women, seem to have unique symptoms and fare worse upon having a heart attack than do others. For a variety of reasons, women are more likely to die after a first heart attack than men are.[30] (See the Health in a Diverse World box for more information on women and heart attacks.)

When heart blockage is more severe, however, the body is unable to adapt on its own, and outside lifesaving support is critical. See the Skills for Behavior Change box to learn what to do in case of a heart attack.

Angina Pectoris

Angina pectoris is a symptom of CHD that occurs when there is not enough oxygen to supply the heart muscle. Nearly 8 million people in the United States suffer from angina symptoms, ranging from indigestion or heartburn-like symptoms to palpitations and crushing chest pain.[31] Although angina pectoris is not a heart attack, it is an indicator of underlying heart

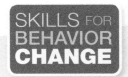
disease. Mild cases may be treated with rest. Drugs such as *nitroglycerin* can dilate veins and provide pain relief. Other medications such as *calcium channel blockers* can relieve cardiac spasms and arrhythmias, lower blood pressure, and slow heart rate. *Beta-blockers* can control potential overactivity of the heart muscle.

Arrhythmias

Over the course of a lifetime, most people experience some type of **arrhythmia**, an irregularity in heart rhythm that occurs when the electrical impulses in the heart that coordinate heartbeat don't work properly. Often described as a heart "fluttering" or racing, these irregularities send many people to the emergency room, only to find they are fine. A racing heart in the absence of exercise or anxiety may be experiencing *tachycardia*, the medical term for abnormally fast heartbeat. On the other end of the continuum is *bradycardia*, or abnormally slow heartbeat. When a heart goes into **fibrillation**, it beats in a sporadic, quivering pattern, resulting in extreme inefficiency in moving blood through the cardiovascular system. If untreated, fibrillation may be fatal.

Not all arrhythmias are life-threatening. In many instances, excessive caffeine or nicotine consumption can trigger an episode. However, severe cases may require drug therapy or external electrical stimulus to prevent serious complications. When in doubt, check with your doctor.

Heart Failure

When the heart muscle is damaged or overworked and lacks the strength to keep blood circulating normally through the body, blood and fluids begin to back up into the lungs and other body tissues, continuing on to the feet, ankles, and legs, along with shortness of breath and tiredness. Known as **heart failure** or **congestive heart failure,** this condition is increasingly common, particularly among those with a history of other heart problems. Nearly 5.7 million adults have heart failure in the United States, with cases estimated to approach 10 million by 2030.[32]

Underlying causes of heart failure may include heart injury from CVD risks, including uncontrolled high blood pressure, rheumatic fever, pneumonia, heart attack, uncontrolled sleep apnea, or other problems. Certain prescription drugs such as NSAIDS and diabetes medications also increase risks, as do chronic drug and alcohol abuse. In some cases, radiation or chemotherapy treatments for cancer cause damage.

Untreated, heart failure can be fatal. However, most cases respond well to treatment that includes *diuretics* ("water pills") to relieve fluid accumulation; drugs, such as *digitalis,* that increase the pumping action of the heart; and drugs called *vasodilators,* which expand blood vessels and decrease resistance, allowing blood to flow more freely and making the heart's work easier.

Stroke

Like heart muscle, brain cells require a continuous supply of oxygen. A **stroke** (also called a *cerebrovascular accident*) occurs when blood supply to the brain is interrupted. Strokes may be either *ischemic* (caused by plaque formation that narrows blood flow or a clot that obstructs a blood vessel) or *hemorrhagic* (due to a weakening of a blood vessel that causes it to bulge or rupture). An **aneurysm** (a widening or bulge in a blood vessel that may become hemorrhagic) is the most well-known of the hemorrhagic strokes. When any of these events occurs, oxygen deprivation kills brain cells.

Some strokes are mild and cause only temporary dizziness or slight weakness or numbness. More serious interruptions in blood flow may impair speech, swallowing, memory, or motor control in the long term. Other strokes affect parts of the brain that regulate heart and lung function, killing within minutes. According to the American Heart Association, nearly 7 million

arrhythmia An irregularity in heartbeat.

fibrillation A sporadic, quivering pattern of heartbeat that results in extreme inefficiency in moving blood through the cardiovascular system.

congestive heart failure (CHF) An abnormal cardiovascular condition that reflects impaired cardiac pumping and blood flow; pooling blood leads to congestion in body tissues.

stroke A condition occurring when the brain is damaged by disrupted blood supply; also called cerebrovascular accident.

aneurysm A weakened blood vessel that may bulge under pressure and, in severe cases, burst.

transient ischemic attacks (TIAs) Brief interruption of the blood supply to the brain that causes only temporary impairment; often an indicator of impending major stroke.

Americans suffer a stroke every year, and almost 129,000 people die as a result, making it the fourth leading cause of death in the United States.[33] Strokes cause countless levels of disability and suffering; depression is often an issue with patients recovering from strokes.

Even scarier, more young people are having strokes than ever before, possibly due to increased obesity and hypertension.[34] Many strokes are preceded days, weeks, or months earlier by **transient ischemic attacks (TIAs)**, brief interruptions of the blood supply to the brain that cause only temporary impairment. Symptoms of TIAs include dizziness, particularly when first rising in the morning, weakness, temporary paralysis or numbness in the face or other regions, temporary memory loss, blurred vision, nausea, headache, slurred speech, or other unusual physiological reactions. Some people may experience unexpected falls or have blackouts; however, others may have no obvious symptoms. TIAs often indicate an impending major stroke. The earlier a stroke is recognized and treatment started (best results are seen if treatment begins within the first 1–2 hours), the more effective that treatment will be. See the Skills for Behavior Change box for tips on recognizing signs and symptoms of a possible stroke.

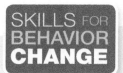

SKILLS FOR BEHAVIOR CHANGE

A SIMPLE TEST FOR STROKE

People often ignore, minimize, or misunderstand stroke symptoms. Starting treatment within just a few hours is crucial for the best recovery outcomes. So if you suspect someone is having a stroke, use the tool many emergency teams use to assess what is happening: think FAST.

▶ Facial droop: Ask the person to smile. It is normal for both sides of the face to move equally, and it is abnormal if one side moves less easily.

▶ Arm weakness: Ask the person to raise both arms. It is normal if both arms move equally (or not at all). It is abnormal if one arm drifts or cannot be raised as high as the other.

▶ Speech difficulty: Have the patient restate a sentence such as, You can't teach an old dog new tricks." It is normal if they can say the sentence correctly, and it is abnormal if they use inappropriate words, slur, or cannot speak.

▶ Time to *act* and call 9-1-1. Don't delay if you note 1–3 above. Time is of the essence.

Source: Centers for Disease Control, "Stroke Signs and Symptoms," April 2015, www.cdc.gov/stroke/signs_symptoms.htm

One of the greatest U.S. medical successes in recent years has been the decline in stroke fatality rates, which have dropped by one third since the 1980s and continue to fall.[35] Greater awareness of stroke symptoms and faster medical attention, improvements in emergency medicine protocols and medicines, and a greater emphasis on fast rehabilitation and therapy after a stroke have helped many survive. Newer treatments, including *tissue plasminogen activator* or *tPA*, the only FDA-approved treatment for ischemic stroke, dissolves clots and improves blood flow to affected areas, resulting in less damage and better chances of recovery. Various surgical techniques and mechanical devices are being tested that may further improve prognosis for future stroke victims.[36]

LO 4 | REDUCING YOUR RISKS

Describe the modifiable and nonmodifiable risk factors for cardiovascular disease and methods of prevention.

Recently, the U.S. Burden of Disease Collaborators determined that greatest contributor to CVD was suboptimal diet, followed by tobacco smoking, high body mass index, high blood pressure, high fasting plasma glucose, and physical inactivity.[37] Newer research indicates that for people aged 12 to 39, smoking, high body fat, and high blood glucose increase the chances of dying from CVD-related complications before age 60.[38] As mentioned previously, hypertension doesn't just

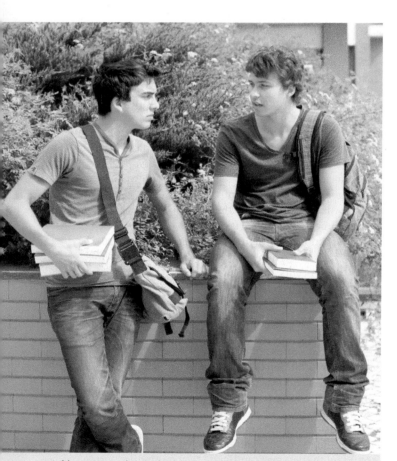

Young men, in particular, are at an elevated risk for stroke.

wreak havoc with your heart and circulatory system; it may eventually lead to cognitive function declines and may increase risk for Alzheimer's disease.[39] **Cardiometabolic risks** are the combined risks that indicate physical and biochemical changes that can lead to both CVD and type 2 diabetes. Some of these risks result from choices and behaviors, and so are modifiable. Others are inherited or intrinsic (such as your age and gender) and cannot be modified.

Metabolic Syndrome: Quick Risk Profile

A cluster of combined cardiometabolic risks, variably labeled as *syndrome X, insulin resistance syndrome,* and, most recently, **metabolic syndrome** are believed to increase the risk for atherosclerotic heart disease by as much as three times the normal rates. Women are more likely than men to have metabolic syndrome overall. Nearly 23 percent of whites, 19 percent of African Americans, and 34.8 percent of Mexican Americans meet the criteria for metabolic syndrome.[40] Although different professional organizations have slightly different criteria for the syndrome, the National Cholesterol Education Program's Adult Treatment Panel (NCEP/ATP III) is most commonly used. According to these criteria, a person with three or more of the following risks is diagnosed with metabolic syndrome:[41]

- Abdominal obesity (waist measurement of more than 40 inches in men or 35 inches in women).
- Elevated blood fat (triglycerides greater than 150) or on drug treatment for elevated triglycerides
- Low levels of HDL ("good") cholesterol (less than 40 in men and less than 50 in women) or on drug treatment for HDL reduction
- Elevated blood pressure greater than 130/85 or on drug treatment for BP reduction
- Elevated fasting glucose greater than 100 mg/dL (a sign of insulin resistance or glucose intolerance) or on drug treatment for elevated glucose

Metabolic syndrome and other, similar terms have been important for highlighting the relationship between the number of risks a person possesses and that person's likelihood of developing CVD and diabetes. Groups such as the AHA and others are giving increased attention to focusing on multiple risks and emphasizing cardiovascular health in lifestyle interventions.

Modifiable Risks

It may surprise you that younger adults are not invulnerable to CVD risks. The reality is that from the first moments of your life, you begin to accumulate increasing numbers of risks. Your past and future lifestyle choices may haunt you as you enter your middle and later years of life. Behaviors you choose today and over the coming decades can actively reduce or promote your risk for CVD.[42]

Avoid Tobacco Today, approximately 21 percent of U.S. adults age 18 and over are regular smokers in spite of massive efforts aimed at prevention and control (see Chapter 8).[43] Just how great a risk is smoking when it comes to CVD? Consider this:[44]

- Smokers are two to four times more likely to develop CHD than nonsmokers.
- Cigarette smoking doubles a person's stroke risk.
- Smokers are over 10 times more likely to develop peripheral vascular diseases than nonsmokers.

Some believe that nicotine in tobacco forces the heart to work harder to obtain sufficient oxygen. Other chemicals in smoke are thought to damage and inflame the lining of the coronary arteries, allowing cholesterol and plaque to accumulate more easily, increasing blood pressure and forcing the heart to work harder.

The good news is that if you stop smoking, your heart begins to mend itself. After 1 year, a former smoker's risk of heart disease drops by 50 percent. Between 5 to 15 years after quitting, the risk of stroke and CHD becomes similar to that of nonsmokers. Younger, college-age students take note: Studies have shown that those who quit smoking at age 30 reduce their chance of dying prematurely from smoking-related diseases by more than 90 percent.[45]

> **cardiometabolic risks** Risk factors that impact both the cardiovascular system and the body's biochemical metabolic processes.
>
> **metabolic syndrome (MetS)** A group of metabolic conditions occurring together that increases a person's risk of heart disease, stroke, and diabetes.

Cut Back on Saturated Fat and Cholesterol

Cholesterol is a fatty, waxy substance found in the bloodstream and in body cells. Although we tend to hear only bad things about it, in truth, cholesterol plays an important role in the production of cell membranes and hormones and in other body functions. However, when blood cholesterol levels get

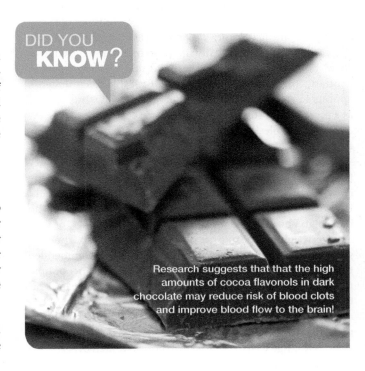

DID YOU **KNOW**?

Research suggests that that the high amounts of cocoa flavonols in dark chocolate may reduce risk of blood clots and improve blood flow to the brain!

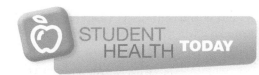
IS CHOLESTEROL SO BAD?

When blood cholesterol levels get too high, the consensus until recently has been that CVD risk escalates. According to new ACC/AHA report, things might not be quite so black and white. In the report:

- Cholesterol is redeemed as *not being the major culprit* in artery clogging atherosclerosis. Instead, the report suggests we should be limiting saturated and avoiding *trans* fats. That means that eggs and shrimp, which are low in fat and high in protein, are taken off the "eat very little" list.

- Fruits and vegetables get a boost as being beneficial for all potential health outcomes.
- A *healthy diet,* including increases in fruits and vegetables, whole grains, low-fat and non-fat (low-sugar) foods, seafood, legumes, and nuts is emphasized.
- Sugar is a "no no." Intake should be limited to 12 teaspoons per day (less than a can of soda!). Right now, Americans consume over double that amount each day.
- Coffee gets a boost due to its antioxidant benefits.

- Salt consumption recommendations are reduced.

Until we learn more, current recommendations are to consume a balanced, plant-based diet such as the Mediterranean diet.

Sources: N.J Stone et al., "ACC/AHA Guidelines on the Treatment of Blood Cholesterol to Reduce Atherosclerotic Cardiovascular Risk in Adult: A Report of the American College of Cardiology/American Heart Association Task force on Practice Guidelines," *Circulation* 129 (2014): S1-S45; N. Stone et al., "Treatment of Blood Cholesterol to Reduce Atherosclerotic Cardiovascular Disease Risk in Adults: Synopsis of the 2013 American College of Cardiology/American Heart Association Cholesterol Guidelines," *Annals of Internal Medicine* 160, no. 5 (2014): 339–43.

---

too high, CVD risk escalates. See **Student Health Today** for info on the gray area around cholesterol.

Seventy-five percent of blood cholesterol is produced by your liver and other cells—mostly out of your control. The other 25 percent comes from the foods you eat. Changing your diet can make real improvements in your overall cholesterol level, even if your total amount is naturally high.

Diets high in saturated fat and *trans* fats are known to raise cholesterol levels, send the body's blood-clotting system into high gear, and make blood more viscous in just a few hours, increasing the risk of heart attack or stroke. Increased blood levels of cholesterol also contribute to atherosclerosis. Total cholesterol level isn't the only level to be concerned about; the type of cholesterol also matters. The two major types of blood cholesterol are *low-density lipoprotein (LDL)* and *high-density lipoprotein (HDL)*. Low-density lipoprotein, often referred to as "bad" cholesterol, is believed to build up on artery walls. In contrast, high-density lipoprotein, or "good" cholesterol, appears to remove cholesterol from artery walls, thus serving as a protector. In theory, if LDL levels get too high or HDL levels too low, cholesterol will accumulate inside arteries and lead to cardiovascular problems.

Triglycerides have also gained increasing attention as a key factor in CVD risk. When you consume extra calories, the body converts them to triglycerides, which are stored in fat cells. High levels of blood triglycerides are often found in people who have high cholesterol levels, heart problems, diabetes, or who are overweight. As people get older, heavier, or both, their triglyceride and cholesterol levels tend to rise. It is recommended that a baseline cholesterol test (known as a lipid panel or lipid profile) be taken at age 20, with follow-ups every 5 years. This test, which measures triglyceride levels as well as HDL, LDL, and total cholesterol levels, requires that you fast for 12 hours prior to the test, are well hydrated, and avoid coffee and tea prior to testing. Men over the age of 35 and women over the age

of 45 should have their lipid profile checked annually, with more frequent tests for those at high risk. See **TABLE 12.2** for current recommended levels of cholesterol and triglycerides.

TABLE **12.2** | Recommended Cholesterol Levels for Lower/Moderate Risk Adults

Total Cholesterol Level (lower numbers are better)	
Less than 200 mg/dL	Desirable
200–239 mg/dL	Borderline high
240 mg/dL and above	High
HDL Cholesterol Level (higher numbers are better)	
Less than 40 mg/dL (for men)	Low
60 mg/dL and above	Desirable
LDL Cholesterol Level (lower numbers are better)	
Less than 100 mg/dL	Optimal
100–129 mg/dL	Near or above optimal
130–159 mg/dL	Borderline high
160–189 mg/dL	High
190 mg/dL and above	Very high
Triglyceride Level (lower numbers are better)	
Less than 150 mg/dL	Normal
150–199 mg/dL	Borderline high
200–499 mg/dL	High
500 mg/dL and above	Very high

Source: Adapted from National Heart, Lung, and Blood Institute, National Institutes of Health, *ATP III Guidelines At-A-Glance Quick Desk Reference,* NIH Publication No. 01-3305, Update on Cholesterol Guidelines, 2004, www.nhlbi.nih.gov

SEE IT! VIDEOS

What habits can you change now to improve your heart health? Watch **Importance of Heart Health in Your Youth,** on MasteringHealth™

In general, LDL (or "bad" cholesterol) is more closely associated with cardiovascular risk than is total cholesterol. Until recently, most authorities agreed that looking only at LDL ignored the positive effects of "good" cholesterol (HDL) and that raising HDL was an important goal. There has been general agreement that the best method of evaluating risk is to examine the ratio of HDL to total cholesterol. If the level of HDL is lower than 35 mg/dL, cardiovascular risk increases dramatically. To reduce risk, the goal has been to manage the ratio of HDL to total cholesterol by lowering LDL levels, raising HDL, or both. New research indicates that trying to raise HDL as a means of preventing negative CVD outcomes may not be as beneficial as once thought.[46]

Drugs that were effective in raising HDL levels had little or no effect on CVD risks or mortality. Regular exercise and a healthy diet low in saturated fat continue to be the best methods for maintaining healthy ratios. See the **Health Headlines** box on page 366 for information about foods and dietary practices that can help maintain healthy cholesterol levels.

About 45 percent of adults aged 20 and over have cholesterol levels at or above 200 mg/dL, and another 16 percent have levels in excess of 240 mg/dL.[47] Over half of all men aged 65 and over and nearly 40 percent of all women aged 65 or older are taking antihyperlipidemia prescription drugs and other medications to reduce blood fats.[48]

Maintain a Healthy Weight Researchers are not sure whether high-fat, high-sugar, high-calorie diets are a direct risk for CVD or whether they invite risk by causing obesity, which strains the heart, forcing it to push blood through the many miles of capillaries that supply each pound of fat. A heart that has to continuously move blood through an overabundance of vessels may become damaged. Overweight people are more likely to develop heart disease and stroke even if they have no other risk factors. This is especially true if you're an "apple" (thicker around your upper body and waist) rather than a "pear" (thicker around your hips and thighs).

Exercise Regularly Even modest levels of low-intensity physical activity—walking, gardening, housework, dancing—are beneficial if done regularly and over the long term. Exercise can increase HDL, lower triglycerides, and reduce coronary risks in several ways.

Control Diabetes Heart disease death rates among adults with diabetes are two to four times higher than the rates for adults without diabetes. At least 65 percent of people with diabetes die of some form of heart disease or stroke.[49] However, through a prescribed regimen of diet, exercise, and medication, they can control much of their increased risk for CVD. (See **Focus On: Minimizing Your Risk for Diabetes** starting on page 386 for more on preventing and controlling diabetes.)

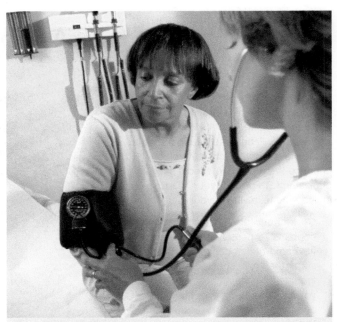

While many behavioral and environmental factors contribute to a person's risk for cardiovascular diseases, research suggests hereditary culprits, too. Find out your family history of CVD and have regular blood pressure and blood cholesterol screenings, as well as avoid lifestyle risks.

Control Your Blood Pressure In general, the higher your blood pressure, the greater your risk for CVD. Key factors in increasing blood pressure include obesity, lack of exercise, atherosclerosis, kidney damage from diabetes complications, and other factors.[50] Treatment of hypertension can involve dietary changes (avoiding high sodium and processed foods and cutting calories when appropriate),[51] medication, regular exercise, controlling stress, and getting enough sleep.

Manage Stress In recent years, scientists have shown compelling evidence that both acute and chronic stress may trigger acute cardiac events or even sudden cardiac death, as well as increase risks of hypertension, stroke, and elevated cholesterol levels.[52] Financial stressors, pressure to succeed in college and get a great job, pressure to find a partner, and pressure to please significant others can have a tsunamis-like effect on people young and old.[53] See Chapter 3 for more on effects of and coping with stress.

Nonmodifiable Risks

Unfortunately, not all risk factors for CVD can be prevented or controlled. The most important are the following:

- **Race and ethnicity.** African Americans tend to have the highest overall rates of CVD and hypertension and the lowest rates of physical activity. Mexican Americans have the highest percentage of adults with cholesterol levels exceeding 200 mg/dL and the highest rates of obesity and overweight.[54]

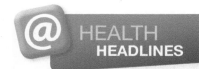
HEART-HEALTHY SUPER FOODS

The foods you eat play a major role in your CVD risk. While many foods can increase your risk, several have been shown to reduce the chances that cholesterol will be absorbed in the cells, reduce levels of LDL cholesterol, or enhance the protective effects of HDL cholesterol. To protect your heart, include the following in your diet:

- **Dark chocolate.** Dark chocolate contains 70 percent or more of flavonoid-rich cocoa, and much less sugar than milk chocolate. If you must indulge, buy the highest percent cocoa you can find, and savor the 1 to 2 ounces a bit at a time. Moderation is the key.
- **Fish high in omega-3 fatty acids.** Consumption of fish such as salmon, sardines, and herring may help reduce blood pressure and the inflammation that leads to plaque formation; however, new research is showing conflicting results about the benefits of omega-3s.
- **Olive oil.** Using monounsaturated fats in cooking, particularly extra virgin olive oil, helps lower total cholesterol and raise your HDL levels. Canola oil; margarine labeled *trans* fat–free; and cholesterol-lowering margarines such as Benecol, Promise Activ, or Smart Balance are also excellent choices.
- **Whole grains and fiber.** Getting enough fiber each day in the form of 100 percent whole wheat, steel cut oats, oat bran, flaxseed, fruits, and vegetables helps lower LDL or bad cholesterol. Soluble fiber, in particular, seems to keep cholesterol from being absorbed in the intestines.

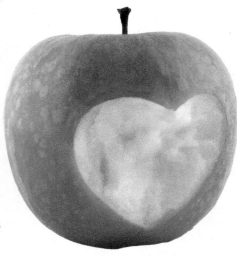

While an "apple a day" may not keep the proverbial doctor away, making sure that fruits and vegetables are part of a balanced diet is key to risk reduction for CVD and other health issues.

- **Plant sterols and stanols.** These essential components of plant membranes are found naturally in vegetables, fruits, and legumes. In addition, many food products, including juices and yogurt, are now fortified with them. These compounds are believed to benefit your heart health by blocking cholesterol absorption in the bloodstream, thus reducing LDL levels.
- **Nuts.** Long maligned for being high in calories, walnuts, almonds, and other nuts are naturally high in omega-3 fatty acids, which are important in lowering cholesterol and good for the blood vessels themselves.
- **Green tea.** Several studies have indicated that green tea may reduce LDL cholesterol. The flavonoids in it act as powerful antioxidants that may protect the cells of the heart and blood vessels;

however, other studies indicate that the FDA should *not* endorse health claims for green tea. Research in support is methodologically weak, and there are safety issues with the wide range of unfiltered tea available on the market.

- **Red wine.** In recent years, many observational studies have indicated that one glass of red wine may be protective and reduce your risk of CHD. Although the research is promising, the American Heart Association is slow to endorse drinking alcohol to reduce CVD risk and instead recommends dietary modification, exercise, and stress reduction, while supporting additional research. While one drink of red wine might be protective, adding additional doses of wine won't help and, in fact, is likely to be harmful.

Sources: L. Hooper, C. Kay, A. Abdelhamid et al., "Effects of Chocolate, Cocoa, and Flavan-3-ols on Cardiovascular Health: A Systematic Review and Meta-Analysis of Randomized Trials," *American Journal of Clinical Nutrition* 95, no. 3 (2012): 740–51; American Heart Association, "Alcoholic Beverages and Cardiovascular Disease," 2014, www.heart.org/HEARTORG/GettingHealthy/Nutrition-Center/HealthyEating/Alcohol-and-Heart-Health_UCM_305173_Article.jsp; P. Ronksley, S. Brien, B. Turner et al., "Association of Alcohol Consumption with Selected Cardiovascular Disease Outcomes: A Systematic Review and Meta-Analysis," *British Medical Journal* 342 (2011): 671–81; S. Kalesi, J. Sun, and N. Buys, "Green Tea Catechins and Blood Pressure: A Systematic Review and Meta Analysis of Randomized Controlled Trials," *European Journal of Nutrition,* May 2014, doi: 10.1007/s00394-014-0720-1; M. Murray, C. Walcuk, M. Suh, and P. J. Jones, "Green Tea Catechins and Cardiovascular Risk Factors. Should a Health Claim be Made by U.S. FDA?," *Trends in Food Science and Technology* 41, no. 2 (2015): 188–97; American Heart Association, "Fish and Omega 3 Fatty Acids," May 14, 2014, www.heart.org/HEARTORG/General/Fish-and-Omega-3-Fatty-Acids_UCM_303248_Article.jsp

- **Heredity.** A family history of heart disease increases risk of CVD significantly. The amount of cholesterol you produce, tendencies to form plaque, and other factors seem to have genetic links. The difficulty comes in sorting out genetic influences from the modifiable factors shared by family members, such as environment, stress, dietary habits, and so on. Newer research has focused on studying the interactions between nutrition and genes (*nutrigenetics*) and the role that diet may play in increasing or decreasing risks among certain genetic profiles.[55]

- **Age.** Although cardiovascular disease can affect all ages, over 68 percent of those aged 60 to 79 and 85 percent of those over 80 have one or more CVD issue.[56] Increasing age ups the risk of CVD for all.
- **Gender.** Men are at greater risk for CVD until about age 60, when women begin to catch up, taking the lead at age 80. Otherwise healthy women under age 35 have a fairly low risk, although oral contraceptive use and smoking increase risks. After menopause, or after estrogen levels are otherwise reduced (for example, because of hysterectomy), women's

LDL levels tend to go up, which increases the chance for CVD. Women also have poorer health outcomes and higher death rates than men when they have a heart attack.[57]

Other Risk Factors Being Studied

Although risk factors for CVD are widely known, most people who die suddenly of a heart attack don't have obvious symptoms before it happens. New tests and emerging risk factors are being studied. Two fairly new CVD risks include high levels of inflammation in the vessels and homocysteine levels.

Inflammation and C-Reactive Protein
Occurring when tissues are injured by bacteria, trauma, toxins, or heat, among other things, inflammation is increasingly being considered a culprit in atherosclerotic plaque formation. Injured vessel walls are more prone to plaque formation. To date, several factors, including cigarette smoke, high blood pressure, high LDL cholesterol, diabetes mellitus, certain forms of arthritis, gastrointestinal problems, and exposure to toxic substances have all been linked to increased risk of inflammation. However, the greatest risk appears to be from certain infectious disease pathogens, most notably *Chlamydia pneumoniae*, a common cause of respiratory infections; *Helicobacter pylori* (a bacterium that causes ulcers); herpes simplex virus (a virus that most of us have been exposed to); and *Cytomegalovirus* (another herpes virus infecting most Americans before the age of 40). During an inflammatory reaction, **C-reactive proteins** tend to be present at high levels. A recent meta-analysis of over 38 studies with nearly 170,000 subjects has shown a strong association between C-reactive proteins in the blood and increased risks for atherosclerosis and CVD.58 Blood tests can test these proteins using a highly sensitive assay called *hs-CRP* (high-sensitivity C-reactive protein); if levels are high, action could be taken to reduce inflammation.

The FDA recently approved a new, nonfasting blood test that predicts heart attack in people with no history of heart disease. Known as *PLAC,* the test measures activity of inflammatory enzymes in the blood, which cause plaque to form. More inflammatory enzymes mean more plaque in vessels—and greater risk. The PLAC test could increase our ability to spot and treat potential heart attacks early in the process.[59]

Fish oil, flax, and other foods high in omega-3 have been recommended by the AHA and other groups for their anti-inflammatory properties, but newer research raises questions about the role of omega-3 in reducing risk of CHD and other cardiovascular problems.[60] In spite of conflicting reports, major professional organizations continue to recommend dietary omega-3 supplementation for risk reduction.[61] More research is necessary to determine the actual role that inflammation plays in increased risk of CVD or if there is something unique about inflammation that omega-3 may work to counter.[62]

Homocysteine In the last decade, an increasing amount of attention has been given to the role of **homocysteine**—an amino acid normally present in the blood—in increased risk for CVD. When present at high levels, homocysteine may be related to higher risk of coronary heart disease, stroke, and peripheral artery disease. Although more research is needed, scientists hypothesize that homocysteine works like C-reactive proteins—inflaming the inner lining of the arterial walls, promoting fat deposits on the damaged walls, and encouraging blood clot development.[63] When early studies indicated that folic acid and other B vitamins may help break down homocysteine in the body, food manufacturers responded by adding folic acids to a number of foods and touting the CVD benefits. With conflicting research, the jury is still out on the role of folic acid in CVD risk reduction. In fact, professional groups such as the American Heart Association do not currently recommend taking folic acid supplements to lower homocysteine levels and prevent CVD.[64] For now, a healthy diet is the best preventive action.

> **C-reactive protein (CRP)** A protein whose blood levels rise in response to inflammation.
>
> **homocysteine** An amino acid normally present in the blood that, when found at high levels, may be related to higher risk of cardiovascular disease.
>
> **electrocardiogram (ECG)** A record of the electrical activity of the heart; may be measured during a stress test.

LO 5 | DIAGNOSING AND TREATING CARDIOVASCULAR DISEASE

Examine current strategies for diagnosis and treatment of cardiovascular disease.

Today, CVD patients have many diagnostic, treatment, prevention, and rehabilitation options that were not available a generation ago. Medications can strengthen heartbeat, control arrhythmias, remove fluids, reduce blood pressure, improve heart function, and reduce pain. Among the most common groups of drugs are *statins*, chemicals used to lower blood cholesterol levels; *ACE inhibitors*, which cause the muscles surrounding blood vessels to contract, thereby lowering blood pressure; and *beta-blockers*, which reduce blood pressure by blocking the effects of the hormone epinephrine. New treatment procedures and techniques are saving countless lives. Even long-standing methods of cardiopulmonary resuscitation (CPR) have been changed to focus primarily on chest compressions rather than mouth-to-mouth breathing. The thinking behind this is that people will be more likely to do CPR if the risk for exchange of body fluids is reduced—and any effort to save a person in trouble is better than inaction.

Techniques for Diagnosing Cardiovascular Disease

Several techniques are used to diagnose CVD, including electrocardiogram, angiography, and positron emission tomography scans. An **electrocardiogram (ECG)** is a record of the electrical activity of the heart. Patients may undergo a *stress test*—standard exercise on a stationary bike or treadmill with an electrocardiogram and no injections—or a *nuclear stress test,* which involves injecting a radioactive dye and taking images of the heart to reveal problems with blood flow. In **angiography** (often referred to as *cardiac catheterization*), a needle-thin tube called a *catheter* is threaded through heart arteries, a dye is injected, and an X-ray image is taken to discover which areas are blocked. *Positron emission tomography (PET)* produces three-dimensional images of the heart as blood flows through it. Other tests include the following:

- **Magnetic resonance imaging (MRI).** This test uses powerful magnets to look inside the body. Computer-generated pictures can help physicians identify damage from a heart attack and evaluate disease of larger blood vessels such as the aorta.
- **Ultrafast computed tomography (CT).** This is an especially fast form of X-ray imaging of the heart designed to evaluate bypass grafts, diagnose ventricular function, and measure calcium deposits.
- **Cardiac calcium score.** This test measures the amount of calcium-containing plaque in the coronary arteries, a marker for overall atherosclerotic buildup. The greater amount of calcium, the higher your calcium score and the greater   your risk of heart attack. Concerns have been raised over higher than average exposure to radiation from these tests.

angiography A technique for examining blockages in heart arteries.

coronary bypass surgery A surgical technique whereby a blood vessel taken from another part of the body is implanted to bypass a clogged coronary artery.

angioplasty A technique in which a catheter with a balloon at the tip is inserted into a clogged artery; the balloon is inflated to flatten fatty deposits against artery walls and a stent is typically inserted to keep the artery open.

thrombolysis Injection of an agent to dissolve clots and restore some blood flow, thereby reducing the amount of tissue that dies from ischemia.

5-year survival rates The percentage of people in a study or treatment group who are alive 5 years after they were diagnosed with or treated for cancer.

remission A temporary or permanent period when cancer is responding to treatment and under control. This often leads to the disappearance of the signs and symptoms of cancer.

Bypass Surgery, Angioplasty, and Stents

Coronary bypass surgery has helped many patients who suffered coronary blockages or heart attacks. In a coronary artery bypass graft (CABG), referred to as a "cabbage," a blood vessel is taken from another site in the patient's body (usually the saphenous vein in the leg or the internal thoracic artery in the chest) and implanted to bypass blocked coronary arteries and transport blood to heart tissue.

Another procedure, **angioplasty** (sometimes called *balloon angioplasty*), carries fewer risks. As in angiography, a thin catheter is threaded through blocked heart arteries. The catheter has a balloon at the tip, which is inflated to flatten fatty deposits against the artery walls, allowing blood to flow more freely. A stent (a mesh-like stainless steel tube) may be inserted to prop open the artery. Although highly effective, stents can lead to inflammation and tissue growth in the area that can actually lead to more blockage and problems. In about 30 percent of patients, the treated arteries become clogged again within 6 months. Newer stents are usually medicated to reduce this risk. Nonetheless, some surgeons argue that given this high rate of recurrence, bypass may be a more effective treatment. Newer forms of laser angioplasty and *atherectomy*, a procedure that removes plaque, are being done in several clinics.

Aspirin and Other Drug Therapies

Although aspirin has been touted for its blood-thinning qualities and possibly reducing risks for future heart attacks among those who already have had MI events, the benefits of an aspirin regimen for otherwise healthy adults remains in question. New research and government recommendations seems to indicate that once daily, low-dose aspirin for otherwise healthy adults may not reduce CVD risk and, in fact, may do more harm than good. The FDA indicates it may be helpful to those who have had a heart attack or stroke in preventing a recurrence; however, it shouldn't be taken forever.[65] Furthermore, once a patient has taken aspirin regularly for possible protection against CHD, stopping this regimen may, in fact, increase his or her risk.[66]

If a victim reaches an emergency room and is diagnosed fast enough, a form of clot-busting therapy called **thrombolysis** can be performed. Thrombolysis involves injecting an agent such as *tissue plasminogen activator* (*tPA*) to dissolve the clot and restore some blood flow to the heart (or brain), thereby reducing the amount of tissue that dies from ischemia.[67] These drugs must be administered within 1 to 3 hours after a cardiovascular event.

LO 6 | CANCER: AN EPIDEMIOLOGICAL OVERVIEW

Describe the impact of cancer on people in the United States and compare it to other major health problems in terms of morbidity/mortality, costs, and overall effectiveness of prevention and control.

After heart disease, cancer is the greatest killer in the United States.[68] Although there were over 589,000 deaths in 2015, the **5-year survival rates** (the relative rates for survival in persons living 5 years after diagnosis) are up dramatically from the virtual death sentences of many cancers in the early 1900s. Of course, there are often differences in stage of diagnosis, age of survivor, and other factors that may increase or decrease chances of survival. Today, of the approximately 1.7 million people diagnosed each year, nearly 68 percent will still be alive 5 years from now—an increase of nearly 20 percent since the 1970s—and survival rates for people diagnosed with many cancers in early stages approach 90 to 95 percent.[69] Some cancers will enter **remission**, which means the cancer is responding to treatment and under control. Others will be considered "cured," meaning that the people have no subsequent cancer in their bodies and can expect to live long and productive lives. Lifestyle, follow-up by health care providers, preventive treatments, environmental conditions, immune system functioning, and several other factors can influence the course of any cancer.

Lifetime risk of cancer refers to the probability that a person will develop or die from cancer. Although treatments and survival statistics have improved, nearly 1 in every 2 men and nearly 1 in 3 women will develop cancer in America.[70] In the following sections, we provide an overview of factors that increase risk of cancer and discuss ways to reduce them.

LO 7 | WHAT IS CANCER?

Describe cancer, how it develops, and key risks for cancers overall.

Cancer is the general term for a large group of diseases characterized by the uncontrolled growth and spread of abnormal cells. If these cells aren't stopped, they can impair vital functions of the body and lead to death. When something interrupts normal cell function, uncontrolled growth and abnormal cellular development result in a **neoplasm,** a new growth of tissue serving no physiological function. This neoplasmic mass often forms a clumping of cells known as a **tumor.**

Not all tumors are **malignant** (cancerous); in fact, most are **benign** (noncancerous). Benign tumors are generally harmless unless they grow to obstruct or crowd out normal tissues. A

benign tumor of the brain, for instance, is life threatening when it grows enough to restrict blood flow and cause a stroke. The only way to determine whether a tumor is malignant is through **biopsy,** or microscopic examination of cell development.

Benign and malignant tumors differ in several key ways. Benign tumors generally consist of ordinary-looking cells enclosed in a fibrous shell or capsule that prevents their spreading to other body areas. Malignant tumors are usually not enclosed in a protective capsule and can therefore spread to other organs (**FIGURE 12.5**). This process, known as **metastasis,** makes some forms of cancer particularly aggressive. By the time they are diagnosed, malignant tumors have frequently metastasized throughout the body, making treatment extremely difficult. Unlike benign tumors, which merely expand to take over a given space, malignant cells invade surrounding tissue, emitting clawlike protrusions that disturb the RNA and DNA within

lifetime risk The probability that a person will develop or die from cancer.

cancer A large group of diseases characterized by the uncontrolled growth and spread of abnormal cells.

neoplasm A new growth of tissue that serves no physiological function and results from uncontrolled, abnormal cellular development.

tumor A neoplasmic mass that grows more rapidly than surrounding tissue.

malignant Very dangerous or harmful; refers to a cancerous tumor.

benign Harmless; refers to a noncancerous tumor.

biopsy Microscopic examination of tissue to determine whether a cancer is present.

metastasis Process by which cancer spreads from one area to different areas of the body.

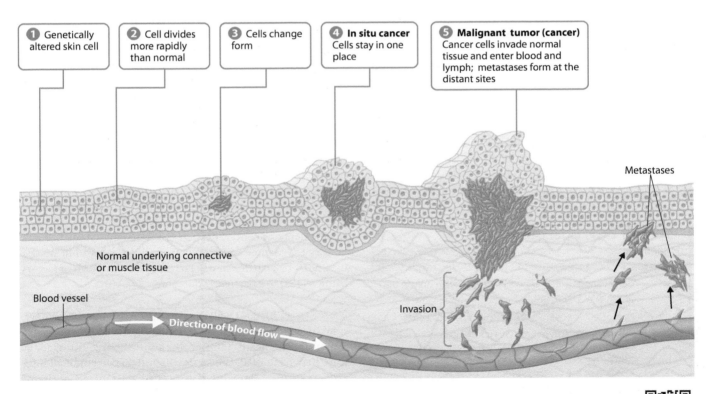

FIGURE 12.5 Metastasis A mutation to the genetic material of a skin cell triggers abnormal cell division and changes cell formation, resulting in a cancerous tumor. If the tumor remains localized, it is considered in situ cancer. If the tumor spreads, it is considered a malignant cancer.

VIDEO TUTOR
Metastasis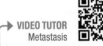

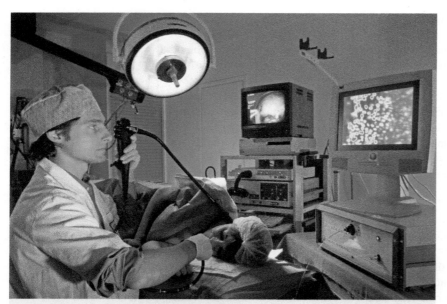

Physicians usually order biopsies of tumors, in which sample cells are taken from the tumor and studied under a microscope to determine whether they are cancerous. Newer techniques, like the minimally invasive "optical biopsy" shown here, allow for the microscopic examination of tissue without doing a physical biopsy.

normal cells. Disrupting these substances, which control cellular metabolism and reproduction, produces **mutant cells** that differ in form, quality, and function from normal cells.

Cancer staging is a classification system that describes how much a cancer has spread at the time it is diagnosed; it helps doctors and patients decide on appropriate treatments and estimate a person's life expectancy. Cancers are often staged based on the *TNM system* (**T**, the extent of the primary tumor, type of cells, size, and reach; **N**, the extent of spread to regional lymph nodes; and **M**, metastasis, the number of tumors, and grade/abnormality of cells). The most commonly known staging system assigns the numbers zero to four (see **TABLE 12.3**). However, some cancers, such as

mutant cells Cells that differ in form, quality, or function from normal cells.

cancer staging A classification system that describes how far a person's disease has advanced.

carcinogens Cancer-causing agents.

TABLE **12.3** | Cancer Stages

Stage	Definition
0	Early cancer, when abnormal cells remain only in the place they originated.
I	Higher numbers indicate more extensive disease:
II	Larger tumor size and/or spread of the cancer
III	beyond the organ in which it first developed to nearby lymph nodes and/or organs adjacent to the location of the primary tumor.
IV	Cancer has spread to other organs.

Source: National Cancer Institute, National Institutes of Health, "Fact Sheet, Cancer Staging, 2015," January 6, 2015, www.cancer.gov/cancertopics/diagnosis-staging/staging/staging-fact-sheet

bone cancers and lymphomas are staged based on grade. Typically, the lower the stage and grade, the better the prognosis.[71]

LO **8** | **WHAT** CAUSES CANCER?

Explain the suspected causes of cancer, and describe your own risks, based on genetics and lifestyle.

Causes of cancer are generally divided into two categories of risk factors: *hereditary* and *acquired* (environmental). Where hereditary factors cannot be modified, we have control over some environmental and behavioral factors, such as tobacco use, nutrition, physical activity, obesity, inflammation, certain infectious agents, certain medical treatments, drug and alcohol consumption, excessive sun exposure, and exposures to **carcinogens** (cancer-causing agents) in food. Where we live, the water we drink, the air we breathe and exposures in the workplace are often part of broader life choices.

Lifestyle Risks

Anyone can develop cancer; however, most cases affect adults beginning in middle age. In fact, 78 percent of cancers are diagnosed at age 55 and above.[72] In order to determine why some people get cancer and others do not, scientists examine specific risks. *Relative risk* is a measure of the strength of the relationship between risk factors and a particular cancer. Basically, relative risk compares your risk if you engage in certain known risk behaviors with that of someone who does not engage in such behaviors. For example, men and women who smoke have 25 times the risk of lung cancer of a nonsmoker—a relative risk of 25.[73]

Over the years, researchers have found that diet, a sedentary lifestyle (and resultant obesity), overconsumption of alcohol, tobacco use, stress, and other lifestyle factors play a role in the incidence of cancer. Keep in mind that a high relative risk does not guarantee cause and effect, but it does indicate the likelihood of a particular risk factors or combination of factors being related to a particular outcome.

Tobacco Use Of all the potential risk factors for cancer, smoking is among the greatest. In the United States, tobacco is responsible for nearly 1 in 5 deaths annually, accounting for at least 30 percent of all cancer deaths and 80 percent of all lung cancer deaths.[74]. Smoking is associated with increased risk of at least 15 different cancers, including those of the nasopharynx, nasal cavity, paranasal sinuses, lip, oral cavity, pharynx, larynx, lung, esophagus, pancreas, uterine cervix, kidney, bladder, and stomach, and acute myeloid leukemia.

1/3

OF THE **CANCER** CASES THAT OCCUR IN DEVELOPED COUNTRIES ARE RELATED TO OVERWEIGHT OR OBESITY, PHYSICAL INACTIVITY, AND/OR POOR NUTRITION.

Surprisingly, women who smoke today have a greater risk of dying from lung cancer than during past decades. Several factors contribute to this risk, including women smoking more cigarettes, smoked over more years (*pack years*). Evidence also suggests that newly designed ventilated filters and increased levels of some chemicals in cigarettes may be factors in this increased risk.[75]

Poor Nutrition, Physical Inactivity, and Obesity
Mounting scientific evidence suggests that about one third of the cancer deaths that occur in the United States each year may be due to lifestyle factors such as overweight or obesity, physical inactivity, and poor nutrition.[76] Dietary choices—particularly high-calorie, high-fat, and high-animal-protein diets—and physical activity are the most important modifiable determinants of cancer risk (besides not smoking). Several studies indicate a relationship between a high body mass index (BMI) and death rates from cancers of the esophagus, colon, rectum, liver, stomach, kidney, pancreas, and others.[77]

Just how great is the risk for someone with a high BMI? Women who gain 55 pounds or more after age 18 have almost a 50 percent greater risk of breast cancer compared to those who maintain their weight.[78] The relative risk of colon cancer in men is 40 percent higher for obese men than it is for non-obese men. The relative risks of gallbladder and endometrial cancers are five times higher in obese individuals than in individuals of healthy weight.[79] Numerous other studies support the link between various forms of cancer and obesity.[80]

Genetic and Physiological Risks

Although there is still much uncertainty, scientists believe that between 5 and 10 percent of all cancers are strongly hereditary; some people may be more predisposed to the malfunctioning of genes that ultimately cause cancer.[81] Suspected cancer-causing genes are called **oncogenes.** While these genes are typically dormant, certain conditions such as age, stress, and exposure to carcinogens, viruses, and radiation may activate them. Once activated, they cause cells to grow and reproduce uncontrollably. Scientists are uncertain whether only people who develop cancer have oncogenes or whether we all have genes that can become oncogenes under certain conditions.

Certain cancers, particularly those of the breast, stomach, colon, prostate, uterus, ovaries, and lungs, are among those most likely to run in families. For example, a woman runs a much higher risk of breast cancer and/or ovarian cancer if her mother or sisters (primary relatives) have had the disease or if she inherits the breast cancer susceptibility genes (*BRCA1* or *BRCA2*). Hodgkin's disease and certain leukemias show similar familial patterns. The complex interaction of hereditary predisposition, lifestyle, and environment on the development of cancer makes it a challenge to determine a single cause. Even among those predisposed to genetic mutations, avoiding risks may decrease chances of cancer development.

Reproductive and Hormonal Factors The effects of reproductive factors on breast and cervical cancers have been well documented. Increased numbers of fertile or menstrual cycle years (early menarche, late menopause), not having children or having them later in life, recent use of birth control pills or hormone replacement therapy, and opting not to breast-feed, all appear to increase risks of breast cancer.[82] While the above factors appear to play a significant role in increased risk for non-Hispanic white women, they do not appear to have as strong an influence on Hispanic women, who may have more protective reproductive patterns (an overall lower age at first birth and greater number of births). They also use less hormone replacement therapy and have a lower utilization rate for mammograms, making comparisons difficult.[83]

Inflammation and Cancer Risks In recent years, several researchers have theorized that chronic inflammation can lead to increased risks for cancer, particularly cancer of the colon and digestive system. Theories hold that inflammation can damage cellular DNA, cause cells to divide more rapidly, and lead to an immune system that is weakened by having to cope with chronic inflammatory bombardment; infectious viruses, bacteria and parasitic invaders, and exposure to environmental irritants may lead to the inflammation that serves to initiate and/or promote cancer development.[84]

Although promising, more research is necessary to determine the exact role and mechanism that inflammation plays in cancer initiation and development, whether inflammation is the culprit or if other factors converge to increase risk.

Occupational and Environmental Risks

Overall, workplace hazards account for only a small percentage of all cancers. However, various substances are known to cause cancer when exposure levels are high or prolonged. One is asbestos, a fibrous material once widely used in the construction, insulation, and automobile industries. Nickel, chromate, and chemicals such as benzene, arsenic, and vinyl chloride have been shown definitively to be carcinogens for humans. People who routinely work with certain dyes and radioactive substances may also have increased risks for cancer. Working with coal tars, as in mining, or with inhalants, as in the auto-painting business, is hazardous. So is working with herbicides and pesticides, although evidence is inconclusive for low-dose exposures. Several federal and state

> **oncogenes** Suspected cancer-causing genes.

agencies are responsible for monitoring such exposures and ensuring that businesses comply with standards designed to protect workers.

Radiation Ionizing radiation (IR)—radiation from X-rays, radon, cosmic rays, and ultraviolet radiation (primarily ultraviolet B, or UVB, radiation)—is the only form of radiation proven to cause human cancer. Evidence that high-dose IR causes cancer comes from studies of atomic bomb survivors, patients receiving radiotherapy, and certain occupational groups (e.g., uranium miners). Virtually any part of the body can be affected by IR, but bone marrow and the thyroid are particularly susceptible. Radon exposure in homes can increase lung cancer risk, especially in cigarette smokers. To reduce the risk of harmful effects, diagnostic medical and dental X-rays are set at the lowest dose levels possible.

Nonionizing radiation produced by radio waves, cell phones, microwaves, computer screens, televisions, electric blankets, and other products has been a topic of great concern in recent years, but research has not proven excess risk to date. A wide range of studies has been conducted, and there is limited evidence (as compared to no evidence) that newer phones used for longer periods may increase cancer risks, particularly in children. Most of the key policymaking and health organizations have indicated that existing research does not support a cell phone–cancer link. Stay tuned; more studies are under way.[85] (See Chapter 15 for more on the potential environmental and health hazards of radiation.)

Chemicals in Foods

Much of the concern about chemicals in foods centers on the possible harm caused by pesticide and herbicide residues. Although some of these chemicals cause cancer at high doses in experimental animals, the very low concentrations found in some foods are well within established government safety levels. Continued research regarding pesticide and herbicide use is essential, and scientists and consumer groups stress the importance of a balance between chemical use and the production of high-quality food products. Prevention efforts should focus on policies to protect consumers, develop low-chemical pesticides and herbicides, and reduce environmental pollution.

Infectious Diseases and Cancer

Between 15 and 20 percent of cancers globally are believed to be caused by infectious viruses, bacteria, and parasites, particularly in the developing world.[86] Viruses are believed to inject their genes into host cells and cause them to grow uncontrollably. *Helicobacter pylori* (*H. pylori*) bacteria has long been associated with increased risk of stomach cancer.[87] Other pathogens can lead to inflammation that may prime cells for cancer development or overcome the immune system, leaving cells vulnerable to cancer growth.[88] (See **Focus On: Reducing Risks and Coping with Chronic Diseases and Conditions** for more on the role of infections in specific chronic diseases.)

Hepatitis B, Hepatitis C, and Liver Cancer

Viruses such as hepatitis B (HBV) and C (HCV) are believed to stimulate the growth of cancer cells in the liver because they are chronic diseases that inflame liver tissue—potentially priming the liver for cancer or making it more hospitable for cancer development. Global increases in hepatitis B and C rates and concurrent rises in liver cancer rates seem to provide evidence of such an association.

Human Papillomavirus and Cervical Cancer

Nearly 100 percent of women with cervical cancer have evidence of human papillomavirus (HPV) infection—a virus believed to be a major cause of cervical cancer. Fortunately, only a small percentage of HPV cases progress to cervical cancer.[89] Today, a vaccine is available to help protect young women from becoming infected with HPV and developing cervical cancer. (For more on the HPV vaccine, see the discussion in Chapter 13.)

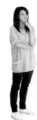

WHICH PATH WOULD YOU TAKE ?
Scan the QR code to see how different health choices YOU make today can affect your risk for developing cardiovascular disease and cancer.

LO 9 | TYPES OF CANCERS

Describe symptoms, populations at risk, and key methods of prevention for the most common types of cancer.

Cancers are grouped into four broad categories based on the type of tissue from which each arise.

- **Carcinomas.** Epithelial tissues (tissues covering body surfaces and lining most body cavities) are the most common sites for cancers called *carcinomas*. These cancers affect the outer layer of the skin and mouth as well as the mucous membranes. They metastasize through the circulatory or lymphatic system initially and form solid tumors.
- **Sarcomas.** Sarcomas occur in the mesodermal, or middle, layers of tissue—for example, in bones, muscles, and general connective tissue. They metastasize primarily via the blood in the early stages of disease. These cancers are less common but generally more virulent than carcinomas. They also form solid tumors.
- **Lymphomas.** Lymphomas develop in the lymphatic system—the infection-fighting regions of the body—and metastasize through the lymphatic system. Hodgkin's disease is an example. Lymphomas also form solid tumors.
- **Leukemias.** Cancer of the blood-forming parts of the body, particularly the bone marrow and spleen, is called leukemia. A nonsolid tumor, leukemia is characterized by an abnormal increase in the number of white blood cells.

Estimated New Cases of Cancer *		Estimated Deaths from Cancer *	
Female	**Male**	**Female**	**Male**
Breast 231,840 (29%)	**Prostate** 220,800 (26%)	**Lung & bronchus** 71,660 (26%)	**Lung & bronchus** 86,380 (28%)
Lung & bronchus 105,590 (13%)	**Lung & bronchus** 115,610 (14%)	**Breast** 40,290 (15%)	**Prostate** 27,540 (9%)
Colon & rectum 47,200 (6%)	**Colon & rectum** 45,890 (5%)	**Colon & rectum** 23,600 (9%)	**Colon & rectum** 26,100 (8%)
Uterine corpus 54,870 (8%)	**Urinary bladder** 56,3920 (6%)	**Pancreas** 19,850 (7%)	**Pancreas** 20,710 (7%)
Thyroid 47,230 (6%)	**Melanoma of the skin** 42,670 (5%)	**Ovary** 14,180 (5%)	**Liver & intrahepatic bile duct** 17,030 (5%)
Non-Hodgkin lymphoma 32,000 (4%)	**Kidney & renal pelvis** 38,270 (5%)	**Leukemia** 10,240 (4%)	**Leukemia** 14,210 (5%)
Melanoma of the skin 31,200 (4%)	**Non-Hodgkin lymphoma** 39,850 (5%)	**Uterine corpus** 10,170 (4%)	**Esophagus** 12,600 (4%)
Kidney & renal pelvis 23,290 (3%)	**Oral cavity & pharynx** 32,670 (4%)	**Non-Hodgkin lymphoma** 490 (1%)	**Urinary bladder** 11,510 (4%)
Pancreas 24,120 (3%)	**Leukemia** 30,900 (4%)	**Liver & intrahepatic bile duct** 7,520 (3%)	**Non-Hodgkin lymphoma** 11,480 (4%)
Leukemia 23,370 (3%)	**Pancreas** 24,840 (3%)	**Brain & other nervous system** 6,380 (2%)	**Kidney & renal pelvis** 9,070 (3%)
All Sites 810,170 (100%)	**All Sites** 848,200 (100%)	**All Sites** 277,280 (100%)	**All Sites** 312,150 (100%)

*Excludes basal and squamous cell skin cancers and in situ carcinoma except urinary bladder. Percentages may not total 100% due to rounding.

FIGURE 12.6 Leading Sites of New Cancer Cases and Deaths, 2015 Estimates

Source: Data from American Cancer Society, *Cancer Facts & Figures 2015* (Atlanta, GA: American Cancer Society, Inc.), table on page 9.

FIGURE 12.6 shows the most common sites of cancer and the estimated number of new cases and deaths from each type in 2015. A comprehensive discussion of the many different forms of cancer is beyond the scope of this book, but we will discuss the most common types in the next sections.

Lung Cancer

Lung cancer is the leading cause of cancer deaths for both men and women in the United States. Even as rates have decreased in recent decades, it still killed an estimated 221,200 Americans in 2015.[90] Since 1987, more women have died each year from lung cancer than from breast cancer, which over the previous 40 years had been the leading cause of cancer deaths in women. Although past reductions in smoking rates bode well for cancer and CVD statistics, there is growing concern about the number of youth, particularly young women and persons of low income and low educational level, who continue to pick up the habit. There is also concern about the increase in lung cancers among those who have never smoked—representing as many as 15 percent of all lung cancers. This type of lung cancer is believed to be related to exposure to secondhand smoke, radon gas, asbestos, wood-burning stoves, and aerosolized oils caused by cooking with oil and deep fat frying.[91]

Detection, Symptoms, and Treatment

Symptoms of lung cancer include a persistent cough, blood-streaked sputum, chest pain, and recurrent attacks of pneumonia or bronchitis. Treatment depends on the type and stage of the cancer. Surgery, radiation therapy, and chemotherapy are all options. If the cancer is localized, surgery is usually the treatment of choice. If it has spread, surgery is combined with radiation and chemotherapy. Despite advances in medical technology, survival rates 1 year after diagnosis are only 44 percent overall. The 5-year survival rate for all stages combined is only 17 percent.[92] Newer tests, such as low-dose CT scans, molecular markers in sputum, and improved biopsy techniques, have helped improve diagnosis, but we still have a long way to go.

Risk Factors and Prevention

Smokers, especially those who have smoked for more than 20 years, and people who have been exposed to secondhand smoke and industrial substances such as arsenic and asbestos or to radiation, are at the highest risk for lung cancer. Quitting smoking does reduce the risk,[93] but exposure to both secondhand cigarette smoke and radon gas is also believed to play an important role in lung cancer development.[94]

Breast Cancer

Women have about a 1 in 8 chance of developing breast cancer in their lifetime. For women from birth to age 39, the chance is about a 1 in 202, with significantly higher rates after menopause.[95] In 2015, approximately 232,000 women and 2,400 men in the United States were diagnosed with invasive breast cancer for the first time. In addition, 60,000 new cases of in situ breast cancer, a more localized cancer, were diagnosed.

About 41,000 (and 440 men) died, making breast cancer the second leading cause of cancer death for women.[96] The good news is that death rates have dropped nearly 35 percent from peak rates in the 1990s. Earlier diagnosis and improved treatment are key factors in this decline.[97]

Detection, Symptoms, and Treatment

The earliest signs of breast cancer are usually observable on mammograms, often before lumps can be felt. However, mammograms are not fool-proof and accuracy for younger women with dense breasts is lower.[98] Although mammograms detect between 80 and 90 percent of breast cancers in women without symptoms, a newer form of MRI appears to be more accurate, particularly in women with genetic risks for tumors.[99] In addition, MRIs may pick up an early form of *atypical hyperplasia* (also referred to as breast cancer *atypia*), in which precancerous cells are growing abnormally but would not show up in routine testing.

For decades monthly breast self-exams were also recommended for cancer screening. However, recent studies indicate that breast self-exams may lead to unnecessary worry, unnecessary tests, and increased health care costs. As a result, several groups downgraded the recommendation about breast self-exams from "do them and do them regularly" to "learn how to do them, and if you desire, do them to know your body and be able to recognize changes." FIGURE 12.7 describes how to do a breast self-exam.

Once breast cancer has grown enough that it can be felt by palpating the area, many women will recognize the threat and seek medical care. Symptoms may include persistent breast changes, such as a lump in the breast or surrounding lymph nodes, thickening, dimpling, skin irritation, distortion,

WHY SHOULD I CARE?

In the United States, breast cancer accounts for 1 in every 3 cancer diagnoses in women. You can reduce your risk by maintaining a healthy weight, drinking less than one alcoholic beverage daily, and exercising regularly.

retraction or scaliness of the nipple, nipple discharge, or tenderness.

Treatments range from a lumpectomy to radical mastectomy to various combinations of radiation or chemotherapy. Among nonsurgical options, promising results have been noted among women using *selective estrogen-receptor modulators (SERMs)* such as tamoxifen and raloxifene, particularly women whose cancers appear to grow in response to estrogen. These drugs, as well as new *aromatase inhibitors,* work by blocking estrogen. The 5-year survival rate for people with localized breast cancer is 98 percent today; for higher stage cancer, the 5-year survival rate drops dramatically.[100]

Risk Factors and Prevention

The incidence of breast cancer increases with age. Risk factors well supported by research include family history of breast cancer, menstrual periods that started early and ended late in life, weight gain after the age of 18, obesity after menopause, recent use of oral contraceptives or postmenopausal hormone therapy, never having children or having a first child after age 30, consuming two or more alcoholic drinks per day, and physical inactivity. Women with dense breasts, high bone mineral density, and exposure to high-dose radiation are also at increased risk.[101] Women who possess *BRCA1* and *BRCA2* gene mutations have a 60 to 80 percent risk of developing breast cancer by age 70, whereas women without the mutations have a 7 percent risk. Because these genes are rare, routine screening for them is not recommended unless there is a strong family history of breast cancer.[102]

International differences in breast cancer incidence correlate with variations in diet, especially fat intake, although a causal role for these dietary factors has not been firmly

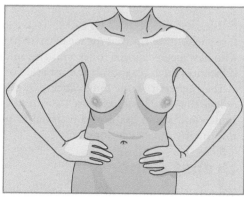

❶ Face a mirror and check for changes in symmetry.

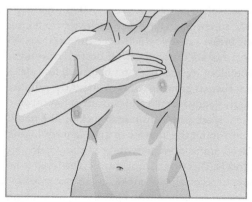

❷ Either standing or lying down, use the pads of the three middle fingers to check for lumps. Follow an up and down pattern on the breast to ensure all tissue gets inspected.

FIGURE 12.7 Breast Self-Exam

Source: Adapted from Breast Self-Exam Illustration Series, National Cancer Institute Visuals Online Collection, U.S. National Institutes of Health, 1984.

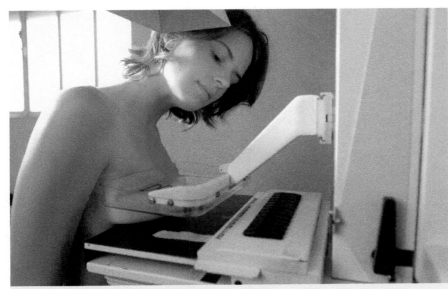

Early detection using the latest equipment with the lowest radiation exposure greatly increases a woman's chance of surviving breast cancer.

established. Sudden weight gain has also been implicated. Research also shows that regular exercise can reduce risk,[103] as may increasing dietary fiber intake.[104]

Colon and Rectal Cancers

Colorectal cancers (cancers of the colon and rectum) continue to be the third most common cancer in both men and women, with just over 93,000 cases of colon and nearly 40,000 cases of rectal cancer diagnosed in the United States in 2013 and 49,700 deaths. Most cases occur in persons age 50 and over; however, new cases can occur at any age.[105] Younger men and women have approximately a 1 in 300 risk of developing colon and rectal cancer from birth to age 49. At age 50, risk for men is about 1 in 148 and 1 in 193 for women, increasing to about 1 in 26 by age 70.[106]

Detection, Symptoms, and Treatment

Because colorectal cancer tends to spread slowly, the prognosis is quite good if it is caught in the early stages. While later stages may have symptoms such as stool changes, bleeding, cramping or pain in the lower abdomen, and unusual fatigue, colorectal cancers usually have no early symptoms. Regular screenings, such as colonoscopy or barium enemas, are recommended for those at high risk. Late in 2014, the FDA approved the first at home, noninvasive colon cancer test that detects blood and DNA mutations that indicate pre-cancer or cancer with over 90 percent accuracy; it may significantly increase early diagnosis and improve outcomes.[107] Treatment often consists of radiation or surgery. Chemotherapy, although not used extensively in the past, is increasingly used.

Risk Factors and Prevention

Anyone can get colorectal cancer, but people over age 50, who are obese, smoke, who have a family history of colon and rectal cancer,

a personal or family history of polyps (benign growths) in the colon or rectum, or who have type 2 diabetes or inflammatory bowel problems such as colitis are at increased risk. Protective factors, such as increased physical activity, aspirin use, hormone replacement therapy, and removal of polyps appear to decrease risk of colon cancer. However, other factors, such as use of nonsteroidal anti-inflammatory drugs (NSAIDS), diet, vitamins, and calcium have shown conflicting results in studies.[108]

Skin Cancer

Skin cancer is the most common form of cancer in the United States; however, since it is not reported, exact numbers are difficult to assess for the two most common, most curable forms of skin cancer—basal cell and squamous cell carcinoma—although estimates of 3.5 million cases are common.[109] **Malignant melanoma** affects nearly 74,000 Americans each year and kills over 10,000 per year, compared to 3,400 deaths for other forms of skin cancer.[110]

Detection, Symptoms, and Treatment

Many people do not know what to look for when examining themselves for skin cancer. Fortunately, potentially cancerous growths are often visible as abnormalities on the skin. Basal and squamous cell carcinomas can be a recurrent annoyance, showing up most commonly on the face, ears, neck, arms, hands, and legs as warty bumps, colored spots, or scaly patches. Bleeding, itchiness, pain, or oozing are other symptoms that warrant attention.[111] Surgery may be necessary to remove them, but they are seldom life threatening.

> **malignant melanoma** A virulent cancer of the melanocytes (pigment-producing cells) of the skin.

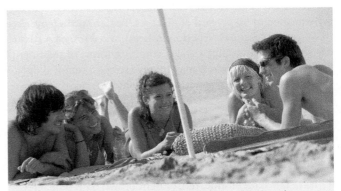

There is no such thing as a "safe" tan, because a tan is visible evidence of UV-induced skin damage. According to the American Cancer Society, tanned skin provides only about the equivalent of sun protection factor (SPF) 4 sunscreen—much too weak to be considered protective.

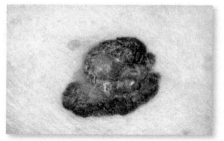 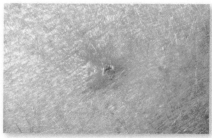 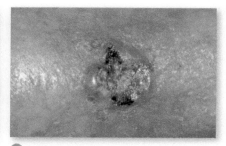

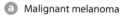 Malignant melanoma ⓑ Basal cell carcinoma ⓒ Squamous cell carcinoma

FIGURE 12.8 Types of Skin Cancers Preventing skin cancer includes keeping a careful watch for any new pigmented growths and for changes to any moles. The ABCD warning signs of melanoma **(a)** include *asymmetrical* shapes, irregular *borders*, *color* variation, and an increasein *diameter*. Basal cell carcinoma **(b)** and squamous cell carcinoma **(c)** should be brought to your physician's attention, but are not as deadly as melanoma.

Melanoma, in contrast, is an invasive killer that may appear as a skin lesion that changes size, shape, or color and that spreads throughout organs of the body. While melanoma is less common than basal and squamous cell carcinomas, it is responsible for the majority of skin cancer deaths. Women are more likely to develop melanoma before age 50. After age 65, men have twice the risk of women.[112] Recreational sun exposure and occupational exposure are key risks. This is one of the few cancers that develops frequently in younger people, however, education and improved sunscreens appear to be factors in declining rates.[113] FIGURE 12.8 shows melanoma compared to basal cell and squamous cell carcinomas. A simple *ABCD* rule outlines the warning signs of melanoma:

- **Asymmetry.** One half of the mole or lesion does not match the other half.
- **Border irregularity.** The edges are uneven, notched, or scalloped.
- **Color.** Pigmentation is not uniform. Melanomas may vary in color from tan to deeper brown, reddish black, black, or deep bluish black.
- **Diameter.** The diameter is greater than 6 millimeters (about the size of a pea).

Treatment of skin cancer depends on its seriousness. Surgery is performed in 90 percent of all cases. Radiation therapy, *electrodesiccation* (tissue destruction by heat), and *cryosurgery* (tissue destruction by freezing) are also common forms of treatment. For melanoma, treatment may involve surgical removal of the regional lymph nodes, radiation, or chemotherapy.

Risk Factors and Prevention Anyone overexposed to ultraviolet radiation without adequate protection is at risk for skin cancer. The risk is greatest for people who fit the following categories:

- Have fair skin; blonde, red, or light brown hair; blue, green, or gray eyes
- Always burn before tanning or burn easily and peel readily
- Don't tan easily but spend lots of time outdoors
- Use no or low sun protection factor (SPF) sunscreens or old, expired suntan lotions

- Have previously been treated for skin cancer or have a family history of skin cancer
- Have experienced severe sunburns during childhood

Preventing skin cancer is a matter of limiting exposure to harmful UV rays found in sunlight. What happens when you expose yourself to sunlight? Biologically, the skin responds to photodamage by increasing its thickness and the number of pigment cells (melanocytes), which produce the "tan" look. The skin's cells that ward off infection are also prone to photodamage, lowering the normal immune protection of our skin and priming it for cancer. Photodamage also causes wrinkling by impairing the elastic substances (collagens) that keep skin soft and pliable. Stay safe in the sun by limiting sun exposure when its rays are strongest, between 10:00 AM and 4:00 PM, and by applying an SPF 15 or higher sunscreen before going outside.

Despite the risk of skin cancer, many Americans are still "working on a tan," and many tanning salon patrons incorrectly believe that tanning booths are safer than sitting in the sun. The truth is that there is no such thing as a safe tan from *any* source! Every time you tan, you are exposing your skin to harmful UV light rays. All tanning lamps emit UVA rays, and most emit UVB rays as well; both types can cause long-term skin damage and contribute to cancer. Even worse, some salons do not calibrate the UV output of their tanning bulbs properly, which can cause more or less exposure than you paid for.

WHAT DO YOU THINK?

How do we determine whether a behavior or substance is a risk factor for a disease? Should programs be enacted to reduce the risk or stop the behavior?

- Do you think that there should be legislation banning tanning booths in all 50 states? Why or why not? Would you favor such a bill if it banned tanning for minors only?

Prostate Cancer

Cancer of the prostate is the most frequently diagnosed cancer in American males today, excluding skin cancer, and is the second leading cause of cancer deaths in men after lung cancer. In 2015, about 221,000 new cases of prostate cancer were diagnosed in the United States, causing 27,500 deaths.[114] Fortunately, most cases of prostate cancer are diagnosed in earlier stages, resulting in survival rates of nearly 99 percent.[115]

Detection, Symptoms, and Treatment The prostate is a muscular, walnut-sized gland that surrounds part of a man's urethra, the tube that transports urine and sperm out of the body. As part of the male reproductive system, its primary function is to produce seminal fluid. Symptoms of prostate cancer include weak or interrupted urine flow; difficulty starting or stopping urination; feeling the urge to urinate frequently; pain upon urination; blood in the urine; or pain in the low back, pelvis, or thighs. Many men have no symptoms in the early stages.

Men over the age of 40 should have an annual digital rectal prostate examination. Another screening method for prostate cancer is the **prostate-specific antigen (PSA) test,** which is a blood test that screens for an indicator of prostate cancer. However, in 2011, a governmental panel called the United States Preventive Services Task Force made the recommendation that healthy men no longer receive the PSA test; overall, it does not save lives and may lead to painful, unnecessary cancer treatments. If you have a family history or other symptoms, consult with your physician.

Risk Factors and Prevention Chances of developing prostate cancer increase dramatically with age. More than 60 percent of prostate cancers are diagnosed in men over the age of 65, and 97 percent occur in men 50 or older.[116] The disease is discovered because it has progressed to the point of displaying symptoms, or more likely, men are seeing a doctor for other problems and get a screening test or PSA test.

Race is also a risk factor in prostate cancer. The highest prostate cancer incidence rates in the world are found in African American men and Jamaican men of African descent. They are also more likely to be diagnosed at more advanced stages than other racial groups.[117]

Having a father or brother with prostate cancer more than doubles a man's risk of getting prostate cancer. Risk is higher for men with an affected brother than it is for those with an affected father.[118]

Eating more fruits and vegetables, particularly those containing lycopene, a pigment found in tomatoes and other red fruits, may lower the risk of prostate cancer. The best advice is to follow the national dietary recommendations and maintain a healthy weight.

Ovarian Cancer

Ovarian cancer is the fifth leading cause of cancer deaths for women, with about 21,300 diagnoses in 2015 and just over 14,000 deaths.[119] Ovarian cancer causes more deaths than any other cancer of the reproductive system because women tend not to discover it until the cancer is at an advanced stage, when 5-year survival is only 27 percent. Younger women (under the age of 65) are much more likely to survive 5 years compared to those 65 or older. For all stages, the 5-year survival is 45 percent.[120]

Ovarian cancer symptoms are often not obvious, and it is common for women to have no early symptoms at all. A woman may complain of feeling bloated, having pain in the pelvic area, feeling full quickly, or feeling the need to urinate more frequently. Some may experience persistent digestive disturbances, while other symptoms include fatigue, pain during intercourse, unexplained weight loss, unexplained changes in bowel or bladder habits, and incontinence.

Primary relatives (mother, daughter, sister) of a woman who has had ovarian cancer are at increased risk, as are those with a family or personal history of breast or colon cancer. Women who have never been pregnant are more likely to develop ovarian cancer than those who have had a child, and the use of fertility drugs may also increase a woman's risk.

General prevention strategies such as focusing on a healthy diet, exercise, sleep, stress management, and weight control are good ideas to lower your risk for any of the diseases discussed in this chapter. Getting annual pelvic examinations is important, and women over the age of 40 should have a cancer-related checkup every year.

> **prostate-specific antigen (PSA)** An antigen found in prostate cancer patients.
>
> **Pap test** A procedure in which cells taken from the cervical region are examined for abnormal activity.

Cervical and Endometrial (Uterine) Cancer

Most uterine cancers develop in the body of the uterus, usually in the *endometrium* (lining). The rest develop in the cervix, located at the base of the uterus. In 2015, an estimated 12,900 new cases of cervical cancer and 54,870 cases of endometrial cancer were diagnosed in the United States, with nearly 10,200 deaths.[121] Increased estrogen levels as a result of menopausal estrogen therapy, being overweight/obese, and never having children may dramatically increase risk for endometrial cancer. In addition, risks are increased by treatment with tamoxifen for breast cancer, metabolic syndrome, late menopause, a history of polyps in the uterus or ovaries, a history of other cancers, and race (white women are at higher risk). Pregnancy, use of oral contraceptives or intrauterine devices, and physical activity are associated with reduced risk.

The overall incidence of cervical cancer has been declining steadily over the past decade, whereas the incidence of endometrial cancer has been increasing by nearly 2 percent per year.[122] The decline in cervical cancer may be due to more regular screenings of younger women using the **Pap test,** a procedure in which cells taken from the cervical region are examined for abnormal cellular activity.

magnetic resonance imaging (MRI) A device that uses magnetic fields, radio waves, and computers to generate an image of internal tissues of the body for diagnostic purposes without the use of radiation.

Although very effective for detecting early-stage cervical cancer, Pap tests are less effective for detecting cancers of the uterine lining. Early warning signs of uterine cancer include bleeding outside the normal menstrual period or after menopause or persistent unusual vaginal discharge. As of 2015, it is recommended women get a Pap test every 2 years beginning at age 21. Between ages 30 and 65, women should have an HPV and Pap test every 5 years and a Pap test alone every 3 years. Those with parents and/or siblings with breast cancer should talk with their doctor about having tests more frequently.

The primary cause of cervical cancer is infection with certain types of the human papillomavirus (HPV). Having sex at a young age and having multiple partners and unprotected sex can increase risks dramatically. Progression to cancer appears to be related to a weakened immune system, multiple births, cigarette smoking, and using oral contraceptives. Today, both young men and women have the option of getting vaccinated with either *Gardasil* or *Cervarix,* designed to protect against the two types of HPV that cause over 70 percent of cervical cancers. (See **Focus On: Reducing Risks and Coping with Chronic Diseases and Conditions** for more on these vaccines). Other sexually transmitted infections such as herpes may also increase risks.[123]

Testicular Cancer

Testicular cancer is one of the most common types of solid tumors found in young adult men, affecting nearly 8,450 young men in 2015.[124] The average age at diagnosis is 33; however, teens and middle-aged men are often affected.[125] Still, with a 96 percent 5-year survival rate, it is one of the most curable forms of cancer. Although the cause of testicular cancer is unknown, several risk factors have been identified. Men with undescended testicles appear to be at greatest risk; HIV and a family history of testicular cancer are also possible risks.[126]

In general, testicular tumors first appear as an enlargement of one or both of the testis, a lump or thickening in testicular tissue. Some men report a heavy feeling, dull ache, or pain that extends to the lower abdomen or groin area. Testicular self-exams have long been recommended as a means of detecting testicular cancer (**FIGURE 12.9**). However, recent studies discovered that findings from monthly self-exams result in testing for noncancerous conditions and thus are not cost-effective. For this reason, the U.S. Preventive Services Task Force stopped recommending self-exams. Regardless, most cases of testicular cancer are discovered through self-exam; there is currently no other screening test for the disease.

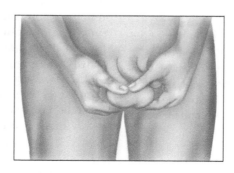

FIGURE 12.9 Testicular Self-Exam

Source: From Michael Johnson, *Human Biology: Concepts and Current Issues*, 3rd ed. Copyright © 2006. Reprinted with permission of Pearson Education, Inc.

The testicular self-exam is best done after a hot shower, which relaxes the scrotum. Standing in front of a mirror, hold the testicle with one hand while gently rolling its surface between the thumb and fingers of your other hand. Feel underneath the scrotum for the tubes of the epididymis and blood vessels that sit close to the body. Repeat with the other testicle. Look for any lump, thickening, or pea-like nodules, paying attention to any areas that may be painful over the entire surface of the scrotum. When done, wash your hands with soap and water. Consult a doctor if you note anything that is unusual.

Pancreatic Cancer: Deadly and on the Rise

Pancreatic cancer is one of the deadliest forms of cancer, with only 28 percent of patients surviving 1 year after diagnosis, and only 5 to 7 percent surviving 5 years.[127] Although most cases occur after age 50, there are increasing numbers of cases at earlier ages. Overall, rates are higher in men than women, in African Americans, and in populations with lower socioeconomic status and education levels.

Tobacco use appears to be a key risk factor, as is obesity, consumption of high levels of red meat, and high-fat diet. Family history, possible genetic links, and a history of chronic inflammation of the pancreas over the years (*pancreatitis*), seem to increase risk. Also, there appears to be a greater risk among diabetics and those who have had infections with hepatitis B and C and the *Helicobacter* bacteria. Because pancreatic cancer has few early symptoms, there is no reliable test to detect it in its early stages. Often, by the time it is diagnosed via CT or MRI examinations, it is too advanced to treat effectively.

LO 10 | FACING CANCER

Discuss cancer diagnosis and treatment, including radiotherapy and chemotherapy, and describe more recent developments in detection and treatment.

The earlier cancer is diagnosed, the better the prospect for survival. Make a realistic assessment of your own risk factors; avoid behaviors that put you at risk; and increase healthy behaviors, such as improving your diet and exercise levels, reducing stress, and getting regular checkups. Even if you have significant risks, there are factors you can control. Do you have a family history of cancer? If so, what types? Make sure you know which symptoms to watch for, avoid known carcinogens—such as tobacco—and other environmental hazards, and follow the recommendations for self-exams and medical checkups outlined in **TABLE 12.4** on the next page.

The use of several high-tech imaging systems to detect cancer has become standard. **Magnetic resonance imaging (MRI)** uses a huge electromagnet to

TABLE 12.4 | Screening Guidelines for the Early Detection of Cancer in Average-Risk Asymptomatic People

Cancer Site	Screening Procedure	Age and Frequency of Test
Breast	Mammograms	The National Cancer Institute recommends that women in their forties and older have mammograms every 1 to 2 years. Women who are at higher-than-average risk of breast cancer should talk with their health care provider about whether to have mammograms before age 40 and how often to have them.
Cervix	Pap test (Pap smear)	Women should begin having Pap tests 3 years after they begin having sexual intercourse or when they reach age 21 (whichever comes first). Most women should have a Pap test at least once every 3 years.
Colon and rectum	*Fecal occult blood test:* Sometimes cancer or polyps bleed. This test can detect tiny amounts of blood in the stool. *Sigmoidoscopy:* Checks the rectum and lower part of the colon for polyps. *Colonoscopy:* Checks the rectum and entire colon for polyps and cancer.	People aged 50 and older should be screened. People who have a higher-than-average risk of cancer of the colon or rectum should talk with their doctor about whether to have screening tests before age 50 and how often to have them Note: Although not part of recommendations, a new "at-home" blood/cancer DNA test is now FDA approved.
Prostate	Prostate-specific antigen (PSA) test	Some groups encourage yearly screening for men over age 50, and some advise men who are at a higher risk for prostate cancer to begin screening at age 40 or 45. Others caution against routine screening and encourage checking with your doctor. Currently, Medicare provides coverage for an annual PSA test for all men age 50 and older.

Sources: National Cancer Institute, National Institutes of Health, "What You Need to Know About Cancer Screening," 2014, www.cancer.gov; National Cancer Institute, Fact Sheet, Prostate-Specific Antigen (PSA) Test, 2014, www.cancer.gov

detect hidden tumors by mapping the vibrations of the various atoms in the body on a computer screen. Another key weapon is the **computed tomography scan (CT scan)**, which uses X-rays to examine parts of the body. In both of these painless, noninvasive procedures, cross-sectioned pictures can reveal a tumor's shape and location more accurately than can conventional X-ray images. Exciting new tests are being explored for widespread use. These offer the promise of much earlier diagnosis and improved treatment for early cancer recurrence. New 3D mammogram machines offer significant improvements in imaging and breast cancer detection, but deliver nearly double the radiation risk of conventional mammograms.

Cancer Treatments

Cancer treatments vary according to the type of cancer and the stage in which it is detected. Surgery, in which the tumor and surrounding tissue are removed, is one common treatment. New **stereotactic radiosurgery**, also known as **gamma knife surgery**, uses a targeted dose of gamma radiation to zap tumors with pinpoint accuracy without blood loss or need for a scalpel. **Radiotherapy** (the use of radiation) or **chemotherapy** (the use of drugs) to kill cancerous cells are also used. When cancer has spread throughout the body, chemotherapy is necessary.

Whether used alone or in combination, virtually all cancer treatments have side effects, including nausea, nutritional deficiencies, hair loss, and general fatigue. The more aggressive the cancer, the more likely there will be side effects from powerful drugs and invasive procedures. In the process of killing malignant cells, some healthy cells are also destroyed, and long-term damage to the cardiovascular system, kidneys, liver, and other body systems can be significant.

New ways of killing tumors and new chemotherapeutic drug cocktails are being developed regularly. Promising areas of research include *immunotherapy,* which enhances the body's own disease-fighting mechanisms, *cancer-fighting vaccines* to combat abnormal cells, *gene therapy* to increase the patient's immune response, and treatment with various substances that block cancer-causing events along the cancer pathway. Another promising avenue of potential treatment is *stem cell research,* although controversy around the use of stem cells continues to slow research. Because our knowledge of cancer treatment is constantly evolving, those who have been diagnosed with cancer and their loved ones should do their best to access information on the best cancer centers for specific types of cancer, new treatments being developed, and whether or not they are eligible for new clinical trials and experimental treatments that might be available for particularly aggressive cancers.

> **computed tomography scan (CT scan)** A scan by a machine that uses radiation to view internal organs not normally visible on X-ray images.
>
> **stereotactic radiosurgery** A type of radiation therapy that can be used to zap tumors. Also known as *gamma knife surgery.*
>
> **radiotherapy** Use of radiation to kill cancerous cells.
>
> **chemotherapy** Use of drugs to kill cancerous cells.

ASSESS | YOURSELF

CVD and Cancer: What's Your Personal Risk?

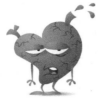

1 Evaluating Your CVD Risk

Complete each of the following questions and total your points in each section.

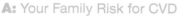

A: Your Family Risk for CVD

	Yes (1 point)	No (0 point)	Don't Know
1. Do any of your primary relatives (parents, grandparents, siblings) have a history of heart disease or stroke?	○	○	○
2. Do any of your primary relatives have diabetes?	○	○	○
3. Do any of your primary relatives have high blood pressure?	○	○	○
4. Do any of your primary relatives have a history of high cholesterol?	○	○	○
5. Would you say that your family consumed a high-fat diet (lots of red meat, whole dairy, butter/margarine) during your time spent at home?	○	○	○

Total points: _____

B: Your Lifestyle Risk for CVD

1. Is your total cholesterol level higher than it should be?	○	○	○
2. Do you have high blood pressure?	○	○	○
3. Have you been diagnosed as prediabetic or diabetic?	○	○	○
4. Would you describe your life as being highly stressful?	○	○	○
5. Do you smoke?	○	○	○

Total points: _____

C: Your Additional Risks for CVD

1. How would you best describe your current weight?
   a. Lower than what it should be for my height and weight (0 points)
   b. About what it should be for my height and weight (0 points)
   c. Higher than it should be for my height and weight (1 point)

2. How would you describe the level of exercise that you get each day?
   a. Less than what I should be exercising each day (1 point)
   b. About what I should be exercising each day (0 points)
   c. More than what I should be exercising each day (0 points)

3. How would you describe your dietary behaviors?
   a. Eating only the recommended number of calories each day (0 points)
   b. Eating less than the recommended number of calories each day (0 points)
   c. Eating more than the recommended number of calories each day (1 point)

4. Which of the following best describes your typical dietary behavior?
   a. I eat from the major food groups, especially trying to get the recommended fruits and vegetables. (0 points)
   b. I eat too much red meat and consume too much saturated and *trans* fats from meat, dairy products, and processed foods each day. (1 point)
   c. Whenever possible, I try to substitute olive oil or canola oil for other forms of dietary fat. (0 points)

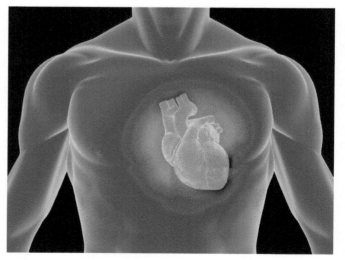

5. Which of the following (if any) describes you?

   a. I watch my sodium intake and try to reduce stress in my life. (0 points)

   b. I have a history of chlamydia infection. (1 point)

   c. I try to eat 5 to 10 mg of soluble fiber each day and try to substitute a non-animal source of protein (beans, nuts, soy) in my diet at least once each week. (0 points)

Total points: _____

Scoring Part 1

If you scored between 1 and 5 in any section, consider your risk. The higher the number, the greater your risk will be. If you answered Don't Know for any question, talk to your parents or other family members as soon as possible to find out if you have any unknown risks.

2 Evaluating Your Cancer Risk

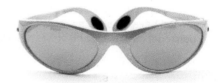

Read each question and circle the number corresponding to each with Yes or No. Individual scores for specific questions should not be interpreted as a precise measure of relative risk, but the totals in each section give a general indication of risk.

A: Cancers in General

	Yes	No
1. Do you smoke cigarettes on most days of the week?	2	1
2. Do you consume a diet that is rich in fruits and vegetables?	1	2
3. Are you obese, or do you lead a primarily sedentary lifestyle?	2	1
4. Do you live in an area with high air pollution levels or work in a job where you are exposed to several chemicals on a regular basis?	2	1
5. Are you careful about the amount of animal fat in your diet, substituting olive oil or canola oil for animal fat whenever possible?	1	2
6. Do you limit your overall consumption of alcohol?	1	2
7. Do you eat foods rich in lycopenes (such as tomatoes) and antioxidants?	1	2
8. Are you "body aware" and alert for changes in your body?	1	2
9. Do you have a family history of ulcers or of colorectal, stomach, or other digestive system cancers?	2	1
10. Do you avoid unnecessary exposure to radiation and microwave emissions?	1	2

Total points: _____

B: Skin Cancer

	Yes	No
1. Do you spend a lot of time outdoors, either at work or at play?	2	1
2. Do you use sunscreens with an SPF rating of 15 or more when you are in the sun?	1	2
3. Do you use tanning beds or sun booths regularly to maintain a tan?	2	1
4. Do you examine your skin once a month, checking any moles or other irregularities, particularly in hard-to-see areas such as your back, genitals, neck, and under your hair?	1	2
5. Do you purchase and wear sunglasses that adequately filter out harmful sun rays?	1	2

Total points: _____

C: Breast Cancer

	Yes	No
1. Do you check your breasts at least monthly using breast self-exam procedures?	1	2
2. Do you look at your breasts in the mirror regularly, checking for any irregular indentations/lumps, discharge from the nipples, or other noticeable changes?	1	2
3. Has your mother, sister, or daughter been diagnosed with breast cancer?	2	1
4. Have you ever been pregnant?	1	2
5. Have you had a history of lumps or cysts in your breasts or underarm?	2	1

Total points: _____

D: Cancers of the Reproductive System

Men

	Yes	No
1. Do you examine your penis regularly for unusual bumps or growths?	1	2
2. Do you perform regular testicular self-examinations?	1	2
3. Do you have a family history of prostate or testicular cancer?	2	1
4. Do you practice safe sex and wear condoms during every sexual encounter?	1	2
5. Do you avoid exposure to harmful environmental hazards such as mercury, coal tars, benzene, chromate, and vinyl chloride?	1	2

Total points: _____

Women

	Yes	No
1. Do you have regularly scheduled Pap tests?	1	2
2. Have you been infected with HPV, Epstein-Barr virus, or other viruses believed to increase cancer risk?	2	1
3. Has your mother, sister, or daughter been diagnosed with breast, cervical, endometrial, or ovarian cancer (particularly at a young age)?	2	1
4. Do you practice safer sex and use condoms with every sexual encounter?	1	2
5. Are you obese, taking estrogen, or consuming a diet that is very high in saturated fats?	2	1

Total points: _____

Scoring Part 2

Look carefully at each question for which you received a 2. Are there any areas in which you received mostly 2s? Did you receive total points of 11 or higher in A? Did you receive total points of 6 or higher in B through D? If so, you have at least one identifiable risk. The higher the score, the more risks you may have.

YOUR PLAN FOR CHANGE

ASSESS YOURSELF activities evaluated your risk of heart disease and cancer. Based on your results, you may need to take steps to reduce your risk for these diseases and improve your future health.

TODAY, YOU CAN:

☐ Get up and move! Take a walk in the evening, use the stairs, or ride your bike to class. Think of ways to incorporate more physical activity into your daily routine.

☐ Improve your dietary habits by reading labels and choosing low-sodium foods, low-fat foods, and nutrient-dense fruits and vegetables. Replace meat and processed foods with a serving of fresh fruit or soy-based protein and green leafy vegetables several times per week. Eat more monounsaturated fat and foods with lower cholesterol counts. Watch your total calorie consumption.

☐ Assess your personal risks for specific cancers, looking at lifestyle as well as your genetic risks. For which cancers might you be most at risk?

WITHIN THE NEXT TWO WEEKS, YOU CAN:

☐ Buy a bottle of broad-spectrum sunscreen (with SPF 15 or higher). Apply it liberally as part of your daily routine. (Be sure to check the expiration date, particularly on sale items!) Also, stay in the shade when the sun is strongest, from 10 AM to 4 PM.

☐ Find out your family health history. Talk to your parents, grandparents, or an aunt or uncle to find out if family members have developed cancer or CVD. Ask if they know their latest cholesterol LDL/HDL levels. Do you have a family history of diabetes?

☐ Begin a regular exercise program. Set small goals and try to meet them. (See Chapter 9 for ideas.)

☐ Practice a new stress management technique. (See Chapter 3 for ideas for managing stress.)

☐ Make sure you get at least 8 hours of sleep per night.

BY THE END OF THE SEMESTER, YOU CAN:

☐ Get a full lipid panel for yourself and have your blood pressure checked. Once you know your levels, you'll have a better sense of what risk factors to address. If your levels are high, talk to your doctor about how to reduce them.

☐ Stop smoking, avoid secondhand smoke, and limit your alcohol intake.

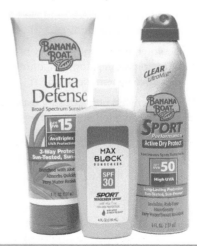

CHAPTER REVIEW

To hear an MP3 Tutor Session, scan here or visit the Study Area in MasteringHealth.

LO 1 | Cardiovascular Disease in the United States

- Cardiovascular disease is the leading cause of death in the United States, and it puts a huge economic burden on our society. African Americans have the highest rates of CVD deaths out of any other group in the United States. CVD is also a leading cause of death globally and is an increasing threat in the developing world.

LO 2 | Understanding the Cardiovascular System

- The cardiovascular system consists of the heart and circulatory system and is a carefully regulated, integrated network of vessels that supplies the body with the nutrients and oxygen necessary to perform daily functions.

LO 3 | Key Cardiovascular Diseases

- Cardiovascular diseases include atherosclerosis, coronary artery disease, peripheral artery disease, coronary heart disease, stroke, hypertension, angina pectoris, arrhythmias, congestive heart failure, and congenital and rheumatic heart disease.

LO 4 | Reducing Your Risks

- *Cardiometabolic risks* refer to combined factors that increase a person's chances of CVD and diabetes. A person who possesses three or more cardiometabolic risk factors may have metabolic syndrome. Metabolic syndrome is increasing at all levels—among young and old, rich and poor, and in all ethnicities.
- Many risk factors for cardiovascular disease can be modified, such as cigarette smoking, high blood cholesterol and triglyceride levels, hypertension, lack of exercise, poor diet, obesity, diabetes, and emotional stress. Some risk factors, such as age, gender, and heredity, cannot be modified. The more risks you have; the greater your chances of developing CVD.

LO 5 | Diagnosing and Treating Cardiovascular Disease

- Coronary bypass surgery is an established treatment for heart blockage; increasing numbers of angioplasty procedures and stents are being used with great success. Increasing numbers of pharmacological interventions such as statins are being used to reduce risk and prevent problems. Drug therapies can be used to prevent and treat CVD.

To hear an MP3 Tutor Session, scan here or visit the Study Area in MasteringHealth.

LO 6 | Cancer: An Epidemiological Overview

- Cancer is the second most common cause of death in the United States. The current 5-year survival rates for cancer have greatly increased from those of previous generations.

LO 7 | What Is Cancer?

- Cancer is a group of diseases characterized by uncontrolled growth and spread of abnormal cells. These cells may create tumors. Benign (noncancerous) tumors grow in size but do not spread; malignant (cancerous) tumors spread to other parts of the body.

LO 8 | What Causes Cancer?

- Lifestyle factors for cancer include smoking and obesity as well as poor diet, lack of exercise, and other factors. Biological factors include inherited genes, age, and gender. Potential environmental carcinogens include asbestos, radiation, preservatives, and pesticides. Infectious agents may increase your risks for cancer; those that appear most likely to cause cancer are chronic hepatitis B and C, human papillomavirus, and genital herpes.

LO 9 | Types of Cancers

- Each type of cancer poses different risks, depending on several factors. Common cancers include that of the lung, breast, colon and rectum, skin, prostate, testis, ovary, and uterus; leukemia; and lymphomas. Each has different strategies for prevention.

LO 10 | Facing Cancer

- The most common treatments for cancer are surgery, chemotherapy, and radiation; newer therapies, including biologicals, smart drugs, and immunotherapy show promising results and should always be considered.
- Early diagnosis improves survival rate. Self-exams for breast, testicular, and skin cancer aid early diagnosis.

POP QUIZ

Visit MasteringHealth to personalize your study plan with Chapter Review Quizzes and Dynamic Study Modules.

LO 1 | Cardiovascular Disease in the United States

1. Which of the following is true about CVD?
   a. It's only a problem in developed nations.
   b. It claims the lives of more men than women every year.
   c. Risk factors are only an issue starting at age 50.
   d. It's the leading cause of death in America.

LO 2 | Understanding the Cardiovascular System

2. Which type of blood vessels carry oxygenated blood away from the heart?
   a. Ventricles
   b. Arteries
   c. Pulmonary arteries
   d. Venules

3. A stroke results
   a. when a heart stops beating.
   b. when cardiopulmonary resuscitation has failed to revive the stopped heart.
   c. when blood flow in the brain has been compromised, either due to blockage or hemorrhage.
   d. when blood pressure rises above 120/80 mm Hg.

LO **4** | **Reducing Your Risks**

4. The "bad" type of cholesterol found in the bloodstream is known as
   a. high-density lipoprotein (HDL).
   b. low-density lipoprotein (LDL).
   c. total cholesterol.
   d. triglyceride.

LO **5** | **Diagnosing and Treating Cardiovascular Disease**

5. The surgery in which a blood vessel is taken from another site in the patient's body and implanted to bypass the blocked artery and transport blood to the heart is called
   a. atherosclerosis surgery.
   b. thrombolysis.
   c. coronary bypass surgery.
   d. angioplasty.

LO **6** | **Cancer: An Epidemiological Overview**

6. Overall, which cancer has the worst 5-year survival rate today?
   a. Prostate
   b. Pancreas
   c. Melanoma
   d. Breast

LO **7** | **What Is Cancer?**

7. When cancer cells have *metastasized,*
   a. it has grown into a malignant tumor.
   b. it has spread to other parts of the body.

   c. the cancer is retreating and cancer cells are dying off.
   d. the tumor is localized and considered in situ.

LO **8** | **What Causes Cancer?**

8. One of the biggest factors in increased risk for cancer is
   a. increasing age.
   b. not having children.
   c. being of long-lived parents.
   d. increased consumption of fruits and vegetables.

LO **9** | **Types of Cancers**

9. The cancer that causes the most deaths for men and women in the United States is
   a. colorectal cancer.
   b. pancreatic cancer.
   c. lung cancer.
   d. stomach cancer.

LO **10** | **Facing Cancer**

10. Which of the following treatment methods uses drugs to kill cancerous cells?
    a. Radiotherapy
    b. Chemotherapy
    c. Stem cell therapy
    d. Stereotactic radiosurgery

Answers to the Pop Quiz can be found on page A-1. If you answered a question incorrectly, review the section identified by the learning outcome. For even more study tools, visit MasteringHealth.

THINK ABOUT IT!

LO **1** | **Cardiovascular Disease in the United States**

1. Why do you think hypertension rates are rising among today's college students?

LO **2** | **Understanding the Cardiovascular System**

2. What can your resting heart rate tell you about your overall health? What are some reasons a person's

resting heart rate might be higher or lower than the median?

LO **3** | **Key Cardiovascular Diseases**

3. List the different types of CVD. Compare and contrast their symptoms, risk factors, prevention, and treatment.

LO **4** | **Reducing Your Risks**

4. Discuss the role that exercise, stress management, dietary changes, medical checkups, sodium reduction, and other factors can play in reducing risk for CVD. What role might infectious diseases play in CVD risk?

LO **5** | **Diagnosing and Treating Cardiovascular Disease**

5. Describe some of the diagnostic, preventive, and treatment alternatives for CVD. If you had a heart attack today, which treatment would you prefer? Explain why.

LO **6** | **Cancer: An Epidemiological Overview**

6. What are some of the factors that account for the great increase in 5-year survival rates for people with cancer in recent years?

LO **7** | **What Is Cancer?**

7. What is cancer? How does it spread? What is the difference between a benign tumor and a malignant tumor?

LO **8** | **What Causes Cancer?**

8. List the likely causes of cancer. Which of these causes would be a risk for you, in particular? What can you do to reduce these risks? What risk factors do you share with family members? Friends?

LO 9 | Types of Cancers

9. What are the differences between carcinomas, sarcomas, lymphomas, and leukemia? Which is the most common? Least common? Why is it important that you know the stage of your cancer?

LO 10 | Facing Cancer

10. Why are breast and testicular self-exams especially important for college students? What factors keep you from doing your own self-exams? What could you do to make sure you do regular self-exams?

ACCESS YOUR HEALTH ON THE INTERNET

The following websites explore further topics and issues related to CVD and cancer. For links to the websites below, visit MasteringHealth.

American Heart Association. This is the home page of the leading private organization dedicated to heart health. This site provides information, statistics, and resources regarding cardiovascular care, including an opportunity to test your risk for CVD. www.heart.org

National Heart, Lung, and Blood Institute. This valuable resource provides information on all aspects of cardiovascular health and wellness. www.nhlbi.nih.gov

Global Cardiovascular Infobase. This site contains epidemiological data and statistics for cardiovascular diseases for countries throughout the world, with a focus on developing nations. www.cvdinfobase.ca

American Cancer Society. This private organization is dedicated to cancer prevention. Here you'll find information, statistics, and resources regarding cancer. www.cancer.org

National Cancer Institute. On this site you will find valuable information on cancer facts, results of research, new and ongoing clinical trials, and the Physician Data Query (PDQ), a comprehensive database of cancer treatment information. www.cancer.gov

Oncolink. Sponsored by the University of Pennsylvania Cancer Center, this site educates cancer patients and their families by offering information on support services, cancer causes, screening, prevention, and common questions. www.oncolink.com

Susan G. Komen for the Cure. Up-to-date information about breast cancer, issues in treatment, and support groups are presented here, as well as a wealth of videos and information. This site is especially useful for diagnosed patients looking for additional support and advice. www.komen.org

National Coalition for Cancer Survivorship. Cancer survivors share their experiences advocating for themselves during and after cancer treatment. www.canceradvocacy.org

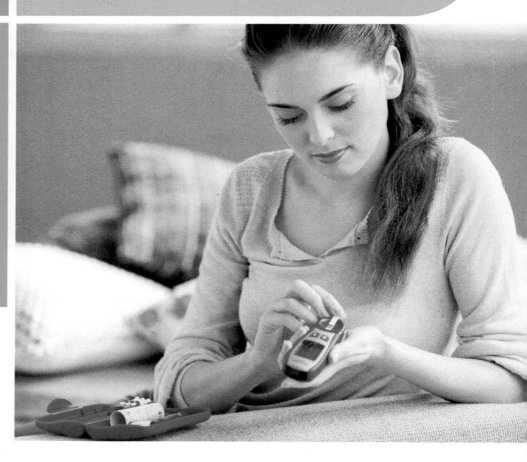

FOCUS ON | Minimizing Your Risk for Diabetes

Your genetics play a key role in risk for diabetes, along with learned dietary patterns from parents and your own health behaviors.

LEARNING OUTCOMES

1 Differentiate among types of diabetes and identify common risk factors.
2 Describe the symptoms of, complications associated with, and main tests for diabetes.
3 Explain how diabetes can be prevented and treated.

Nora is overweight. She used to figure it was no big deal; but last week her mom called to tell Nora that she'd just been diagnosed with type 2 diabetes. Her voice sounded shaky as she reminded Nora about her own mother's death from kidney failure—a complication of diabetes—at age 52. Later, Nora searched online for information about her risk for diabetes. Her Hispanic ethnicity, family history, high stress level and lack of sleep, excessive weight, and sedentary lifestyle made her a prime candidate.

Nora made an appointment for a diabetes screening. She was instructed to fast the night before. At her visit, the nurse practitioner took a blood sample. A few days later, she called to tell Nora that her blood glucose was elevated, and

although she wasn't diabetic yet, she needed to make changes to her diet and lifestyle to reduce her risk for developing type 2 diabetes, like her mom.

Over the past two decades, diabetes rates in the United States have increased dramatically[1] (see FIGURE 1). The Centers for Disease Control and Prevention (CDC) estimates that nearly 30 million people—almost 10 percent of the U.S. population—have diabetes, and another 86 million have *prediabetes*.[2] Experts predict that at current rates, more than 1 in 3 Americans will have diabetes by 2050. Diabetes kills more Americans each year than breast cancer and AIDS combined, and millions suffer the physical, emotional, and economic burdens of dealing with this difficult disease.[3]

Diabetes rates increase as age and weight increase. Among persons aged 20–44 years, approximately 4.1 percent have diabetes, compared to roughly 16.2 percent of those aged 45–64 and over 25.9 percent of those aged 65–74.[4] The economic burden of diagnosed diabetes, gestational diabetes, undiagnosed diabetes, and prediabetes was over $322 billion in 2012.[5] Costs for diagnosed diabetics averages nearly $11,000 per person per year, while undiagnosed diabetes averages just over $4,000.[6] For an explanation of the personal financial toll that comes with diabetes, read the Money & Health box on page 388.

LO 1 | WHAT IS DIABETES?

Differentiate among types of diabetes and identify common risk factors.

Diabetes mellitus is a group of diseases, each with its own mechanism, all characterized by a persistently high level of glucose, a type of sugar, in the blood. One sign of diabetes is the production of an abnormal level of glucose in the urine, a fact reflected in its name: *Diabetes* derives from a Greek word meaning "to flow through," and *mellitus* is the Latin word for "sweet." The high blood glucose levels—or **hyperglycemia**—seen in diabetes can lead to serious health problems and premature death.

In a healthy person, the digestive system breaks down the carbohydrates we eat into glucose—one of our main energy sources—which it releases into the bloodstream for use by body cells. Our red blood cells can only use glucose to fuel functioning, and brain and other nerve cells prefer glucose over other fuels. When glucose levels drop below normal, you may feel unable to concentrate, and certain mental functions may be impaired. When more glucose is available than required to meet immediate needs, the excess is stored as glycogen in the liver and muscles for later use.

Glucose can't simply cross cell membranes on its own. Instead, cells have structures that transport glucose across in response to a signal generated by the **pancreas,** an organ located just beneath

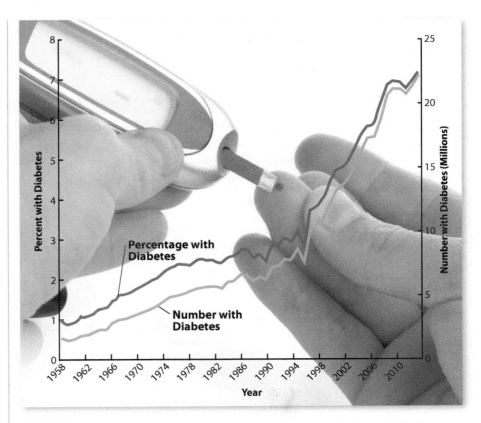

FIGURE 1 Percentage and Number of U.S. Population with Diagnosed Diabetes, 1958–2013 Notice that these data are for diagnosed cases. Estimates of actual prevalence are higher.

Source: CDC, "Long-Term Trends in Diabetes," October 2014, www.cdc.gov/diabetes/statistics/slides/long_term_trends.pdf

the stomach. Whenever a surge of glucose enters the bloodstream, the pancreas secretes a hormone called **insulin.** Insulin stimulates cells to take up glucose from the bloodstream and carry it into the cell, where it's used for immediate energy. Conversion of glucose to glycogen for storage in the liver and muscles is also assisted by insulin. When levels of glucose fall, the pancreas stops secreting insulin—until the next influx of glucose arrives.

Type 1 Diabetes

The more serious and less prevalent form of diabetes, called **type 1 diabetes** (or insulin-dependent diabetes), is an autoimmune disease in which the individual's immune system attacks and destroys the insulin-making cells in the pancreas. Destruction of these cells causes a dramatic reduction, or total cessation, of insulin production. Without insulin, cells cannot take up glucose, leaving blood glucose levels

permanently elevated. Only about 5 percent of diabetic cases are type 1.[7] European ancestry, a genetic predisposition, and certain viral infections all increase the risk.[8]

People with type 1 diabetes require daily insulin injections or infusions and must carefully monitor their diet and exercise levels. Often they face unique challenges as the "lesser known" diabetic type, with fewer funds available for research and fewer options for treatment.

diabetes mellitus A group of diseases characterized by elevated blood glucose levels.

hyperglycemia Elevated blood glucose level.

pancreas Organ that secretes digestive enzymes into the small intestine and hormones, including insulin, into the bloodstream.

insulin Hormone secreted by the pancreas and required by body cells for the uptake and storage of glucose.

type 1 diabetes Form of diabetes mellitus in which the pancreas is not able to make insulin, and therefore blood glucose cannot enter the cells to be used for energy.

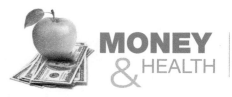

MONEY & HEALTH

DIABETES
At What Cost?

One in every 5 health care dollars is spent on diabetes care today: fees for doctor visits, testing supplies, laboratory results, medicines to control glucose and others to control side effects, as well as the costs for other necessities often only partially covered, even for those with insurance. If you are underinsured or uninsured, the *diabetes drain* on your bank account could be major.

Costs of treatment varies tremendously; whether you have insurance, the nature of your deductibles and co-pays, proximity to pharmacies with a supply of generics, and the number and dosage of drugs necessary to control your blood glucose are all factors. What is known is that costs for diabetic drugs are on a rapid rise. Newer drugs may not be more effective, yet they may cost significantly more. Often, after a person takes one drug for a period of time, the drug becomes less effective

and additional drugs are necessary. To give you an idea of what it might cost someone who is diagnosed with type 2 diabetes and who doesn't have insurance, consider these very conservative monthly estimates.

The American Diabetes Association estimates costs of between $350 and $900 per month for the typical type 2 diabetic. However, insulin-dependent diabetics may have costs that are two to three times higher.

Diabetic Health Care Need	Estimated Monthly Cost
Doctor visit for monitoring and testing	$200
Lab tests: Fasting glucose blood test, glucose tolerance, A1C tests	$35–$200
Home glucose meter, test strips	Meter= $35–$50 Test strips = roughly $1 each. Average = $100/month
Lancets and lancing devices, alcohol wipes	$5–$10/month
Oral medications like *metformin* (depends on dosage and type); *Actos* (depends on dosage); *Januvia* (depends on dosage)	*Metformin:* $13–$15 at low end per month. Less at big box stores, more for different dosage; *Actos:* $220–$370/month; *Januvia:* $265/month

Sources: American Diabetes Association, "Fast Facts: Data and Statistics about Diabetes," 2014, http://professional.diabetes.org/ResourcesForProfessionals.aspx?cid=91777; American Diabetes Association, "What Are My Options," March 2015, www.diabetes.org/living-with-diabetes/treatment-and-care/medication/oral-medications/what-are-my-options.html

Type 2 Diabetes

Type 2 diabetes (non–insulin-dependent diabetes) accounts for 90–95 percent of all cases.[9] In type 2, either the pancreas does not make sufficient insulin, or body cells are resistant to its effects—a condition called **insulin resistance**—and don't use it efficiently (**FIGURE 2**).

Development of Type 2 Diabetes

Type 2 diabetes usually develops slowly. In early stages, cells throughout the body begin to resist the effects of insulin; Over time, the body may not produce enough insulin. An overabundance of free fatty acids concentrated in a person's fat cells (as may be the case in an

obese individual) inhibit glucose uptake by body cells and suppress the liver's sensitivity to insulin. As a result, the liver's ability to self-regulate its conversion of glucose into glycogen begins to fail, and blood levels of glucose gradually rise.

The pancreas attempts to compensate by producing more insulin, but it cannot maintain hyperproduction indefinitely. More and more pancreatic insulin-producing cells become nonfunctional, insulin output declines, and blood glucose levels rise high enough to warrant a diagnosis of type 2 diabetes.

Nonmodifiable Risk Factors

Type 2 diabetes is associated with a cluster of nonmodifiable risk factors including age, ethnicity, and genetic and biological factors.

One in four adults over age 65 has type 2 diabetes. Although it used to be referred to as *adult-onset diabetes*, today it is increasingly diagnosed among children

and teens.[10] Currently, diabetes is one of the leading chronic diseases in youth, affecting over 208,000 people under the age of 20, or 1 in every 400 youth.[11]

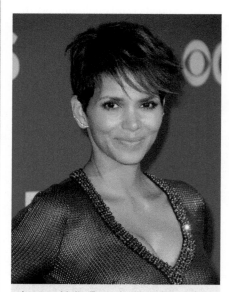

Actress Halle Berry is one of many Americans diagnosed with type 2 diabetes.

type 2 diabetes Form of diabetes mellitus in which the pancreas does not make enough insulin or the body is unable to use insulin correctly.

insulin resistance State in which body cells fail to respond to the effects of insulin; obesity increases the risk that cells will become insulin resistant.

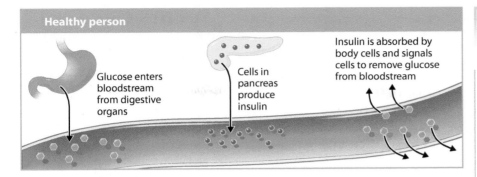

Healthy person

Glucose enters bloodstream from digestive organs

Cells in pancreas produce insulin

Insulin is absorbed by body cells and signals cells to remove glucose from bloodstream

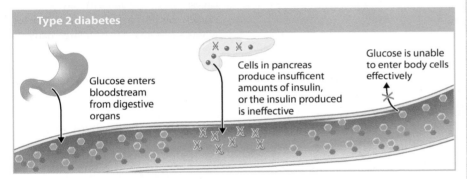

Type 1 diabetes

Glucose enters bloodstream from digestive organs

Pancreas produces little or no insulin because cells have been destroyed

Glucose is not removed from bloodstream

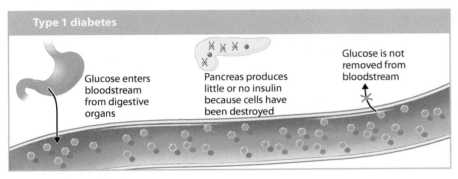

Type 2 diabetes

Glucose enters bloodstream from digestive organs

Cells in pancreas produce insufficent amounts of insulin, or the insulin produced is ineffective

Glucose is unable to enter body cells effectively

FIGURE 2 Diabetes: What It Is and How It Develops
In a healthy person, a sufficient amount of insulin is produced and released by the pancreas and used efficiently by the cells. In type 1 diabetes, the pancreas makes little or no insulin. In type 2 diabetes, either the pancreas does not make sufficient insulin, or cells are resistant to insulin and are not able to use it efficiently.

➤ **VIDEO TUTOR**
How Diabetes Develops

Non-Hispanic whites, Native Americans, and non-Hispanic black youth have the highest rates, while Asian/Pacific Islanders have the lowest.[12] Having a close relative with type 2 diabetes is a significant risk factor. Most experts believe that type 2 diabetes is caused by a complex interaction between environmental factors, lifestyle, and genetic susceptibility. Although numerous genes have been identified as likely culprits in increased risk, the mechanisms by which inherited diabetes develops remains poorly understood.[13]

Modifiable Risk Factors

Body weight, dietary choices, level of physical activity, sleep patterns, and stress level are all diabetes-related factors people have some control over. Type 2 diabetes is linked to overweight and obesity. In adults, a body mass index (BMI) of 25 or greater increases risks, with significantly higher risks for each 5 kg/m² increase.[14] In particular, excess weight carried around the waistline—a condition called *central adiposity*—and measured by waist circumference is a significant risk factor

prediabetes Condition in which blood glucose levels are higher than normal, but not high enough to be classified as diabetes.

for older women.[15] People with type 2 diabetes who lose weight and increase their physical activity can significantly improve their blood glucose levels.

Inadequate sleep may contribute to the development of both obesity and type 2 diabetes, possibly due to the fact that sleep-deprived people tend to engage in less physical activity.[16] People routinely sleep-deprived are also at higher risk for *metabolic syndrome* (discussed shortly), a cluster of risk factors that include poor glucose metabolism.[17] Recent data provides evidence of a link between diabetes and psychological or physical stress; however, a recent analysis of studies focused on the role of work-related stress on type 2 diabetes development showed mixed results.[18]

Prediabetes

An estimated 86 million Americans age 20 or older—37 percent of the population over 20—and 51 percent of those over 65—have **prediabetes**, a condition involving higher than normal blood glucose levels, but not high enough to be classified as diabetes. Nine out of ten people with prediabetes do not know they have it.[19] Current rates of prediabetes in college students are unknown; however, results from small studies as well as known increases in the rates of obesity, sedentary lifestyle, and metabolic risks point to a likely rise of rates on campus.[20]

Often, prediabetes is one of the risk factors linked to overweight and obesity that together constitute *metabolic syndrome*. Of the six conditions, prediabetes and central adiposity appear to be most dominant.[21] A person who has metabolic syndrome is five times more likely

WHAT DO YOU THINK?

Why do you think type 2 diabetes is increasing in the United States?

- Why is it increasing among young people?
- Do you think young people are generally aware of what diabetes is and their own susceptibility for it?

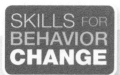

SKILLS FOR BEHAVIOR CHANGE
REDUCING YOUR RISK FOR DIABETES

Maintain a healthy weight, and lose weight if you need to.

▶ Eat smaller portions and choose foods with less fat, salt, and added sugars. Keep calories equal to energy expended. Eat more fruits, vegetables, and complex carbohydrates, and make sure you consume lean protein.

▶ Get your body moving. At least 30 minutes of moderate activity 5 days a week is a minimum recommendation.

▶ Quit smoking. In addition to cancer and heart disease, smoking increases blood glucose levels.

▶ Reduce or eliminate alcohol consumption. It's high in calories and can interfere with blood glucose regulation.

▶ Get enough sleep. Inadequate sleep may contribute to the development of type 2 diabetes.

▶ Inoculate yourself against stress. Learn to take yourself less seriously, find time for fun, develop a strong support network, and use relaxation skills.

▶ If you have a family history, or several risk factors, get regular checkups.

Sources: Centers for Disease Control and Prevention, "National Diabetes Prevention Program," 2015, www.cdc.gov/diabetes/prevention/recognition/curriculum.htm; ADA, "Living with Type 2 Diabetes Program Plan." https://donations.diabetes.org/site/SPageServer/?pagename=LWT2D_English&loc=dorg_diabetes-myths&s_src=dorg&s_subsrc=diabetes-myths

SEE IT! VIDEOS
Could fewer, larger meals be better for people with diabetes? Watch **Two Meals a Day Could Help Diabetics Control Blood Sugar** in the Study Area of MasteringHealth™

to develop type 2 diabetes than is a person without it.[22] Overall, Mexican Americans have the highest rates of metabolic syndrome, with white Americans and African Americans not far behind.[23] Women with uterine fibroids or ovarian cysts also are at increased risk.[24]

Without weight loss and increases in moderate physical activity, 15–30 percent of those with prediabetes will develop type 2 diabetes within 5 years.[25] Lack of knowledge—9 out of 10 people with prediabetes don't know they have it—poses a major challenge to slowing increasing diabetes rates.[26] A prediabetes diagnosis represents an opportunity to adjust your lifestyle. Increasing physical activity, improving diet, and losing weight can all prevent or delay a diabetes diagnosis.[27] See tips for halting or slowing the progression of diabetes in the Skills for Behavior Change box.

Gestational Diabetes

Gestational diabetes is a state of high blood glucose levels during pregnancy, posing risks for both mother and child. Thought to be associated with metabolic stresses that occur in response to changing hormonal levels, as many as 18 percent of pregnancies are affected by gestational diabetes.[28] Between 40 and 50 percent of gestational diabetics may develop type 2 diabetes within a decade of initial diagnosis if they don't lose weight, improve diet, and exercise. If excess weight is never lost, higher "normal" weight increases risk of progression to type 2 diabetes with subsequent births.[29]

Women with gestational diabetes also have increased risk of high blood pressure, high blood acidity, increased infections, and death.[30] A result of the excess fat accumulation that is a hallmark sign of gestational diabetes, women can give birth to large babies—increasing the risk of birth injuries and the need for caesarean sections. High blood sugar and excess weight in a pregnant woman can trigger high insulin levels and blood sugar fluctuations in the newborn. Babies born to women

gestational diabetes Form of diabetes mellitus in which women who have never had diabetes have high blood sugar (glucose) levels during pregnancy.

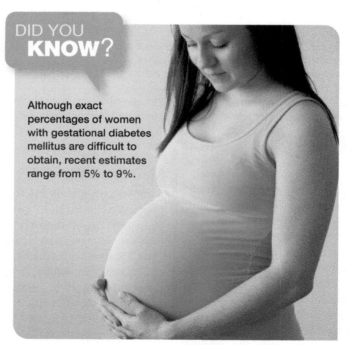

DID YOU KNOW?

Although exact percentages of women with gestational diabetes mellitus are difficult to obtain, recent estimates range from 5% to 9%.

Source: C. Desisto et al., "Prevalence Estimates of Gestational Diabetes in the United States. Pregnancy Risk Assessment Monitoring System (PRAMS) 2007–2010," *Preventing Chronic Disease* 11 (2014): 130415, doi: http:11dx.doi.org/10.5888/pcd 11.130415

with gestational diabetes are also at risk for malformations of the heart, nervous system, and bones; respiratory distress; and fetal death.[31]

LO 2 | WHAT ARE THE SYMPTOMS OF DIABETES?

Describe the symptoms of, complications associated with, and main tests for diabetes.

The symptoms of diabetes are similar for both type 1 and type 2, including:

- **Thirst.** Kidneys filter excessive glucose by diluting it with water. This can pull too much water from the body and result in dehydration.
- **Excessive urination.** For the same reason, increased need to urinate occurs.
- **Weight loss.** Because so many calories are lost in the glucose that passes into urine, a person with diabetes often feels hungry. Despite eating more, he or she typically loses weight.
- **Fatigue.** When glucose cannot enter cells, fatigue and weakness occur.
- **Nerve damage.** A high glucose concentration damages the smallest blood vessels of the body, including those supplying nerves in the hands and feet. This can cause numbness and tingling.
- **Blurred vision.** Too much glucose causes body tissues to dry out—particularly damaging to the eyes.
- **Poor wound healing and increased infections.** High levels of glucose can affect the body's ability to ward off infections and may affect overall immune system functioning.

Complications of Diabetes

The main complications of poorly controlled diabetes include:[32]

- **Diabetic coma.** A coma from high blood acidity known as *diabetic ketoacidosis*

WHY SHOULD I CARE?

You may think you are too young to worry about developing diabetes, but the statistics say otherwise. In the past decade, cases of type 2 diabetes in people under age 20 have risen to the tens of thousands. Each year, 5,089 people under 20 are diagnosed with type 2 diabetes. Overall, the risk of death among people with diabetes is about twice that of people of similar age without diabetes.

can occur when, in the absence of glucose, body cells break down stored fat for energy. The process produces acidic molecules called *ketones*. Too many ketones can raise blood acid level dangerously high. The diabetic person slips into a coma and, without medical intervention, will die.

- **Cardiovascular disease.** Because many diabetics are also overweight or obese, hypertension is often present. Blood vessels become damaged as glucose-laden blood flows sluggishly and essential nutrients and other substances are not transported as effectively.
- **Kidney disease.** Diabetes is the leading cause of kidney failure. The kidneys become scarred by

overwork and the high blood pressure in their vessels. More than 240,000 Americans are currently living with kidney failure caused by diabetes.[33] In fact, 35 percent of those 20 years or older with diabetes have kidney failure.[34] Many of these people are on dialysis or waiting for a kidney transplant that may never come.

- **Amputations.** An impaired immune response combined with damaged blood vessels and neuropathy in hands and feet makes it easier for people with diabetes to not notice injury until damage is extensive. Lack of circulation to the area increases risk of infection and difficulty of treatment, leading to tissue death and amputation. More than 60 percent of nontraumatic amputations of legs, feet, and toes are due to diabetes[35] (see FIGURE 3a). In fact, each year nearly 73,000 nontraumatic lower-limb amputations are performed on people with diabetes (180 per day).[36]
- **Eye disease and blindness.** High blood glucose levels damage microvessels in the eye, leading to vision loss. Nearly 7.7 million people over the age of 40 have early-stage retinopathy, swelling of capillaries in the eye, which could lead to blindness without treatment (FIGURE 3b).[37]
- **Infectious diseases.** Persons with diabetes have increased risk of poor

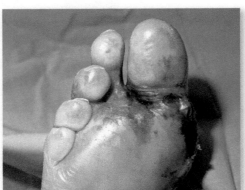

ⓐ Infections in the feet and legs are common in people with diabetes, and healing is impaired; thus, amputations are often necessary.

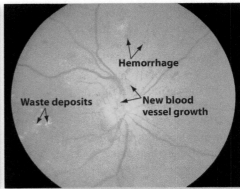

ⓑ Uncontrolled diabetes can damage the eye, causing swelling, leaking, and rupture of blood vessels; growth of new blood vessels; deposits of wastes; and scarring. All of these can progress to blindness.

Hemorrhage

Waste deposits

New blood vessel growth

FIGURE 3 Complications of Uncontrolled Diabetes: Amputation and Eye Disease

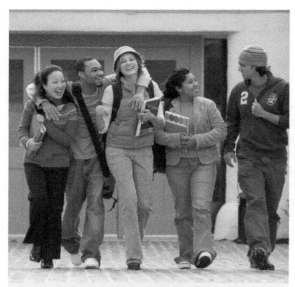

About 208,000 people younger than age 20 have type 1 or type 2 diabetes, with thousands more estimated to have prediabetes.

Source: American Diabetes Association, "Fast Facts: Data and Statistics about Diabetes," 2014, http://professional.diabetes.org

wound healing and greater susceptibility to infectious diseases, particularly influenza and pneumonia. Once infection occurs, it may be more difficult to treat.

■ **Tooth and gum diseases.** Research indicates that persons with diabetes are more susceptible to bacterial infections of the mouth that can lead to *gingivitis* (an early stage of gum disease) and *periodontitis*—a more serious inflammation of the gums that can lead to decay, tooth loss, and a variety of other health risks.[38] Emerging research suggests that the relationship between diabetes and gum disease may be a two way street, with those who have gum disease being more susceptible to problems with blood glucose control, increasing the risk of progression to diabetes.[39]

■ **Other complications.** Diabetics may have foot neuropathy and chronic pain that makes walking,

driving, and simple tasks more difficult. Persons with diabetes are more likely to suffer from depression, making intervention and treatment more difficult. Depressed individuals are 60 percent more likely to develop type 2 diabetes.

Diagnosing Diabetes

Diabetes and prediabetes are diagnosed when a blood test reveals elevated blood glucose levels. Generally, a physician orders one of the following blood tests:

■ The *fasting plasma glucose (FPG) test* requires a patient to fast for 8 to 10 hours. Then, a small sample of blood is tested for glucose concentration. An FPG level greater than or equal to 100 mg/dL indicates prediabetes, and a level greater than or equal to 126 mg/dL indicates diabetes (**FIGURE 4**).

■ The *oral glucose tolerance test (OGTT)* requires the patient to drink

concentrated glucose. A sample of blood is drawn for testing 2 hours after drinking. A reading greater than or equal to 140 mg/dL indicates prediabetes; a reading greater than or equal to 200 mg/dL indicates diabetes.

■ A third test, *A1C* or *glycosylated hemoglobin test (HbA1C)*, doesn't require fasting and gives the average value of a patient's blood glucose over the past 2 to 3 months, instead of at one moment in time. In general, an A1C of 5.7 to 6.4 means high risk for diabetes or being prediabetic. If A1C is 6.5 or higher, then diabetes may be diagnosed.[40] **Estimated average glucose (eAG)** shows how A1C numbers correspond to blood glucose numbers. For example, someone with an A1C value of 6.1 would be able to look at a chart and see that his or her average blood glucose was around 128—a high level that should encourage healthy lifestyle modifications.

People with diabetes need to check blood glucose levels several times each day to ensure they stay within their target range. To check blood glucose, diabetics must prick their finger to obtain a drop of blood. A handheld glucose meter can then evaluate the blood sample.

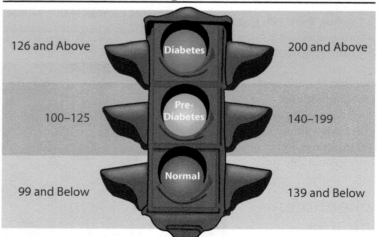

FIGURE 4 Blood Glucose Levels in Prediabetes and Untreated Diabetes The fasting plasma glucose (FPG) test measures levels of blood glucose after a person fasts overnight. The oral glucose tolerance test (OGTT) measures levels of blood glucose after a person consumes a concentrated amount of glucose.

Source: American Diabetes Association, "Diagnosing Diabetes and Learning about Prediabetes," March 2014, www.diabetes.org/diabetes-basics/diagnosis

estimated average glucose (eAG) A method for reporting A1C test results that gives the average blood glucose levels for the testing period using the same units (milligrams per deciliter [mg/dL]) that patients are used to seeing in self-administered glucose tests.

LO 3 | TREATING DIABETES

Explain how diabetes can be prevented and treated.

Treatment options for people with pre-diabetes and diabetes vary according to type and progression of the disease.

Lifestyle Changes

Studies have shown that lifestyle changes can prevent or delay the development of type 2 diabetes by up to 58 percent.[41] Even for people with type 2 diabetes, lifestyle changes can sometimes prevent or delay the need for medication or insulin injections.

Losing Weight

A landmark clinical trial, the *Diabetes Prevention Program (DPP)* study, showed that a loss of as little as 5 to 7 percent of current body weight and regular physical activity significantly lowered the risk of progressing to diabetes.[42] If you have diabetes, weight loss and exercise can improve your blood glucose and other health indicators.[43]

Adopting a Healthy Diet

To prevent surges in blood sugar, people with diabetes must pay attention to the glycemic index and glycemic load of the foods they eat. Glycemic index compares the potential of foods containing the same amount of carbohydrate to raise blood glucose. The concept of glycemic load was developed by scientists to simultaneously describe the quality (glycemic index) and quantity of carbohydrate in a meal.[44] By learning to combine high—and low—glycemic index foods to avoid surges in blood glucose, diabetics can help control average blood glucose levels throughout the day.

35%

OF THOSE 20 YEARS OLD OR OLDER WITH DIABETES HAVE **KIDNEY FAILURE**.

Researchers have studied a variety of specific foods for their effect on blood glucose levels. Here is a brief summary of their findings:

- **Whole grains.** A diet high in whole grains may reduce a person's risk of developing type 2 diabetes.[45]
- **High-fiber foods.** Recent research indicates that eating high-fiber foods may reduce diabetes risk.[46]
- **Fatty fish.** An impressive body of evidence has linked the consumption of fish high in omega-3 fatty acids with decreased progression of insulin resistance.[47] However, newer research has called omega-3's beneficial effects into question. More research is necessary to determine the role fatty acids play in diabetes risk reduction.[48]

Increasing Physical Fitness

The DPP and other organizations recommend at least 30 minutes of physical activity 5 days a week to reduce your risk of type 2 diabetes.[49] Exercise increases sensitivity to insulin. The more muscle mass you have and the more you use your muscles, the more efficiently cells use glucose for fuel, meaning there will be less glucose circulating in the bloodstream. For most people, activity of moderate intensity can help keep blood glucose levels under control.

Medical Interventions

Lifestyle changes are not always sufficient to control diabetes. Sometimes medication is necessary. In cases where medications are less effective, bariatric surgery may be an option for slowing or halting the progression of prediabetes and type 2 diabetes.

Oral Medications

When lifestyle changes fail to control type 2 diabetes, oral medications may be prescribed. Some medications reduce glucose production by the liver, whereas others slow the absorption of carbohydrates from the small intestine. Other medications increase insulin production by the pancreas, whereas still others work to increase the insulin sensitivity of cells. The newest class of diabetes drugs is known as SGLT2

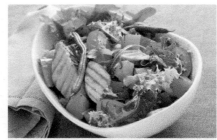

People with diabetes can occasionally indulge in sweets in moderation, particularly if they balance carbohydrates with protein. However, meals low in saturated and *trans* fats and high in fiber, like this salad of salmon and fresh vegetables, are recommended for helping to control blood glucose and body weight.

inhibitors. These drugs cause the kidneys to excrete more glucose, lowering levels of glucose circulating in the body.

Some people use diabetes medications without altering lifestyle, thinking the drugs are taking care of the problem. With time, medications become less effective and treatment options increasingly scarce. It is best to follow American Diabetes Association recommendations on diet, exercise, and lifestyle, in general.

Weight Loss Surgery

People who undergo gastric/bariatric surgery for weight loss have shown remarkable reductions in blood glucose and diabetes symptoms for 2 to 3 years after surgery.[50] Those who combined gastric bypass or sleeve gastrectomy with intensive medical therapy had similar outcomes.[51] In many cases, former diabetics can stop taking medications for some of their cardiovascular risks, and stop diabetes symptoms altogether. Many professional groups are pushing for wider use of these more drastic weight loss methods.[52] Gastric bypass surgeries are not without risks, however, and can include death and serious complications. (See Chapter 10 for more on gastric bypass surgeries.)

Insulin Injections

For people with type 1 diabetes, insulin injections or infusions are absolutely essential for daily functioning, because

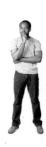

WHICH **PATH** WOULD YOU TAKE **?**

Scan the QR code to see how different health choices YOU make today can affect your risk for developing diabetes.

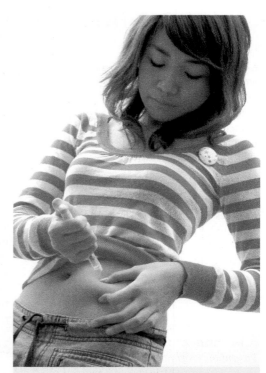

Some type 2 diabetics can control their condition with changes in diet and lifestyle habits or with oral medications. However, some type 2 diabetics and all type 1 diabetics require insulin injections or infusions.

their pancreases can no longer produce adequate amounts of insulin. In addition, people with type 2 diabetes whose blood glucose levels cannot be adequately controlled with other treatment options require insulin injections. Because insulin is a protein and would be digested in the gastrointestinal tract, it cannot be taken orally, and must be injected into the fat layer under the skin; from there, it is absorbed into the bloodstream.

People with diabetes used to need two or more daily insulin injections. Now, many use an *insulin infusion pump* to deliver minute amounts of insulin throughout the day. The external portion is only about the size of an MP3 player and can easily be hidden by clothes, while a thin tube and catheter is inserted under the patient's skin. Infusion over time is less painful and more effective than a few larger doses of insulin.

To overcome current insulin therapy limitations, researchers are working to link glucose monitoring and insulin delivery by developing an artificial pancreas. An artificial pancreas would mimic, as closely as possible, the way a healthy pancreas detects changes in blood glucose levels, responding automatically to secrete appropriate amounts of insulin. Although the first prototype devices received FDA approval, they cannot yet do the job of a fully functional pancreas.[53]

Are You at Risk for Diabetes?

Certain characteristics place people at greater risk for diabetes. Nevertheless, many people remain unaware of the symptoms of diabetes until after the disease has begun to progress. Take the following quiz to help determine your risk for diabetes. If you answer yes to three or more of these questions, consider seeking medical advice.

		Yes	No
1.	Do any of your primary relatives (parents, siblings, grandparents) have diabetes?	○	○
2.	Are you overweight or obese?	○	○
3.	Do you smoke?	○	○
4.	Have you been diagnosed with high blood pressure?	○	○
5.	Are you typically sedentary (seldom, if ever, engage in vigorous aerobic exercise)?	○	○
6.	Have you noticed an increase in your craving for water or other beverages?	○	○
7.	Have you noticed that you have to urinate more frequently than you used to during a typical day?	○	○
8.	Have you noticed any tingling or numbness in your hands and feet, which might indicate circulatory problems?	○	○
9.	Do you often feel a gnawing hunger during the day, even though you usually eat regular meals?	○	○
10.	Are you often so tired that you find it difficult to stay awake?	○	○
11.	Have you noticed that you are losing weight but don't seem to be doing anything in particular to make this happen?	○	○
12.	Have you noticed that you have skin irritations more frequently and that minor infections don't heal as quickly as they used to?	○	○
13.	Have you noticed any unusual changes in your vision (blurring, difficulty in focusing, etc.)?	○	○
14.	Have you noticed unusual pain or swelling in your joints?	○	○
15.	Do you often feel weak or nauseated when you wake in the morning or if you wait too long to eat a meal?	○	○
16.	If you are a woman, have you had several vaginal yeast infections during the past year?	○	○

YOUR PLAN FOR CHANGE

If the results of the ASSESS YOURSELF activity "Are You at Risk for Diabetes?" indicate you need to take further steps to decrease your risks, then follow this plan.

TODAY, YOU CAN:

☐ Talk to your parents and find out if there is a history of prediabetes or diabetes mellitus in your family.

☐ Take stock of other risk factors you may have for diabetes—do you exercise regularly and watch your weight? Do you eat healthfully? Have you ever had your blood glucose measured?

WITHIN THE NEXT TWO WEEKS, YOU CAN:

☐ Make an appointment with your health care provider to have your blood glucose levels tested.

☐ If you smoke, begin devising a plan to quit. (Chapter 8 can give you some ideas.)

BY THE END OF THE SEMESTER, YOU CAN:

☐ Pay attention to what you eat; increase your intake of whole grains, fruits, and vegetables; and decrease your consumption of saturated fats, *trans* fats, and sugar.

☐ Make physical activity and exercise part of your daily routine, aiming for at least 30 minutes 5 days a week.

CHAPTER REVIEW

 To head an MP3 Tutor Session, scan here or visit the Study Area in **MasteringHealth**.

LO 1 | What Is Diabetes?

- *Diabetes mellitus* is a group of diseases, each with its own mechanics. All are characterized by a persistently high level of glucose, a type of sugar, in the blood.
- Complications can range from cardiovascular disease to visual and gum problems, neuropathy, poor wound healing, and a host of other health problems.

LO 2 | What Are the Symptoms of Diabetes?

- Symptoms of diabetes vary, but may include *polydypsia* (increased thirst), *polyphagia* (increased hunger), *polyuria* (increased urination), fatigue, blurred vision, nausea and light-headedness, slow wound healing, numbness or tingling in hands and feet, frequent infections of the skin, tendency to bruise easily, among others.
- Key tests for diabetes include a fasting plasma glucose test taken after an 8- to 10-hour fast, an oral glucose tolerance test, taken 2 hours after consuming a concentrated glucose drink, and an estimated average glucose test.

LO 3 | Preventing and Treating Diabetes

- Prevention of diabetes include lifestyle changes such as a healthy/balanced diet, healthy weight, regular exercise, sufficient sleep, and stress reduction.
- Treatment of diabetes may include oral or injectable medications such as insulin, use of infusion pumps and other technologies, appropriate visits to the doctor, monitoring of glucose levels, and possible weight loss surgery.

POP QUIZ

Visit **MasteringHealth** to personalize your study plan with Chapter Review Quizzes and Dynamic Study Modules.

LO 1 | What Is Diabetes?

1. Which of the following is *not* correct?
   a. Type 1 diabetes is an autoimmune disease in which the body does not produce insulin.
   b. Type 2 diabetes is a disease in which the body may not produce sufficient amounts of insulin, or it may not be utilized properly.
   c. Gestational diabetes is only a problem for the mother while she is pregnant.
   d. Increased weight gain, high stress, lack of sleep, and sedentary lifestyle are key contributors to risks for type 2 diabetes.

LO 2 | What Are the Symptoms of Diabetes?

2. Which of the following is *not* an accurate match between blood glucose level and diabetes-related problems in adults?
   a. A fasting blood glucose of 100–126 mg/dL indicates prediabetes.
   b. A fasting blood glucose of 50–70 mg/dL is an ideal blood glucose level.
   c. A fasting blood glucose of less than 90–99 mgdL is normal.
   d. An A1C test of 5.7 is normal.

LO 3 | Treating Diabetes

3. Which of the following statements is *correct*?
   a. People with type 2 diabetes must eliminate sweets or high sugar foods from their diets.
   b. Skipping meals and eating two high-protein meals/no-carbohydrate meals per day is the best way to control blood sugar.
   c. Regular exercise, weight control, a balanced diet, adequate sleep, and stress management are key factors in blood glucose prevention and control.
   d. Most people with prediabetes know they have it.

Answers to the Pop Quiz questions can be found on page A-1. If you answered a question incorrectly, review the section identified by the Learning Outcome. For even more study tools, visit MasteringHealth.

APPENDIX A ANSWERS TO POP QUIZ QUESTIONS

Chapter 9

1. a; 2. b; 3. b; 4. a; 5. c; 6. b; 7. a; 8. d; 9. b; 10. d

Chapter 10

1. b; 2. a; 3. c; 4. c; 5. b; 6. c; 7. b; 8. a; 9. d; 10. a

Focus On: Enhancing Your Body Image

1. a; 2. b; 3. d

Chapter 11

1. d; 2. c; 3. c; 4. b; 5. b; 6. b; 7. a; 8. c; 9. b; 10. a

Chapter 12

1. d; 2. b; 3. c; 4. b; 5. c; 6. b; 7. b; 8. a; 9. c; 10. b

Focus On: Minimizing Your Risk for Diabetes

1. c; 2. b; 3. c

REFERENCES

Chapter 1: Accessing Your Health

1. K.D. Kochanek et al., "Mortality in the United States, 2013," *NCHS Data Brief,* No. 178 (2014), Available at www.cdc.gov/nchs/data/databriefs/db178.pdf

2. Centers for Disease Control and Prevention, "Achievements in Public Health, 1900–1999: Control of Infectious Diseases," *Morbidity and Mortality Weekly Report* 48, no. 29 (1999): 621–29, www.cdc.gov/mmwr/preview/mmwrhtml/mm4829a1.htm

3. Organization for Economic Cooperation and Development, *Health at a Glance 2013: OECD Indicators* (2013), doi:10.1787/health_glance-2013-en, Available at www.oecd.org/els/health-systems/Health-at-a-Glance-2013.pdf; S. H. Woolf and Laudan Aron, eds., *US Health in International Perspective: Shorter Lives, Poorer Health,* (Washington, DC: National Academies Press, 2013), Available at www.iom.edu/~/media/Files/Report%20Files/2013/US-Health-International-Perspective/USHealth_Intl_PerspectiveRB.pdf

4. U.S. Department of Health and Human Services (DHHS), *Healthy People 2020,* (Washington, DC: U.S. Government Printing Office, January 8, 2015), Available at www.healthypeople.gov/2020/topics-objectives/topic/health-related-quality-of-life-well-being

5. Centers for Disease Control and Prevention, "Adult Obesity Facts," September 2014, www.cdc.gov/obesity/data/adult.html.

6. World Health Organization (WHO), "Constitution of the World Health Organization," *Chronicles of the World Health Organization* (Geneva: WHO, 1947), www.who.int/governance/eb/constitution/en/index.html

7. R. Dubos, *So Human an Animal: How We Are Shaped by Surroundings and Events* (New York: Scribner, 1968), 15.

8. DHHS, *Healthy People 2020,* 2015.

9. Ibid.

10. Centers for Disease Control and Prevention, "Chronic Disease Prevention and Health Promotion," May 2014, www.cdc.gov/chronicdisease/overview/index.htm#2

11. U.S. Burden of Disease Collaborators, "The State of US Health, 1990–2010: Burden of Diseases, Injuries, and Risk Factors," *Journal of the American Medical Association* 310, no. 6 (2013): 591–606, doi:10.1001/jama.2013.13805; Centers for Disease Control and Prevention, "Alcohol Use and Health Fact Sheets," November 2014, www.cdc.gov/alcohol/fact-sheets/alcohol-use.htm; Centers for Disease Control and Prevention, "Smoking and Tobacco Use Fast Facts," February 2014, www.cdc.gov/tobacco/data_statistics/fact_sheets/fast_facts/

12. U.S. Burden of Disease Collaborators, "The State of US Health, " 2013.

13. Ibid.

14. CDC, "Alcohol Use and Health Fact Sheets," 2014.

15. CDC, "Smoking and Tobacco Use Fast Facts," 2014.

16. N.K. Mehta, J.S. House, and M.R. Elliott, "Dynamics of Health Behaviours and Socioeconomic Differences in Mortality in the USA," *Journal of Epidemiology and Community Health* (2015), doi: 10.1136/jech-2014-204248

17. U.S. DHHS, *Healthy People* 2020, 2015.

18. Agency for Healthcare Research and Quality, "2013 National Healthcare Disparities Report," *AHRQ Publication* No. 14-0006 (2014), Available at www.ahrq.gov/research/findings/nhqrdr/nhdr13/2013nhdr.pdf

19. M.P. Doescher et al, "The Built Environment and Utilitarian Walking in Small U.S. Towns," *Preventive Medicine* 69 (2014): 80–86, doi: 10.1016/j.ypmed.2014.08.027; J. Sallis et al., "Role of Built Environments in Physical Activity, Obesity, and Cardiovascular Disease," *Circulation* 125 (2012): 729–37, Available at https://circ.ahajournals.org/content/125/5/729.full

20. J. A. Wasserman et al., "A Multi-Level Analysis Showing Associations between School Neighborhood and Child Body Mass Index," *International Journal of Obesity* 38, no. 7 (2014): 912–18, doi: 10.1038/ijo.2014.64; M. J. Trowbridge and T. L. Schmid, "Built Environment and Physical Activity Promotion: Place-Based Obesity Prevention Strategies," *Journal of Law, Medicine & Ethics,* Weight of the Nation Supplement, (Winter, 2013): 46–51, Available at www.aslme.org/media/downloadable/files/links/j/l/jlme-41-4-supp_trowbridge.pdf

21. S. Lindsay et al., "Monetary Matched Incentives to Encourage the Purchase of Fresh Fruits and Vegetables at Farmers Markets in Underserved Communities," *Preventing Chronic Disease* 10 (2013), doi: 10.5888/pcd10.130124; E. Weinstein et al., "Impact of a Focused Nutrition Educational Intervention Coupled with Improved Access to Fresh Produce on Purchasing Behavior and Consumption of Fruits and Vegetables in Overweight Patients with Diabetes Mellitus," *Diabetes Education* 40, no. 1 (2014): 100–106, doi: 10.1177/0145721713508823

22. The Commonwealth Fund, "Gaining Ground: Americans' Health Insurance Coverage and Access to Care After the Affordable Care Act's First Open Enrollment Period," July 10, 2014, www.commonwealthfund.org/publications/issue-briefs/2014/jul/health-coverage-access-aca

23. The Commonwealth Fund, "Are Americans Finding Affordable Coverage in the Health Insurance Marketplaces?" September 18, 2014, www.commonwealthfund.org/publications/issue-briefs/2014/sep/affordable-coverage-marketplace

24. The Commonwealth Fund, "Too High a Price: Out-of-Pocket Health Care Costs in the United States. Findings from the Commonwealth Fund Health Care Affordability Tracking Survey. September-October 2014," November 13, 2014, www.commonwealthfund.org/publications/issue-briefs/2014/nov/out-of-pocket-health-care-costs

25. I. Rosenstock, "Historical Origins of the Health Belief Model," *Health Education Monographs* 2, no. 4 (1974): 328–35.

26. A. Bandura, "Human Agency in Social Cognitive Theory," *American Psychologist* 44, no. 9 (1989): 1175–84.

27. P.J. Morgan, et al. "Associations between Program Outcomes and Adherence to Social Cognitive Theory Tasks: Process Evaluation of the SHED-IT Community Weight Loss Trial for Men," *International Journal of Behavioral Nutrition and Physical Activity* 11, no. 1 (2014): 89, doi: 10.1186/s12966-014-0089-9

28. M. C. Snead, et al., "Relationship between Social Cognitive Theory Constructs and Self-Reported Condom Use: Assessment of Behaviour in a Subgroup of the Safe in the City Trial," *BMJ Open* 4, no. 12 (2014): e006093, doi: 10.1136/bmjopen-2014-006093

29. J. O. Prochaska and C. C. DiClemente, "Stages and Processes of Self-Change of Smoking: Toward an Integrative Model of Change," *Journal of Consulting and Clinical Psychology* 51 (1983): 390–95.

30. J. Huang, F. J. Chaloupka, and G. T. Fong, "Cigarette Graphic Warning Labels and Smoking Prevalence in Canada: A Critical Examination and Reformulation of the FDA Regulatory Impact Analysis," *Tobacco Control* 23, Supplement 1 (2014): i7–i12, doi: 10.1136/tobaccocontrol-2013-051170

31. K. Simmen-Janevska, V. Brandstatter, and A. Maercker. "The Overlooked Relationship between Motivational Abilities and Posttraumatic Stress: A Review," *European Journal of Psychotraumatology* 10, no. 3 (2012), doi:10.3402/ejpt.v3i0.18560

32. A. Ellis and M. Benard, *Clinical Application of Rational Emotive Therapy* (New York: Plenum, 1985).

33. National Institute on Drug Abuse, "Drugs, Brains, and Behavior: The Science of Addiction: Treatment and Recovery," July 2014, www.drugabuse.gov/publications/drugs-brains-behavior-science-addiction/treatment-recovery

34. American Cancer Society, "Staying Smoke-Free," February 6, 2014, www.cancer.org/healthy/stayawayfromtobacco/guidetoquittingsmoking/guide-to-quitting-smoking-staying-smoke-free

Why Should I Care?

page 3, S.B. Almadani et al., "Effects of Inflammatory Bowel Disease on Students' Adjustment to College," *Clinical Gastroenterology Hepatology* 12, no. 12 (2014), doi: 10.1016/j.cgh.2014.03.032; C.J. Bryan et al., "Depression, Posttraumatic Stress Disorder, and Grade Point Average among Student Service Members and Veterans," *Journal of Rehabilitation Research and Development* 51, no. 7 (2014), doi: 10.1682/JRRD.2014.01.0012.

Pulled Statistics:

page 3, World Health Organization, "Life Expectancy Data by Country," Global Health Observatory Data Repository, 2014, http://apps.who.int/gho/data/node.main.688.

page 10, The Commonwealth Fund, "Gaining Ground: Americans' Health Insurance Coverage and Access to Care After the Affordable Care Act's First Open Enrollment Period," July 10, 2014, www.commonwealthfund.org/publications/issue-briefs/2014/jul/health-coverage-access-aca.

Focus On: Improving Your Financial Health

1. W. Evans, B. Wolfe, and N. Adler, "The Income-Health Gradient," *Institute for Research on Poverty: Focus* 30, no. 1 (2013), Available at www.irp.wisc.edu/publications/focus/pdfs/foc301b.pdf; Institute for Health Metrics and Evaluation, "U.S County Profiles," Accessed February 3, 2015, www.healthdata.org/us-county-profiles

2. World Health Organization, "Social Determinants of Health: Key Concepts," *Commission on Social Determinants of Health, 2005–2008*, Accessed April 2014, www.who.int/social_determinants/thecommission/finalreport/key_concepts/en

3. OECD, *How's Life? 2013: Measuring Well-being* (Paris: OECD Publishing, 2013). doi: http://dx.doi.org/10.1787/9789264201392-en

4. R. Hiscock et al., "Socioeconomic Status and Smoking: A Review," *Annals of the New York Academy of Sciences* 1248, no. 1 (2012): 107–23, doi:10.1111/j.1749-6632.2011.06202.x

5. Ibid.

6. A. Carlsson et al., "Financial Stress in Late Adulthood and Diverse Risks of Incident Cardiovascular Disease and All-Cause Mortality in Women and Men," *BMC Public Health* 14, no. 1 (2014): 17, doi:10.1186/1471-2458-14-17

7. Pruchno et al., "Neighborhood Food Environment and Obesity in Community-Dwelling Older Adults: Individual and Neighborhood Effects," *Journal of Public Health* 104, no. 5 (2014); D. Viola et al., "Overweight and Obesity: Can We Reconcile Evidence about Supermarkets and Fast Food Retailers for Public Health Policy?," *Journal of Public Health Policy* 34, no. 3 (2013): 424–38, doi: 10.1057/jphp.2013.19

8. Centers for Disease Control and Prevention, "Food Deserts," Updated June 2013, www.cdc.gov/healthcommunication/toolstemplates/entertainment/tips/fooddesert.html

9. E. R. Cheng and D. A. Kindig, "Disparities in Premature Mortality Between High- and Low-Income US Counties," *Preventing Chronic Disease* 9 (2012): 110120, doi: http://dx.doi.org/10.5888/pcd9.110120

10. N. Spencer, T. M. Thanh, and S. Louise, "Low Income/Socio-Economic Status in Early Childhood and Physical Health in Later Childhood/Adolescence: A Systematic Review," *Maternal Child Health Journal* 17, no. 3 (2013): 424–31, doi: 10.1007/s10995-012-1010-2

11. College Board, Trends in Higher Education, "Tuition and Fee and Room and Board Charges over Time," Accessed January 2015, http://trends.collegeboard.org/college-pricing/figures-tables/tuition-fees-room-board-time

12. National Survey of Student Engagement, *NSSE Annual Results 2012: Promoting Student Learning and Institutional Improvement: Lessons from NSSE at 13* (Bloomington, IN: Indiana University Center for Postsecondary Research, 2012).

13. American College Health Association, *American College Health Association-National College Health Assessment II (ACHA-NACHA II): Undergraduate Students, Reference Group Data Report, Spring 2014* (Hanover, MD: American College Health Association, 2014).

14. K. Eagan et al., *The American Freshman: National Norms for Fall 2013* (Los Angeles: Higher Education Research Institute, UCLA, 2014).

15. Sallie Mae and Ipsos, *How America Pays for College 2014: A National Study*, Accessed January 2015, http://news.salliemae.com/research-tools/america-pays-2014

16. The White House, Office of the Press Secretary, "FACT SHEET on the President's Plan to Make College More Affordable: A Better Bargain for the Middle Class," August 22, 2013, www.whitehouse.gov/the-press-office/2013/08/22/fact-sheet-president-s-plan-make-college-more-affordable-better-bargain

17. Sallie Mae and Ipsos, *How America Pays for College 2014*, 2015.

18. American Council on Education, "National Study of Non-First-Time Students Shows Disturbing Completion Rates," Accessed February 3, 2015, www.insidetrack.com/2014/10/27/national-study-non-first-time-students-shows-disturbing-completion-rates/

19. National Center for Education Statistics, "Annual Earnings of Young Adults," *The Condition of Education 2014* (NCES 2014-083), May, 2014, http://nces.ed.gov/programs/coe/indicator_cba.asp

20. M. Heron, "Deaths: Leading Causes for 2012, Table 9," *National Vital Statistics Reports* 63, no. 9 (2014), www.cdc.gov/nchs/data/nvsr/nvsr63/nvsr63_09.pdf

21. Healthcare.gov, "Why Should I Have Health Coverage?," Accessed April 2014, www.healthcare.gov/why-should-i-have-health-coverage

22. Bankruptcy Abuse Prevention and Consumer Protection Act of 2005, Pub.L. 109–8, 109th Cong. (2005). Full text available at www.govtrack.us.

23. Federal Reserve Bank of New York, Research and Statistics Group, Microeconomic Studies, "Quarterly Report on Household Debt and Credit," November 2014, www.newyorkfed.org

24. Ibid.

25. Credit Card Accountability Responsibility and Disclosure Act, The CARD Act of 2009, Pub.L. 111–24, 111th Cong. (2009). Full text available at www.gpo.gov.

26. Javelin Strategy & Research, "The 2014 Identity Fraud Report: Card Data Breaches and Inadequate Consumer Password Habits Fuel Disturbing Fraud Trends," February 2014, www.javelinstrategy.com/brochure/314

27. Ibid.

28. Federal Trade Commission, Consumer Information, "Lost or Stolen Credit, ATM, and Debit Cards," August 2012, www.consumer.ftc.gov/articles/0213-lost-or-stolen-credit-atm-and-debit-cards

Pulled Statistics:

page 31, Nerd Wallet, "American Household Credit Card Debt Statistics: 2014," December 2014, www.nerdwallet.com/blog/credit-card-data/average-credit-card-debthousehold

page 33, Javelin Strategy & Research, "The 2014 Identity Fraud Report: Card Data Breaches and Inadequate Consumer Password Habits Fuel Disturbing Fraud Trends," February 2014, www.javelinstrategy.com

Chapter 2: Promoting and Preserving Your Psychological Health

1. K. Neff, *Self Compassion: The Proven Power of Being Kind to Yourself* (New York: Harper Collins, 2011).

2. A. H. Maslow, *Motivation and Personality,* 2nd ed. (New York: Harper and Row, 1970).

3. D. J. Anspaugh and G. Ezell, *Teaching Today's Health*, 10th ed. (Boston: Pearson, 2013).

4. X. Wang et al., "Social Support Moderates Stress Effect on Depression," *International Journal of Mental Health Systems* 8, no. 1 (2014): 1–5; J. Holt-Lunstad, T. B. Smith, and J. B. Layton, "Social Relationships and Mortality Risk: A Meta-Analytic Review," *PLoS Medicine* 7, no. 7 (2010): e1000316, doi: 10.1371/journal.pmed.1000316; N. I. Eisenberger and S. W. Cole, "Social Neuroscience and Health: Neurophysiological Mechanisms Linking Social Ties with Physical Health," *Nature Neuroscience* 15 (2012): 669–74, doi:10.1038/nn.3086; Y. Luo et al., "Loneliness, Health, and Mortality in Old Age: A National Longitudinal Study," *Social Science & Medicine* 74, no. 6 (2012): 907–14.

5. C. Carter, *Raising Happiness: 10 Simple Steps for More Joyful Kids and Happier Parents* (New York: Ballantine Publishing, 2010).

6. X. Wang et al., "Social Support Moderates Stress Effect," 2014; W. Cheng, W. Ickes, and L. Verhofstadt, "How is Family Support Related to Students' GPA Scores? A Longitudinal Study," *Higher Education* 64, no. 3 (2012): 399–420; L. Rice et al., "The Role of Social Support in Students' Perceived Abilities and Attitudes toward Math and Science," *Journal of Youth and Adolescence* 42, no. 7 (2013): 1028–40; J. Cullum et al., "Ignoring Norms with a Little Help from my Friends: Social Support Reduces Normative Influence on Drinking Behavior," *Journal of Social & Clinical Psychology* 32, no. 1 (2013): 17–33; J. Hirsch and A. Barton, "Positive Social Support, Negative Social Exchanges, and Suicidal Behavior in College Students," *Journal of American College Health* 59, no. 5 (2011): 393–98; I. Yalcin, "Social Support and Optimism as Predictors of Life Satisfaction of College Students," *International Journal for the Advancement of Counseling* 33, no. 2 (2011): 79–87.

7. National Cancer Institute, "Spirituality in Cancer Care," Revised 2012, www.cancer.gov/cancertopics/pdq/supportivecare/spirituality/patient

8. M. Seligman, *Helplessness: On Depression, Development, and Death* (New York: W. H. Freeman, 1975).

9. P. Salovey and J. Mayer, "Emotional Intelligence," *Imagination, Cognition, and Personality* 9, no. 3 (1989): 185–211.

10. A. Martins, N. Ramalho, and E. Morin, "A Comprehensive Meta Analysis of the Relationship between Emotional Intelligence and Health," *Personality and Individual Differences* 49, no. 6 (2010): 554–64.

11. D. Goleman, R. Boyatzis, and A. McKee, *Primal Leadership: Unleashing the Power of Emotional Intelligence* (Boston: Harvard Business Review Press, 2013); M. A. Brackett, S. E. Rivers, and P. Salovey, "Emotional Intelligence: Implications for Personal, Social, Academic, and Workplace Success," *Social and Personality Psychology Compass* 5, no. 1 (2011): 88–103.

12. K. Huffman and C. A. Sanderson, *Real World Psychology* (Hoboken, NJ: Wiley, 2014).

13. Ibid.

14. S. Rimer, Harvard School of Public Health, "The Biology of Emotion—And What It May Teach Us about Helping People to Live Longer," 2012, www.hsph.harvard.edu/news/hphr/chronic-disease-prevention/happiness-stress-heart-disease/

15. Ibid; Steptoe, C. de Oliveira, P. Demakakos, and P. Zaninotto, "Enjoyment of Life and Declining Physical Function at Older Ages: A Longitudinal Cohort Study," *Canadian Medical Association Journal* 186, no. 4 (2014): e150–56.

16. Ibid; E. A. Wheeler, "Amusing Ourselves to Health: A Selected Review of Lab Findings," in *Positive Psychology: Advances in Understanding Adult Motivation*, ed. J. D. Sinnott (New York: Springer, 2013).

17. B. Fredrickson, et al., "A Functional Genomic Perspective on Human Well-Being," *Proceedings of the National Academy of Sciences* 110, no. 33 (2013): 13684–89.

18. E. Diener, "Subjective Well-Being: A Primer for Reporters and Newcomers," Accessed February 2015, http://internal.psychology.illinois.edu/~ediener/faq.html; L. Tay, M. Herian, and E. Diener, "The Metrics of Societal Happiness," *Social Indicators Research* 117, no. 2 (2014): 577–600.

19. E. Roysamb et al., "Well-Being: Heritable and Changeable," *Stability of Happiness Theories and Evidence on Whether Happiness Can Change* (San Diego: Academic Press, 2014): 9–35.

20. M. Seligman, *Flourish: A Visionary New Understanding of Happiness and Well-Being* (New York: Free Press, 2011).

21. Medline Plus, "Mental Disorders," February 12, 2015, www.nlm.nih.gov/medlineplus/mentaldisorders.html.

22. Ibid.

23. R. Karg, et al. "Past Year Mental Health Disorders among Adults in the U.S.: Results from the

24. 2008–2012 Mental Health Surveillance Study," *Center for Behavioral Health Statistics and Quality* (2014), Available at www.samhsa.gov/data/sites/default/files/NSDUH-DR-N2MentalDis-2014-1/Web/NSDUH-DR-N2MentalDis-2014.htm

24. National Alliance on Mental Illness, "Mental Illness Factors and Numbers," March 2013, Available at www2.nami.org/factsheet/mentalillness_factsheet.pdf; Substance Abuse and Mental Health Services Administration, "Results from the 2012 National Survey on Drug Use and Health: Mental Health Findings," NSDUH Series H-47, HHS Publication no. (SMA) 13-4805 (Rockville, MD: Substance Abuse and Mental Health Services Administration, 2013).

25. L. Szabo, "Cost of Not Caring: Nowhere to Go," *USA Today*, May 5, 2014, www.usatoday.com/story/news/nation/2014/05/12/mental-health-system-crisis/7746535/; H. A. Whiteford et al., "Global Burden of Disease Attributable to Mental and Substance Use Disorders: Findings from the Global Burden of Disease Study 2010," *The Lancet* 382, no. 9904 (2013): 1575–86.

26. L. Szabo, "Cost of Not Caring," 2014.

27. American Psychological Association, "College Students' Mental Health is a Growing Concern, Survey Finds," June 2013, www.apa.org/monitor/2013/06/college-students.aspx; D. Gruttadaro and D. Crudo, *College Students Speak: A Survey Report on Mental Health* (Arlington, VA: National Alliance on Mental Health, 2012), Available at www.nami.org/Content/NavigationMenu/Find_Support/NAMI_on_Campus1/NAMI_Survey_on_College_Students/collegereport.pdf

28. American College Health Association, *American College Health Association–National College Health Assessment II (ACHA–NCHA II): Reference Group Data Report Spring 2014* (Hanover, MD: American College Health Association, 2014), Available at www.acha-ncha.org/reports_ACHA-NCHAII.html

29. Ibid.

30. National Alliance on Mental Illness, "Mental Illness Factors and Numbers," 2013.

31. R. Karg, et al. "Past Year Mental Health Disorders among Adults in the U.S.," 2014.

32. Ibid.

33. National Institute of Mental Health, "Depression," Accessed February 2014, www.nimh.nih.gov/health/topics/depression/index.shtml

34. Ibid.

35. American College Health Association, *American College Health Association II): Reference Group Data Report Spring 2014*, 2014.

36. HelpGuide.org, "Depression in Men," 2014, www.helpguide.org/mental/depression_men_male.htm

37. A. Shah et al., "Sex and Age Differences in the Association of Depression with Obstructive Coronary Artery Disease and Adverse Cardiovascular Events," Journal of the American Heart Association 3, no. 3 (2014): e000741.

38. R. Karg, et al. "Past Year Mental Health Disorders among Adults," 2014; Mayo Clinic, "Depression in Women: Understanding the Gender Gap," January 19, 2013, www.mayoclinic.org/diseases-conditions/depression/in-depth/depression/art-20047725

39. A. Gurian, "Depression in Adolescence: Does Gender Matter?," *NYU Child Study Center*, Accessed February 23, 2015, www.aboutourkids.org/articles/depression_in_adolescence_does_gender_matter#

40. D. Johnson and M. Whisman, "Gender Differences in Rumination: A Meta-Analysis," *Personality and Individual Differences* 55, no. 4 (2013.): 367–74.

41. R. Uher, "Persistent Depressive Disorder, Dysthymia, and Chronic Depression: Update on Diagnosis, Treatment," *Psychiatric Times*, July 2014, www.psychiatrictimes.com/special-reports/persistent-depressive-disorder-dysthymia-and-chronic-depression/page/0/3

42. WebMD, "Seasonal Depression (Seasonal Affective Disorder)," Accessed February 23, 2015, www.webmd.com/depression/guide/seasonal-affective-disorder

43. American Psychiatric Association, "Seasonal Affective Disorder," Accessed February 23, 2015, www.psychiatry.org/seasonal-affective-disorder; Cleveland Clinic, "Seasonal Depression," Accessed February 2015, http://my.clevelandclinic.org/services/neurological_institute/center-for-behavioral-health/disease-conditions/hic-seasonal-depression

44. SAMHSA, "Mental Disorders: Bipolar and Related Disorders," October 10, 2014, www.samhsa.gov/disorders/mental; R. C. Kessler et al., "Twelve-Month and Lifetime Prevalence and Lifetime Morbid Risk of Anxiety and Mood Disorders in the United States," *International Journal of Methods in Psychiatric Research* 21, no. 3 (2012): 169–84.

45. SAMHSA, "Treatments for Mental Disorders," October 9, 2014, www.samhsa.gov/treatment/mental-disorders

46. Mayo Clinic Staff, MayoClinic.com, "Depression: Causes," 2013, www.mayoclinic.org/diseases-conditions/depression/basics/causes/con-20032977

47. PsychGuides.com, "Mood Disorder Symptoms, Causes and Effects," Accessed 2015, www.psychguides.com/guides/mood-disorder-symptoms-causes-and-effect/

48. SAMSHA, "Mental Disorders: Anxiety Disorders," October 10, 2014, www.samhsa.gov/disorders/mental; R. Karg, et al., "Past Year Mental Health Disorders among Adults in the U.S.," 2014; K. R. Merikangas et al., "Lifetime Prevalence of Mental Disorders in U.S. Adolescents: Results from the National Comorbidity Survey Replication—Adolescent Supplement (NCS-A)," *Journal of the American Academy of Child and Adolescent Psychiatry* 49, no. 10 (2010): 980–89, doi: 10.1016/j.jaac.2010.05.017

49. American College Health Association, *National College Health Assessment III: Reference Group Data Report Spring 2014*, 2014.

50. National Institute of Mental Health, "Anxiety Disorders," Accessed February 2015, www.nimh.nih.gov/health/publications/anxiety-disorders/index.shtml#pub7

51. American College Health Association, *National College Health Assessment II: Reference Group Data Report Spring 2014*, 2014.

52. Mayo Clinic Staff, MayoClinic.com, "Panic Attacks and Panic Disorder: Symptoms," May 31, 2012, www.mayoclinic.org/diseases-conditions/panic-attacks/basics/symptoms/con-20020825

53. Web MD, "Anxiety and Panic Disorders Health Center: Specific Phobias," Accessed February 23, 2015, www.webmd.com/anxiety-panic/specific-phobias

54. Ibid.

55. Mayo Clinic, "Generalized Anxiety Disorder: Causes," Accessed February 2014, www.mayoclinic.org/diseases-conditions/generalized-anxiety-disorder/basics/causes/con-20024562

56. National Institute of Mental Health, "Obsessive Compulsive Disorder: Prevalence," Accessed February 23, 2015, www.nimh.nih.gov/health/statistics/prevalence/obsessive-compulsive-disorder-among-adults.shtml

57. National Institute of Mental Health, "Obsessive Compulsive Disorder," Accessed February 23, 2015, www.nimh.nih.gov/health/topics/obsessive-compulsive-disorder-ocd/index.shtml

58. Anxiety and Depression Association of America, "Facts and Statistics," Accessed February 23, 2015, www.adaa.org/about-adaa/press-room/facts-statistics

59. U.S. Dept. of Veterans Affairs, "PTSD: National Center for PTSD," November 10, 2014, www.ptsd.va.gov/public/PTSD-overview/basics/how-common-is-ptsd.asp; R. H. Pietrzak et al., "Prevalence and Axis I Comorbidity of Full and Partial PTSD in the U.S.: Results from Wave 2 of the National Epidemiologic Survey on Alcohol and Related Conditions," *Journal of Anxiety Disorders* 25, no. 3 (2011): 456–65.

60. U.S. Department of Veterans Affairs, "PTSD: National Center for PTSD," November 10, 2014, www.ptsd.va.gov/public/PTSD-overview/basics/how-common-is-ptsd.asp

61. National Institute of Mental Health, "Post-Traumatic Stress Disorder," Accessed February 23, 2015, www.nimh.nih.gov/health/topics/post-traumatic-stress-disorder-ptsd/index.shtml#part4

62. R. H. Pietrzak et al., "Prevalence and Axis I Comorbidity of Full and Partial PTSD in the U.S.," 2011; J. Gradus, U.S. Department of Veterans Affairs, National Center for PTSD, "Epidemiology of PTSD," January 2014, www.ptsd.va.gov/professional/PTSD-overview/epidemiological-facts-ptsd.asp; S. Staggs, PsychCentral, "Myths and Facts about PTSD," February 2014, http://psychcentral.com/lib/myths-and-facts-about-ptsd

63. American Psychiatric Association, *Diagnostic and Statistical Manual of Mental Disorders (DSM-5)*, 5th ed. (Washington, DC: American Psychiatric Association, 2013).

64. R. A. Sansone and L. A. Sansone, "Personality Disorders: A Nation-Based Perspective on Prevalence," *Innovations in Clinical Neuroscience* 8, no. 4 (2011): 13–18.

65. J. Twenge, *The Narcissism Epidemic: Living in the Age of Entitlement* (San Jose, CA: Atria Books, 2010).

66. American Psychiatric Association, *DSM-5*, 2013.

67. Mayo Clinic Staff, MayoClinic.com, "Borderline Personality Disorder," Accessed February 23, 2015, www.mayoclinic.org/diseases-conditions/borderline-personality-disorder/basics/definition/con-20023204

68. SAMHSA, "Report to Congress on Borderline Personality Disorder," HHS Pub. No. SMA-11-4644, 2011, Available at http://store.samhsa.gov/shin/content//SMA11-4644/SMA11-4644.pdf

69. Ibid.

70. National Institute of Mental Health, "Schizophrenia," Accessed February 23, 2015, www.nimh.nih.gov/health/topics/schizophrenia/index.shtml

71. Ibid.

72. Ibid.

73. World Health Organization, "Preventing Suicide: A Global Imperative," 2014, Available at www.who.int/mental_health/suicide-prevention/world_report_2014/en/)

74. Ibid.

75. Ibid.

76. M. Heron, "Deaths: Leading Causes for 2010," *National Vital Statistics Reports* 62, no. 6 (2013), Available at www.cdc.gov/nchs/data/nvsr/nvsr62/nvsr62_06.pdf

77. Centers for Disease Control and Prevention, "National Suicide Statistics at a Glance," January 2014, www.cdc.gov/violenceprevention/suicide/statistics/index.html

78. A. P. Haas et al., "Suicide and Suicide Risk in Lesbian, Gay, Bisexual, and Transgender Populations: Review and Recommendations," *Journal of Homosexuality* 58, no. 1 (2011): 10–51.

79. D. Reynolds and P. Schneider, "An Overview of Suicide Risks among Lesbian, Gay, Bisexual, Transgender and Questioning (LGBTQ) Youth," Social Workers Help Starts Here, blog, December 9, 2009, www.helpstartshere.org/mind-spirit/suicide-prevention/an-overview-of-suicide-risks-among-lesbian-gay-bisexual-transgender-and-questioning-lgbtq-youth.html

80. Ibid; E. Mereish, C. O'Clerigh, and J. Bradford, "Interrelationships between LGBT-Based Victimization, Suicide, and Substance Use Problems in a Diverse Sample of Sexual and Gender Minority Men and Women," *Psychology, Health & Medicine* 19, no. 1 (2014): 1–13

81. Centers for Disease Control and Prevention, "Suicide Facts at a Glance," 2012, Available at www.cdc.gov/violenceprevention/pdf/Suicide-DataSheet-a.pdf

82. Centers for Disease Control and Prevention, "National Suicide Statistics at a Glance," January 2015, www.cdc.gov/violenceprevention/suicide/statistics/mechanism02.html

83. American Foundation for Suicide Prevention, "Suicide Warning Signs," Accessed February 23, 2015, www.afsp.org/preventing-suicide/suicide-warning-signs

84. Ibid.

85. American Foundation for Suicide Prevention, "Frequently Asked Questions," Accessed February 23, 2015, www.afsp.org/preventing-suicide/frequently-asked-questions

86. Substance Abuse and Mental Health Services Administration, *Results from the 2012 National Survey on Drug Use and Health: Mental Health Findings*, NSDUH Series H-47, HHS Publication No. (SMA) 13-4805, (Rockville, MD: Substance Abuse and Mental Health Services Administration, 2013), Available at www.samhsa.gov/data/sites/default/files/2k12MH_Findings/2k12MH_Findings/NSDUHmhfr2012.pdf

87. Ibid.

88. MentalHealth.gov, "Mental Health Myths and Facts," Accessed February 23, 2015, www.mentalhealth.gov/basics/myths-facts/

89. A. Lasalvia et al., "Global Pattern of Experienced and Anticipated Discrimination Reported by People with Major Depressive Disorder: A Cross-Sectional Survey," *The Lancet* 381, no. 9860 (2013): 55–62, doi: 10.1016/S0140-6736(12)61379-8

90. K. Huffman and C. A. Sanderson, *Real World Psychology* (Hoboken, NJ: Wiley, 2014).

91. Ibid.

92. Mayo Clinic, Cognitive Behavioral Therapy, February 2013, www.mayoclinic.com/health/cognitive-behavioral-therapy/MY00194

93. National Institute of Mental Health, "Antidepressant Medications for Children and Adolescents: Information for Parents and Caregivers," Accessed February 23, 2015, www.nimh.nih.gov/health/topics/child-and-adolescent-mental-health/antidepressant-medications-for-children-and-adolescents-information-for-parents-and-caregivers.shtml

94. B. K. Hölzel et al., "Mindfulness Practice Leads to Increases in Regional Brain Gray Matter Density," *Psychiatry Research: Neuroimaging* 191, no. 1 (2011): 36–43; Mayo Clinic, "St. John's Wort (*Hypericum perforatum*)," November 2013, www.mayoclinic.org/drugs-supplements/st-johns-wort/background/HRB-20060053

Pulled Statistics:

Page 45, Substance Abuse and Mental Health Services Administration, *Results from the 2012 National Survey on Drug Use and Health: Mental Health Findings*, NSDUH Series H-47, HHS Publication no. (SMA) 13-4805 (Rockville, MD: Substance Abuse and Mental Health Services Administration, 2013).

Page 53, National Alliance on Mental Illness, "College Students Speak: A Survey Report on Mental Health," 2012, Available at: www.nami.org/Content/NavigationMenu/Find_Support/NAMI_on_Campus1/collegereport.pdf

Focus On: Cultivating Your Spiritual Health

1. K. Eagan et al., *The American Freshman: National Norms Fall 2014* (Los Angeles: Higher Education Research Institute, UCLA, 2014), Available at http://heri.ucla.edu/monographs/TheAmerican-Freshman2014-Expanded.pdf

2. Ibid.

3. H. G. Koenig, "Religion, Spirituality and Health: The Research and Clinical Implications," *ISRN Psychiatry* (2012), doi: 10.5402/2012/27830

4. K. Eagan et al., *The American Freshman*, 2014.

5. Ibid.

6. B. L. Seaward, *Managing Stress: Principles and Strategies for Health and Well Being*, 7th ed. (Sudbury, MA: Jones and Bartlett, 2012).

7. DanahZohar.com, "Learn the Qs," Accessed January 2014, http://dzohar.com/?page_id=622

8. C. Wigglesworth, "Spiritual Intelligence and Why It Matters," Deep Change, 2011, www.deepchange.com/SpiritualIntelligenceEmotionalIntelligence2011.pdf

9. NIH, NCCIH, Research Results, accessed March 2015, https://nccih.nih.gov/research/results

10. B. C. Bock et al., "Yoga as a Complementary Treatment for Smoking Cessation in Women," *Journal of Women's Health* 21, no. 2 (2012): 240–48; L. Carim-Todd, S. H. Mitchell, and B. S. Oken, "Mind-Body Practices: An Alternative, Drug-Free Treatment for Smoking Cessation? A Systematic Review of the Literature," *Drug and Alcohol Dependence* 132, no. 3 (2013): 399–410; V. Conn, "The Power of Being Present: The Value of Mindfulness Interventions in Improving Health and Well-Being," *Western Journal of Nursing Research* 33 (2011): 993–95; Y. Matchim, J. Armer, and B. Stewart, "Effects of Mindfulness-Based Stress Reduction on Health among Breast Cancer Survivors," *Western Journal of Nursing Research* 33, no. 8 (2011): 996–1016.

11. National Cancer Institute (NCI), "Spirituality in Cancer Care," July 3, 2014, www.cancer.gov/cancertopics/pdq/supportivecare/spirituality/HealthProfessional/page1

12. C. Lysne and A. Wachholtz, "Pain, Spirituality and Meaning Making: What Can We Learn from the Literature?," *Religions*, no. 2 (2011): 1–16, doi:10.3390/rel2010001; H. Koenig and A. Bussing, "Spiritual Needs of Patients with Chronic Diseases." *Religions* 1, no. 1 (2010): 18–27.

13. R. E. Wells et al., "Complementary and Alternative Medicine Use among U. S. Adults with Common Neurological Conditions," *Journal of Neurology* 257, no. 11 (2010): 1822–11, Available at www.ncbi.nlm.nih.gov

14. ClinicalTrials.gov, "Mind–Body Interventions in Cardiac Patients," January 2011, http://clinicaltrials.gov/ct2/show/NCT01270568

15. P. Rajguru et al. "Use of Mindfulness Meditation in the Management of Chronic Pain: A Systematic Review of Randomized Controlled Trials," *American Journal of Lifestyle Medicine* (2014), doi: 10.1177/1559827614522580

16. G. Lucchetti, A. Lucchetti, and H. Koenig, "Impact of Spirituality/Religiosity on Mortality: Comparison with Other Health Interventions," *The Journal of Science and Healing* 7, no. 4 (2011): 234–38.

17. C. Aldwin et al., "Differing Pathways between Religiousness, Spirituality, and Health: A Self-Regulation Perspective," *Psychology of Religion and Spirituality* 6, no. 1 (2014): 9–21.

18. NCI, "Spirituality in Cancer Care," 2014.

19. A. Wachholtz and M. Rogoff, "The Relationship between Spirituality and Burnout among Medical Students," *Journal of Contemporary Medical Education* 1, no. 2 (2013): 83–91, doi: 10.5455/jcme.20130104060612

20. National Center for PTSD, "Spirituality and Trauma: Professionals Working Together," January 3, 2014, www.ptsd.va.gov/professional/provider-type/community/fs-spirituality.asp

21. Ibid.; NCCAM, "Prayer and Spirituality in Health: Ancient Practices, Modern Science," *CAM at the NIH: Focus on Complementary and Alternative Medicine* 12, no. 1 (2005), www.jpsych.com/pdfs/NCCAM%20-%20Prayer%20and%20Spirituality%20in%20Health.pdf; NCI, "Spirituality in Cancer Care," 2014.

22. D. R. Vago and D. A. Silbersweig, "Self-Awareness, Self-Regulation, and Self-Transcendence (S-ART): A Framework for Understanding the Neurobiological Mechanisms of Mindfulness," *Human Neuroscience* 6, no. 269 (2012), Available at www.ncbi.nlm.nih.gov/pmc/articles/PMC3480633/

23. G. Desbordes et al., "Effects of Mindful-Attention and Compassion Meditation Training on Amygdala Response to Emotional Stimuli in an Ordinary, Non-meditative State," *Frontiers in Human Neuroscience* 6, no. 292 (2012), doi: 10.3389/fnhum.2012.00292

24. National Center for Complementary and Integrative Health (NCCIH), "Research Spotlight: Meditation May Increase Empathy," Modified January 2012, https://nccih.nih.gov/research/results/spotlight/060608.htm

25. G. Desbordes et al., "Effects of Mindful-Attention and Compassion Meditation," 2012.

26. F. Zeidan et al., "Neural Correlates of Mindfulness Meditation-Related Anxiety Relief," *Social Cognitive and Affective Neuroscience* 9, no. 6 (2014): 751–59, doi: 10.1093/scan/nst041; G. Desbordes et al, "Effects of Mindful-Attention," 2012; J.C. Ong et al., "A Randomized Controlled Trial of Mindfulness Meditation for Chronic Insomnia," *Sleep* 37, no. 9 (2013): 1553–63; NCCIH, "Research Spotlight," 2014; A. Chiesa and A. Serretti, "Mindfulness-Based Stress Reduction for Stress Management in Healthy People," *Journal of Alternative and Complementary Medicine* 15, no. 5 (2009): 593–600.

27. S. Keng et al. "Effects of Mindfulness on Psychological Health: A Review of Empirical Studies," *Clinical Psychology Review* 31, no. 6 (2011); 1041–1056; E. Hoge et al., "Randomized Controlled Trial of Mindfulness Meditation for Generalized Anxiety Disorder: Effects on Anxiety and Stress Reactivity," *The Journal of Clinical Psychiatry* 74, no. 8 (2013): 786–92; S. Jedel et al., "A Randomized Controlled Trial of Mindfulness-Based Stress Reduction to Prevent Flare-Up in Patients with Inactive Ulcerative Colitis," *Digestion* 89, no. 2 (2014): 142–55.

28. W. Marchand, "Neural Mechanisms of Mindfulness and Meditation: Evidence From Neuroimging Studies," *World Journal of Radiology* 6, no. 7 (2014): 471–70, doi: 10.4329/wjr.v6.i7.471

29. S. Keng et al. "Effects of Mindfulness on Psychological Health," *Clinical Psychology Review* 31, no. 6 (2011); 1041–56.

30. W. Marchand, "Neural Mechanisms of Mindfulness and Meditation," 2014; B. Holzel et al., "Neural Mechanisms of Symptom Improvements in Generalized Anxiety Disorder Following Mindfulness Training," *Neuroimage: Clinical* 2 (2013): 448–58; B. Holzel et al., "Mindfulness Practice Leads to Increases in Regional Brain Gray Matter Density," *Psychiatry Research: Neuroimaging* 191, no. 1 (2011): 36–43; B. Holzel et al., "Stress Reduction Correlates with Structural Changes in the Amygdala," *Social Cognitive and Affective Neuroscience* 5 (2009): 11–17.

31. American Cancer Society, "Spirituality and Prayer," December 2012, www.cancer.org/treatment/treatmentsandsideeffects/complementaryandalternativemedicine/mindbodyandspirit/spirituality-and-prayer; University of Minnesota Center for Spirituality and Healing, "What Is Prayer?," August 2013, www.takingcharge.csh.umn.edu/explore-healing-practices/prayer

32. R. Jahnke et al., "A Comprehensive Review of Health Benefits of Qigong and Tai Chi," *American Journal of Health Promotion* 24, no. 6 (2010): e1–e25, www.ncbi.nlm.nih.gov/pubmed/20594090; American Tai Chi Association, "Psychiatric Expert: Tai Chi and Qigong Can Improve Mood in Older Adults, September 6, 2013, www.americantaichi.net/TaiChiQigongForHealthArticle.asp?cID=2&sID=10&article=chi_201309_1&subject=MentalHealth

33. M. Rudd and J. Aakers, "How to Be Happy by Giving to Others," *Scientific American*, July 8, 2014, www.scientificamerican.com/article/how-to-be-happy-by-giving-to-others/

34. F. Warneken and M. Tomasello, "The Roots of Human Altruism," *British Journal of Psychology* 100, no. 3 (2009): 455–71; C. Carter, *Raising Happiness: 10 Simple Steps for More Joyful Kids and Happier Parents* (New York: Ballantine Publishing, 2010); R. I. Dunbar et al., "Social Laughter Is Correlated with an Elevated Pain Threshold," *Proceedings of the Royal Society,* September 14, 2011, doi: 10.1098/rspb.2011.1373.39%

Pulled Statistics:

Page 61, K. Eagan et al., *The American Freshman: National Norms Fall 2014* (Los Angeles: Higher Education Research Institute, UCLA, 2014), Available at http://heri.ucla.edu/monographs/TheAmericanFreshman2014-Expanded.pdf

Page 63, Higher Education Research Institute, "Attending to Student's Inner Lives," April 2011, Available at http://spirituality.ucla.edu/docs/white%20paper/white%20paper%20final.pdf

Page 67, *Yoga Journal,* "New Study Finds More Than 20 Million Yogis in U.S.," December 5, 2012, http://blogs.yogajournal.com/yogabuzz/2012/12/new-study-find-more-than-20-million-yogis-in-u-s.html

Chapter 3: Managing Stress and Coping with Life's Challenges

1. American Psychological Association, "Stress in America Annual Survey: Are Teens Adopting Adults' Stress Habits?" February 11, 2014, Available at www.apa.org/news/press/releases/stress/2013/stress-report.pdf; American Psychological Association (APA), "Stress in America: Missing the Health Care Connection," February 2013, www.apa.org/news/press/releases/stress/2012/full-report.pdf; S. Bethune, "Health-care Falls Short on Stress Management," *Monitor on Psychology* 44, no. 4 (2013): 22.

2. American Psychological Association, "A Stress Snapshot: Women Continue to Face an Uphill Battle with Stress," Accessed January 30, 2015, http://apa.org/news/press/releases/stress/2013/snapshot.aspx

3. American Psychological Association, "Stress: The Different Kinds of Stress," Accessed February 2014, www.apa.org

4. B. L. Seaward, *Managing Stress: Principles and Strategies for Health and Well-Being,* 8th ed. (Sudbury, MA: Jones and Bartlett, 2013), 8; National Institute of Mental Health (NIMH), "Stress Fact Sheet," Accessed January 2014, www.nimh.nih.gov

5. H. Selye, *Stress without Distress* (New York: Lippincott Williams & Wilkins, 1974), 28–29.

6. W. B. Cannon, *The Wisdom of the Body* (New York: Norton, 1932).

7. M. P. Picard and D. M. Turnbull, "Linking the Metabolic State and Mitochondrial DNA in Chronic Disease, Health and Aging," *Diabetes* 62, no. 3 (2013), Available at http://diabetes.diabetesjournals.org/content/62/3/672.full; S. Cohen et al., "Chronic Stress, Glucocorticoid Receptor Resistance, Inflammation and Disease Risk," *Proceedings of the National Academy of Sciences of the United States of America* 109, no. 16 (2012): 5995–99, doi: 10.1073/pnas.1118355109

8. S. Taylor, *The Tending Instinct: Women, Men and the Biology of Our Relationships* (New York: Time Books, Henry Holt and Company, 2002).

9. C. Cardodosa et al., "Stress-Induced Negative Mood Moderates the Relation between Oxytocin Administration and Trust: Evidence for the Tend-and-Befriend Response to Stress?" *Pschoneuroendocrinology* 38, no. 11 (2013): 2800–804.

10. J. Lee and V. R. Harley, "The Male Fight-Flight Response: A Result of SRY Regulation of Catecholamines?," *BioEssays* 34, no. 6 (2012): 454–57, doi: 10.1002/bies.201100159

11. A. Crum, P. Salovey, and S. Achor, "Rethinking Stress: The Role of Mindsets in Determining the Stress Response," *Journal of Personality and Social Psychology* 104, no. 4 (2013): 716–33.

12. P. Thoits, "Stress and Health: Major Findings and Policy Implications," *Journal of Health and Social Behavior* 51, no. 1, supplement (2010): 554–55, doi: 10.1177/0022146510383499; K. M. Scott et al., "Associations between Lifetime Traumatic Events and Subsequent Chronic Physical Conditions: A Cross-National, Cross-Sectional Study," *PLoS One* 8, no. 11 (2013), doi: 10.1371/journal.pone.0080573

13. K. M. Scott et al., "Associations between Lifetime Traumatic Events and Subsequent Chronic Physical Conditions: A Cross-National, Cross-Sectional Study," *PLoS One* 8, no. 11 (2013), doi: 10.1371/journal.pone.0080573

14. Robert Scaer, *The Body Bears the Burden: Trauma, Dissociation, and Disease,* 3rd ed. (New York: Routledge Press, 2014).

15. A. Steptoe and M. Kivimaki, "Stress and Cardiovascular Disease: An Update on Current Knowledge," *Annual Review of Public Health* 34 (2013): 337–54.

16. N. Aggarwal et al., "Perceived Stress Is Associated with Subclinical Cerebrovacular Disease in Older Adults," *The American Journal of Geriatric Psychiatry* 22, no. 1 (2014): 53–62; A. Steptoe and M. Kivimaki, "Stress and Cardiovascular Disease: An Update on Current Knowledge," *Annual Review of Public Health* 34 (2013): 337–54; S. Richardson et al., "Meta-Analysis of Perceived Stress and Its Association with Incident Coronary Heart Disease," *American Journal of Cardiology* 110, no. 12 (2012): 1711–17; A. Steptoe and M. Kivimaki, "Stress and Cardiovascular Disease," *Nature Reviews Cardiology* 9, no. 6 (2012): 360–70.

17. M. Kivimaki et al., "Job Strain as a Risk Factor for Coronary Heart Disease: A Collaborative Meta-Analysis of Individual Participants," *The Lancet* 380, no. 9852 (2012): 1491–97; E. Mostofsky et al., "Risk of Acute Myocardial Infarction After the Death of a Significant Person on One's Life. The Determinants of Myocardial Infarction Onset Study," *Circulation* 125, no. 3 (2012): 491–96, doi: 10.1161/CIRCULATIONAHA.111.061770

18. K. Scott, S. Melhorn, and R. Sakai. "Effects of Chronic Social Stress on Obesity," *Current Obesity Reports Online First* 1, no. 1 (2012): 16–25, doi: 10.1007/s13679-011-0006-3; F. Ippoliti, N. Canitano, and R. Businare, "Stress and Obesity as Risk Factors in Cardiovascular Diseases: A Neuroimmune Perspective," *Journal of Neuroimmune Pharmacology* 8, no. 1 (2013): 212–26; S. Pagota et al., "Association of Post-Traumatic Stress Disorder and Obesity in a Nationally Representative Sample," *Obesity* 20, no. 1 (2012): 200–205.

19. Mayo Clinic, "Stress and Hair Loss: Are They Related?," January 2014, www.mayoclinic.com/health/stress-and-hair-loss/AN01442

20. American Diabetes Association, "How Stress Affects Diabetes," 2013, www.diabetes.org/living-with-diabetes/complications/mental-health/stress.html; A. Pandy et al., "Alternative Therapies Useful in the Management of Diabetes: A Systematic Review," *Journal of Bioallied Science* 3, no. 4 (2011): 504–12.

21. C. Lee et al., "Increases in Blood Glucose in Older Adults: The Effects of Spousal Health," *Journal of Aging and Health* 26 (2014): 952–68.

22. M. Virtanen et al., "Psychological Distress and Incidence of Type 2 Diabetes in High Risk and Low Risk Populations: The Whitehall II Cohort Study," *Diabetes Care* 37, no. 8 (2014): 2091–97.

23. National Digestive Diseases Information Clearinghouse (NDDIC), "Irritable Bowel Syndrome: How Does Stress Affect IBS?," October 2013, http://digestive.niddk.nih.gov/ddiseases/pubs/ibs/#stress

24. H. F. Herlong, "Digestive Disorders White Paper-2013," *Johns Hopkins Health Alerts,* 2013, www.johnshopkinshealthalerts.com

25. E. Carlsson et al., "Psychological Stress in Children May Alter the Immune Response," *Journal of Immunology* 192, no. 5 (2014): 2071–81; G. Marshall, ed., "Stress and Immune-Based Diseases," *Immunology and Allergy Clinics of North America* 31, no. 1 (2011): 1–148; L. Christian, "Psychoneuroimmunology in Pregnancy: Immune Pathways Linking Stress with Maternal Health, Adverse Birth Outcomes and Fetal Development," *Neuroscience and Biobehavioral Reviews* 36, no. 1 (2012): 350–61, doi: 10.1016/j.neubiorev.2011.07.005; A. Pedersen et al., "Influence of Psychological Stress on Upper Respiratory Infection: A Meta-Analysis of Prospective Studies," *Psychosomatic Medicine* 72, no. 8 (2010): 823–32.

26. M. Kondo, "Socioeconomic Disparities and Health: Impacts and Pathways," *Journal of Epidemiology* 22, no. 1 (2012): 2–6; T. Theorell, "Evaluating Life Events and Chronic Stressors in Relation to Health: Stressors and Health in Clinical Work," *Advances in Psychosomatic Medicine* 32 (2012): 58–71; J. Gouln and J. Kiecolt-Glaser, "The Impact of Psychological Stress on Wound Healing: Methods and Mechanisms," *Immunology and Allergy Clinics of North America* 31, no. 1 (2011): 81–93.

27. American College Health Association (ACHA), *American College Health Association–National College Health Assessment II (ACHA-NCHA II): Reference Group Data Report Spring, 2014* (Hanover, MD: American College Health Association, 2014).

28. Ibid.

29. M. Marin et al., "Chronic Stress, Cognitive Functioning and Mental Health," *Neurobiology of Learning and Memory* 96, no. 4 (2011): 583–95; R. M. Shansky and J. Lipps, "Stress-Induced Cognitive Dysfunction: Hormone-Neurotransmitter Interactions in the Prefrontal Cortex," *Neuroscience and Biobehavioral Reviews* 7 (2013): 123, Available at www.ncbi.nlm.nih.gov/pmc/articles/PMC3617365

30. E. Dias-Ferreira et al., "Chronic Stress Causes Frontostriatal Reorganization and Affects Decision-Making," *Science* 325, no. 5940 (2009): 621–25; D. de Quervan et al., "Glucocorticoids and the Regulation of Memory in Health and Disease," *Frontiers in Neuroendocrinology* 30, no. 3 (2009): 358–70.

31. L. Johansson, "Can Stress Increase Alzheimer's Disease Risk in Women?," *Expert Review of Neurotherapeutics* 14, no. 2 (2014): 123–25, doi: 10.1586/14737175.2014.878651; P. J. Lucassen et al., "Neuropathology of Stress" *Acta Neuropathologica* 127, no. 1 (2014): 109–35.

32. T. Frodi and V. O'Keane, "How Does the Brain Deal with Cumulative Stress? A Review with Focus on Developmental Stress, HPA Axis Function and Hippocampal Structure in Humans," *Neurobiology of Disease* 52 (2013): 24–37; P. S. Nurius, E. Uehara, and D. F. Zatzick, "Intersection of Stress, Social Disadvantage, and Life Course Processes: Reframing Trauma and Mental Health," *American Journal of Psychiatric Rehabilitation* 16 (2013): 91–114; K. Scott et al., "Association of Childhood Adversities and Early-Onset Mental Disorders with Adult-Onset Chronic Physical Conditions," *Archives of General Psychiatry* 68, no. 8 (2011): 833–44.

33. American Psychological Association, "Stress in America: Paying with Our Health," 2015, Accessed April 2015, http://www.apa.org/news/press/releases/stress/2014/stress-report.pdf

34. S. Charles et al., "The Wear and Tear of Daily Stressors on Mental Health," *Psychological Science* 24, no. 5 (2013): 733–41; J. R. Piazza et al., "Affective Reactivity to Daily Stressors and Long-Term Risk of Reporting a Chronic Physical Health Condition," *Annals of Behavioral Medicine* 45, no. 1 (2013): 110–20, doi: 10.1007/s12160-012-9423-0; C. Aldwin et al., "Do Hassles Mediate between Life Events and Mortality in Older Men?: Longitudinal Findings from the VA Normative Aging Study," *Experimental Gerontology* 59 (2014): 74–80.

35. C. Aldwin et al., "Do Hassles Mediate between Life Events and Mortality?," 2014; S. O'Neill et al., "Affective Reactivity to Daily Interpersonal Stressors as a Prospective Predictor of Depressive Symptoms," *Journal of Social and Clinical Psychology* 23, no. 2 (2004): 172–94, doi 10.1521/jscp.23.2.172.31015.

36. K. M. Krajnak, "Potential Contribution of Work-Related Psychosocial Stress to the Development of Cardiovascular Disease and Type II Diabetes: A Brief Review," *Environmental Health Insights* 8, Supplement 1 (2014): 41–45, doi: 10.4137/EHI.S15263.e; N. Vurtanen, S. T. Nyberg, and G. D. Batty, "Perceived Job Insecurity as a Risk Factor for Incident Coronary Heart Disease: Systematic Review and Meta-Analysis," *BMJ* 347 (2013): f4746. doi:10.116/bmj.f4746; K. Toren et al., "A Longitudinal General Population-Based Study of Job Strain and Risk for Coronary Heart Disease and Stroke in Swedish Men," *BMJ Open* 4, no. 3 (2014): e004355, doi: 10:1136/bmjopen-2013-004355

37. American College Health Association, *National College Health Assessment II: Reference Group Data Report Spring, 2014*, 2014.

38. S. Schwartz et al., "Acculturation and Well-Being among College Students from Immigrant Families," *Journal of Clinical Psychology* (2012): 1–21, doi: 10.1002/jclp21847; A. Pieterse et al., "An Exploratory Examination of the Associations among Racial and Ethnic Discrimination, Racial Climate, and Trauma-Related Symptoms in a College Student Population," *Journal of Counseling Psychology* 57, no. 3 (2010): 255–63; A. McAleavey, L. Castonguay, and B. Locke, "Sexual Orientation Minorities in College Counseling: Prevalence, Distress, and Symptom Profiles," *Journal of College Counseling* 14, no. 2 (2011): 127–42.

39. K. Brown, *Predictors of Suicide Ideation and the Moderating Effects of Suicide Attitudes*, Master's thesis, University of Ohio, 2011, http://etd.ohiolink.edu; J. Gomez, R. Miranda, and L Polanco, "Acculturative Stress, Perceived Discrimination and Vulnerability to Suicide Attempts among Emerging Adults," *Journal of Youth and Adolescence* 40, no. 11 (2011): 1465–76.

40. B. L. Seaward, *Managing Stress: Principles and Strategies for Health and Well-Being*, 7th ed. (New York: Barnes and Noble, 2012).

41. J. Twenge, *Generation Me–Revised and Updated: Why Today's Young Americans Are More Confident, Assertive, Entitled and More Miserable Than Ever* (New York, Simon and Schuster, 2014).

42. A. Peng, J. Schaubroeck, and J. Xie, "When Confidence Comes and Goes: How Variation in Self-Efficacy Moderates Stressor–Strain Relationships," *Journal of Occupational Health Psychology*, Jan. 19, 2015: No Pagination Specified, http://dx.doi.org/10.1037/a0038588; R. Fida, et al. "'Yes I can'": The Protective Role of Personal Self Efficacy in Hindering Counterproductive Work Activity Under Stressful Conditions," *Anxiety, Stress and Coping*, 2014: 1–21, doi: 10.1080/10615806.2014.969718

43. A. Peng, J. Schaubroeck, and J. Xie, "When Confidence Comes and Goes," 2015.

44. I. Bragard et al., "Efficacy of a Communication and Stress Management Training on Medical Resident's Self Efficacy, Stressful Communication and Burnout," *Journal of Health Psychology* 15, no. 7 (2010): 1075–84; M. Komarraju and D. Nadler, "Self Efficacy and Academic Achievement: Who Do Implicit Beliefs, Goals and Effort Regulation Matter?," *Learning and Individual Differences* 25 (2013): 67–72.

45. P. N. von der Embse and S. Witmer, "High-Stakes Accountability: Student Anxiety and Large-Scale Testing," *Journal of Applied School Psychology* 30, no. 2 (2014): 132–56, doi: 10.1080/15377903.2014.888529

46. A. Zuffiano et al., "Academic Achievement: The Unique Contribution of Self Efficacy Beliefs in Self-Regulated Learning beyond Intelligence, Personality Traits and Self-esteem," *Learning and Individual Differences* 23 (2013): 158–62.

47. M. Friedman and R. H. Rosenman, *Type A Behavior and Your Heart* (New York: Knopf, 1974).

48. M. Whooley and J. Wong, "Hostility and Cardiovascular Disease," *Journal of the American College of Cardiology* 58, no. 12 (2011): 1228–30; J. Newman et al., "Observed Hostility and the Risk of Incident Ischemic Heart Disease: A Perspective Population Study from the 1995 Canadian Nova Scotia Health Survey," *Journal of the American College of Cardiology* 58, no. 12 (2011): 1222–28; T. Smith et al., "Marital Discord and Coronary Artery Disease: A Comparison of Behaviorally Defined Discrete Groups," *Journal of Consulting and Clinical Psychology* 80, no. 1 (2012): 87–92.

49. G. Mate, *When the Body Says No: Understanding the Stress-Disease Connection* (Hoboken, NJ: John Wiley and Sons, 2011).

50. H. Versteeg, V. Spek, and S. Pedersen, "Type D Personality and Health Status in Cardiovascular Disease Populations: A Meta-Analysis of Prospective Studies," *European Journal of Cardiovascular Prevention and Rehabilitation* 19, no. 6 (2011): 1373–380, doi: 10.1177/1741826711425338; F. Mols and F. J. Denollet, "Type D Personality in the General Population: A Systematic Review of Health Status, Mechanisms of Disease and Work-Related Problems," *Health and Quality of Life Outcomes* 8, no. 9 (2010): 1–10, Available from www.hqlo.com

51. S. Kobasa, "Stressful Life Events, Personality, and Health: An Inquiry into Hardiness," *Journal of Personality and Social Psychology* 37, no. 1 (1979): 1–11.

52. C. D. Schetter and C. Dolbier, "Resilience in the Context of Chronic Stress and Health in Adults," *Social and Personality Psychology Compass* 5, no. 9 (2011): 634–52, doi: 10.1111/j.1751-9004.2011.00379.x

53. C. Ryff et al., "Psychological Resilience in Adulthood and Later Life: Implications for Health," *Annual Review of Gerontology and Geriatrics* 32, no. 1 (2012): 73–92.

54. The American Psychological Association, "The Road to Resilience: What Is Resilience?," Accessed February 2014, www.apa.org/helpcenter/road-resilience.aspx

55. E. Chen et al., "Protective Factors for Adults from Low-Childhood Socioeconomic Circumstances: The Benefits of Shift-and-Persist for Allostatic Load," *Psychosomatic Medicine* 74, no. 2 (2012): 178–86, doi: 10.1097/PSY.0B013e31824206fd

56. Higher Education Research Institute, "A Year of Change: First Year," Accessed January 30, 2015, www.heri.ucla.edu/infographics/YFCY-2014-Infographic.pdf; J. K. Eagen, et al., *The American Freshman: National Norms Fall 2014–Expanded Edition* (Los Angeles: Higher Education Research Institute, 2015),www.heri.ucla.edu/monographs/TheAmericanFreshman2014-Expanded.pdf

57. Ibid.; K. Eagen, *The American Freshman*, 2015.

58. B. L. Seaward, *Managing Stress*, 2012.

59. J. Moskowitz et al., "A Positive Affect Intervention for People Experiencing Health-related Stress: Development and Non-randomized Pilot Test," *Journal of Health Psychology* 17, no. 5 (2012): 676–92, doi: 10.1177/1359105311425275; P. Thoits, "Mechanisms Linking Social Ties and Support to Physical and Mental Health," *Journal of Health and Social Behavior* 52, no. 2 (2011): 145–61; B. Lake and E. Oreheck, "Relational Regulation Theory: A New Approach to Explain the Link between Perceived Social Support and Mental Health," *Psychological Review* 118, no. 3 (2011): 482–95.

60. B. L. Seaward, *Managing Stress*, 2012.

61. M. A. Stults-Kolehmainen and R. Sinha, "The Effect of Stress on Physical Activity and Exercise," *Sports Medicine* 44, no. 1 (2014): 81–121; G. Colom, C. Alcover, C. Sanchez-Curto, and J. Zarate-Osuna, "Study of the Effect of Positive Humour as a Variable That Reduces Stress. Relationship of Humour with Personality and Performance Variables," *Psychology in Spain* 15, no. 1 (2011): 9–21.

62. L. Poole et al., "Associations of Objectively Measured Physical Activity with Daily Mood Ratings and Psychophysiological Stress Responses in Women," *Psychophysiology* 48 (2011): 1165–72, doi: 10.1111/j.1469-8986.2011.01184.x; D. A. Girdano, D. E. Dusek, and G. S. Everly, *Controlling Stress and Tension*, 9th ed. (San Francisco: Benjamin Cummings, 2012), 375.

63. M. A. Stults-Kolehmainen and R. Sinha, "The Effect of Stress on Physical Activity and Exercise," 2014; E. M. Jackson, "Stress Relief: The Role of Exercise in Stress Management," *ACSM Health and Fitness Journal* 17, no. 3 (2013), doi, 10.1249/FIT.0b013e31828cb1c9

64. P. M. Gollwitzer and G. Oettingen, "Implementation Intentions.," in *Encyclopedia of Behavioral Medicine* (Part 9), eds. M. Gellman and J. R. Turner (New York: Springer-Verlag, 2013), 1043–48; C. Stern et al. "Effects of Implementation Intention on Anxiety, Perceived Proximity and Motor Performance," *Personality and Social Psychology Bulletin* 39, no. 5 (2013): 623–35; A. Dalton and S. Spiller, "Too Much of a Good Thing: The Benefits of Implementation Intentions Depend on the Number of Specific Goals," *Journal of Consumer Research* 39, no. 3 (2012): 600–14.

65. National Center for Complementary and Integrative Health."Nationwide Survey reveals widespread use of mind and body practices." February 2015. http://www.nih.gov/news/health/feb2015/nccih-10a.htm

66. NIH Medline Plus, "What Yoga Can and Can't Do for You," December 2013, www.nlm.nih.gov/medlineplus/news/fullstory_143813.html; J. Kiecolt-Glaser et al., "Stress, Inflammation, and Yoga Practice," *Psychosomatic Medicine* 72, no. 2 (2010): 113–21.

67. R. D. Brook et al., "Beyond Medications and Diet: Alternative Approaches to Lowering Blood Pressure: A Scientific Statement from the American Heart Association," *Hypertension* 61, no. 6 (2013): 1360–83.

68. National Center for Complementary and Integrative Health, "Massage Therapy for Health Purposes: What You Need to Know," February 2014, http://nccam.nih.gov/health/massage/massageintroduction.htm

Pulled Statistics:

Page 72, American Psychological Association, "Stress in America: Missing the Health Care Connection," 2013, Accessed January 2015, https://www.apa.org/news/press/releases/stress/2012/full-report.pdf

Page 80, American College Health Association, *American College Health Association-National College*

Health Assessment II: Reference Group Executive Summary Spring, 2014 (Hanover, MD: American College Health Association, 2014), www.acha.org Page 84, American Psychological Association. "Stress in America—Are Teens Adopting Adults' Stress Habits?," 2013, Accessed on January 29, 2015, www.apa.org/news/press/releases/stress/2013/teen-stress.aspx

Focus On: Improving Your Sleep

1. National Heart, Lung, and Blood Institute, "Sleep Disorders & Insufficient Sleep: Improving Health through Research," Accessed January 2015, www.nhlbi.nih.gov/news/spotlight/fact-sheet/sleep-disorders-insufficient-sleep-improving-health-through-research.html

2. The Philips Center for Health and Well-Being, "Philips Index for Health and Well-Being: A Global Perspective Report 2010," October 2011, www.newscenter.philips.com/pwc_nc/main/standard/resources/corporate/press/2010/Global%20Index%20Results/20101111%20Global%20Index%20Report.pdf

3. American College Health Association, *American College Health Association–National College Health Assessment II (ACHA–NCHA II): Reference Group Data Report Spring 2014* (Hanover, MD: American College Health Association, 2014), Available at www.achancha.org/reports_ACHA-NCHAII.html

4. S. Hershner and R. Chevin. "Causes and Consequences of Sleepiness Among College Students," *Nature and Science of Sleep* 6 (2014): 73-84, doi: 10.2147/NSS.S62907; A. Wald et al., "Associations between Healthy Lifestyle Behaviors and Academic Performance in U.S. Undergraduates: A Secondary Analysis of the American College Health Association's National College Health Assessment II," *American Journal of Health Promotion* 28, no. 5 (2014): 298-305, doi: http://dx.doi.org/10.4278/ajhp.120518-QUAN-265; K. Ahrberg et al., "Interaction between Sleep Quality and Academic Performance," *Journal of Psychiatric Research* 46, no. 12 (2012): 1618–22.

5. S. Hershner and R. Chevin. "Causes and Consequences of Sleepiness among College Students," *Nature and Science of Sleep* 6 (2014): 73-84, doi: 10.2147/NSS.S62907; A. Wald et al., "Associations between Healthy Lifestyle Behaviors," 2014.

6. National Sleep Foundation, "2011 Sleep in America Poll: Communications Technology and Sleep," March 2011, www.sleepfoundation.org/article/sleep-america-polls/2011-communications-technology-use-and-sleep

7. National Sleep Foundation, "Excessive Sleepiness," Accessed February 5, 2015, http://sleepfoundation.org/sleep-disorders-problems/excessive-sleepiness

8. Harvard University Radcliff Institute for Advanced Study, "Drowsy Driving," Accessed February 5, 2015, www.radcliffe.harvard.edu/news/radcliffe-magazine/drowsy-driving

9. C-SPAN, "Awake, Alert, Alive: Overcoming the Dangers of Drowsy Driving–NTSB Conference Opening Panel," October 21, 2014, www.c-span.org/video/?322228-1/discussion-combating-drowsy-driving

10. National Sleep Foundation, "Who's at Risk?," Accessed February 5, 2015, http://drowsydriving.org/about/whos-at-risk/

11. L. Culpepper, "The Social and Economic Burden of Shift-Work Disorder," *The Journal of Family Practice* 59, no. 1, Supplement (2010): S3–S11; S. Rajaratname et al., "Sleep Loss and Circadian Disruption in Shift Work: Health Burden and Management," *The Medical Journal of Australia* 199, no. 8 (2013): 11–15; F. P. Cappuccio et al., "Sleep Duration and All-Cause Mortality: A Systematic Review and Meta-Analysis of Prospective Studies," *Sleep* 33, no. 5 (2010): 585–92.

12. National Sleep Foundation, "Who's at Risk?," 2015.

13. G. Hertz et al., "Sleep Dysfunction in Women," *Medscape* (2014), http://emedicine.medscape.com/article/1189087-overview

14. S. Tregear et al., "Obstructive Sleep Apnea and Risk of Motor Vehicle Crash: Systematic Review and Meta-Analysis," *Journal of Clinical Sleep Medicine* 5, no. 6 (2009): 573–81; K. Ward, et al. "Excessive Daytime Sleepiness Increases the Risk of Motor Vehicle Crash in Obstructive Sleep Apnea," *Journal of Clinical Sleep Medicine* 9, no. 10 (2013):1013–21

15. M. Meeker and L. Wu, "How Much Time Do We Really Spend on Our Smartphones Every Day?," *Business Insider,* June 6, 2013, www.businessinsider.com.au/how-much-time-do-we-spend-on-smartphones-2013-6; Marketing Charts, "College Students Own an Average of 7 Tech Devices," June 2013, www.marketingcharts.com/wp/topics/demographics/college-students-own-an-average-of-7-tech-devices-30430

16. Anne-Marie Chang et al., "Evening Use of Light-Emitting eReaders Negatively Affects Sleep, Circadian Time, and Next Morning Alertness," *Proceedings of the National Academy of Sciences* (2014), doi: 10.1073/pnas.1418490112]

17. N. Rod et al., "The Joint Effect of Sleep Duration and Disturbed Sleep on Cause-Specific Mortality: Results from the Whitehall II Cohort Study," *PLoS ONE* 9, no. 4 (2014): e91965, doi:10.1371/journal.pone.0091965; National Heart Lung and Blood Institute, "Why Is Sleep Important?," February 2012, www.nhlbi.nih.gov/health/health-topics/topics/sdd/why.html; F. P. Cappuccio et al., "Sleep Duration and All-Cause Mortality," 2010.

18. K. M. Orzech et al., "Sleep Patterns Are Associated with Common Illness in Adolescents," *Journal of Sleep Research* (2013), doi: 10.1111/jsr.12096; J. M. Krueger and J. A. Majde, "Sleep and Host Defense," in *Principles and Practice of Sleep Medicine,* eds. M. H. Kryger, T. Roth, and W. C. Dement (St. Louis, MO: Saunders 2011), 261–90; M. Manzer and M. Hussein, "Sleep-Immune System Interaction: Advantages and Challenges of Human Sleep Loss Model," *Frontiers of Neurology* 3, no. 2 (2012), doi: 10.3389/fneur.2012.00002

19. X. Yu et al., "TH17 Cell Differentiation Is Regulated by Circadian Clock," *Science* 342, no. 6159 (2013): 727–30; A. Bollinger, A. Bollinger, H. Oster, and W. Scolbach, "Sleep, Immunity and Circadian Clocks: A Mechanistic Model," *Gerontology* 56, no. 6 (2010): 574–80, doi: 10.1159/000281827

20. F. Heredia et al., "Self-Reported Sleep Duration, White Blood Cell Counts and Cytokine Profiles in European Adolescents: The Helena Study," *Sleep Medicine* 15, no. 10 (2014): 1251–58.

21. F. Sofi et al., "Insomnia and Risk of Cardiovascular Disease: A Meta-Analysis," *European Journal of Preventive Cardiology* 21, no. 1 (2014): 57–64; R. Lanfranchi, F. Prince, D. Filipini, and J. Carrier, "Sleep Deprivation Increases Blood Pressure in Healthy Normotensive Elderly and Attenuates the Blood Pressure Response to Orthostatic Challenges," *Sleep* 34, no. 3 (2010): 335–39; F. Cappucio, D. Cooper, and D. Lanfranco, "Sleep Duration Predicts Cardiovascular Outcomes: A Systematic Review and Meta-Analysis of Prospective Studies," *European Heart Journal,* first published online February 7, 2011, doi: 10.1093/eurheart

22. M. A. Miller and F. P. Cappuccio, "Biomarkers of Cardiovascular Risk in Sleep Deprived People," *Journal of Human Hypertension* 27, no. 10 (2013): 583–88; S. Agarwal, N. Bajaj, and C. Bae, "Association between Sleep Duration and Cardiovascular Disease: Results from the National Health and Nutrition Examination Survey (NHANES 2005–2008)," *Journal of the American College of Cardiology* 59, no. 13, Supplement 1 (2012): e1514; F. Sofi et al., "Insomnia and Risk of Cardiovascular Disease: A Meta-Analysis," *European Journal of Preventive Cardiology* 21, no. 1 (2014): 51–67.

23. M. A. Miller et al., "Sustained Short Sleep and Risk of Obesity. Evidence in Children and Adults," in *Handbook of Obesity*, 3rd ed., vol. 1, eds. G. A. Bray and C. Bouchard (Boca Raton, FL: CRC Press, Taylor & Francis Group, 2014), 397–41; Q. Xiao et al., "A Large Prospective Investigation of Sleep Duration, Weight Change and Obesity in the NIH-AARP Diet and Health Study," *American Journal of Epidemiology* 178, no. 11 (2013): 1600–10.

24. M. A. Miller et al., "Sustained Short Sleep and Risk of Obesity," 2014; Q. Xiao et al., "A Large Prospective Investigation of Sleep Duration," 2013; L. Nielson, T. Danielson, and A. Serensen, "Short Sleep Duration as a Possible Cause of Obesity: Critical Analysis of the Epidemiological Evidence," *Obesity Reviews* 12, no. 2 (2011): 78–92; National Sleep Foundation, "Obesity and Sleep," Accessed January 2014, www.sleepfoundation.org/article/sleep-topics/obesity-and-sleep

25. C. L. Jackson et al., "Association between Sleep Duration and Diabetes in Black and White Adults," *Diabetes Care* 36, no. 11 (2013): 3557–65; E. G. Holliday et al., "Short Sleep Duration Is Associated with Risk of Future Diabetes but Not Cardiovascular Disease: A Prospective Study and Meta-Analysis," *PLoS ONE* 8, no. 11 (2013): e82305, doi: 10.1371/journal.pone.0082305; American Diabetes Association, "Too Little Sleep Linked to Higher A1C," January 2014, www.diabetesforecast.org/2014/Jan/too-little-sleep-linked-to.html

26. National Institutes of Health (NIH), "Teacher's Guide–Information about Sleep," Accessed January 2015, http://science.education.nih.gov/supplements/nih3/sleep/guide/info-sleep.htm

27. National Institutes of Health, "Information about Sleep," Accessed January 2015, http://science.education.nih.gov/supplements/nih3/sleep/guide/info-sleep.htm; C. Peri and M. Smith, "What Lack of Sleep Does to Your Mind," WebMD, January 2013, www.webmd.com/sleep-disorders/excessive-sleepiness-10/emotions-cognitive

28. A. Chatburn, et al. "Complex Associative Memory Processing and Sleep: A Systematic Review and Meta-Analysis of Behavioural Evidence and Underlying EEG Mechanisms." *Neuroscience and Biobehavioral Reviews* 47 (2014): 645–55; E. Fortier-Brochu, S. Beauliew-Bonneau, H. Ivers, and C. Morin, "Insomnia and Daytime Cognitive Performance: A Meta-Analysis," *Sleep Medicine Reviews* 16, no. 1 (2011), doi: 10-1016/j.smrv.2011.03.008; W. Klemm, "How Sleep Helps Memory," *Psychology Today*, March 11, 2011, www.psychologytoday.com/blog/memory-medic/201103/how-sleep-helps-memory; M. A. Miller et al., "Chapter: Sleep and Cognition," in *Sleep Disorders* (2014), in press.

29. A. Gomes, J. Tavares, and M. Azevedo, "Sleep and Academic Performance in Undergraduates: A Multi-Measure, Multi-Predictor Approach," *Chronobiology* 28, no. 9 (2011): 786–801, doi:10.3109/07420528.2011.606518; Yu-Chih Chiang, "The Effects of Sleep on Performance of Undergraduate Students Working in the Hospitality Industry as Compared to Those Who Are Not Working in the Industry," 2013, http://lib.dr.iastate.edu/cgi/viewcontent.cgi?article=4067&context=etd

30. Z. Terpening et al., "The Contributors of Nocturnal Sleep to the Consolidation of Motor Skill Learning in Healthy Aging and Parkinson's Disease," *Journal of Sleep Research* 22, no. 4 (2013): 398–405; L. Genzel et al., "Complex Motor Sequence Skills Profit from Sleep," *Neuropsychobiology* 66, no. 4 (2012): 237–43, doi: 10.1159/000341878

31. Centers for Disease Control and Prevention, "Drowsy Driving: Asleep at the Wheel," 2014, Accessed February 2015, http://www.cdc.gov/Features/dsDrowsyDriving/

32. National Sleep Foundation, "Young People More Likely to Drive Drowsy," November 2012, www.sleepfoundation.org/alert/young-people-more-likely-drive-drowsy.

33. Centers for Disease Control and Prevention, "Insufficient Sleep is a Public Health Epidemic," January 13, 2014, www.cdc.gov/features/dssleep/; National Highway Traffic Safety Administration, "Drowsy Driving and Automobile Crashes," February 2014, www.nhtsa.gov/people/injury/drowsy_driving1/Drowsy.html#NCSDR/NHTSA

34. Ibid.; Centers for Disease Control and Prevention, "Drowsy Driving—19 States and the District of Columba. 2009–2010," *Morbidity and Mortality Weekly Report* 61, no. 51 (2013): 1033–37, Available at www.cdc.gov/mmwr/preview/mmwrhtml/mm6151a1.htm

35. H. Oster, "Does Late Sleep Promote Depression?" *Expert Reviews of Endocrinology and Metabolism* 7, no. 1 (2012): 27–29, www.expert-reviews.com/doi/abs/10.1586/eem.11.80;C. Baglioni et al., "Insomnia as a Predictor of Depression: A Meta-Analytic Evaluation of Longitudinal Epidemiological Studies," *Journal of Affective Disorders* 135, no. 1 (2011): 10–19.

36. National Institute of General Medical Sciences, "Circadian Rhythms Fact Sheet," Accessed February 5, 2015, www.nigms.nih.gov/Education/Pages/Factsheet_CircadianRhythms.aspx.

37. E. Carlson et al., "Tick Tock: New Clues About Biological Clocks and Health," *Inside Life Science*, November 1, 2012, http://publications.nigms.nih.gov/insidelifescience/biological-clocks.html; M. Vitaterna, J. Takahashi, and F. Turek, "Overview of Circadian Rhythms," National Institute on Alcohol Abuse and Alcoholism, 2014, http://pubs.niaaa.nih.gov/publications/arh25-2/85-93.htm

38. NIH, "Teacher's Guide–Information about Sleep," Accessed February 2014, http://science.education.nih.gov/supplements/nih3/sleep/guide/info-sleep.htm

39. B. Rasch and J. Born, "About Sleep's Role in Memory," *Physiological Reviews* 93, no. 2 (2013): 681–766.

40. Centers for Disease Control and Prevention, "Insufficient Sleep is a Public Health Epidemic," January 13, 2014, www.cdc.gov/features/dssleep/; F. Cappuccio et al. "Sleep Duration and All-Cause Mortality: Systematic Review," *Sleep* 33, no. 5 (2010): 585–92.

41. NIH, "Teacher's Guide–Information About Sleep," 2014.

42. E. Mezick et al., "Sleep Duration and Cardiovascular Responses to Stress in Undergraduate Men." *Psychophysiology* 51, no. 1 (2014): 88–96.

43. E. Carlson et al., "Tick Tock," 2012; CDC, "Insufficient Sleep Is a Public Health Epidemic," 2014, www.cdc.gov/features/dssleep/

44. N. Rod, M Kumari, and T. Lange et al. "The Joint Effect of Sleep Duration and Disturbed Sleep on Cause-Specific Mortality: Results from the Whitehall II Cohort Study," *PLoS ONE* 9, no. 4 (2014): e91965, doi:10.1371/journal.pone.0091965; Q. Xiao et al., "A Large Prospective Investigation of Sleep Duration, Weight Change, and Obesity in the NIH-AARP Diet and Health Study Cohort," *American Journal of Epidemiology* 178, no. 11 (2013): 1600–10; C .L. Jackson et al., "Association Between Sleep Duration and Diabetes in Black and White Adults," *Diabetes Care* 36, no. 11 (2013): 3557–65; F. Cappuccio et al., "Sleep Duration Predicts Cardiovascular Outcomes: A Systematic Review and Meta-Analysis of Prospective Studies," *European Heart Journal* 32, no. 12 (2011): 1484–92.

45. National Sleep Foundation, "Napping," Accessed February 5, 2015, http://sleepfoundation.org/sleep-topics/napping; National Sleep Foundation, "Drowsy Driving—Is There a Perfect Time to Take a Nap?," Accessed January 15, 2015; B. Faraut et al., "Benefits of Napping and an Extended Duration of Recovery Sleep on Alertness and Immune Cells After Acute Sleep Restriction," *Brain, Behavior and Immunity* 25, no. 1 (2011): 18–24, doi: 10.1016/j.bbi.2010.08.001

46. Vanderbilt University Medical Center Reporter, "Take a Walk in the Sun to Ease Time Change Woes, Sleep Expert Says, " October 30, 2014, http://news.vanderbilt.edu/2014/10/take-a-walk-in-the-sun-to-ease-time-change-woes-says-vanderbilt-sleep-expert/

47. National Sleep Foundation, "Exercise and Sleep," Accessed February 5, 2015, www.sleepfoundation.org/article/sleep-america-polls/2013/exercise-and-sleep

48. National Sleep Foundation, "What You Breathe While You Sleep Can Affect How You Feel the Next Day," Accessed February 5, 2015, http://sleepfoundation.org/bedroom/smell.php

49. E. Carlson et al., "Tick Tock," 2012.

50. American College Health Association, *National College Health Assessment II: Reference Group Data Report Spring 2014*, 2014.

51. National Sleep Foundation, "Caffeine and Sleep," Accessed February 2014, www.sleepfoundation.org; American College Health Association, *National College Health Assessment II: Reference Group Data Report Spring 2014*, 2014.

52. National Sleep Foundation, Insomnia, Accessed February 5, 2015, http://sleepfoundation.org/sleep-disorders-problems/insomnia

53. Ibid.

54. Ibid.

55. Ibid.

56. American College Health Association, *National College Health Assessment II: Reference Group Data Report Spring 2014*, 2014.

57. Society of Behavioral Medicine, "Adult Insomnia," Accessed February 5, 2014, http://www.behavioralsleep.org/adultinsomnia.aspx

58. Y. Chong, C. D. Fryar, and Q. Gu, "Prescription Sleep Aid Use among Adults: United States, 2005–2010," *NCHS Data Brief*, no. 127 (2013), Available at www.cdc.gov/nchs/data/databriefs/db127.htm

59. National Sleep Foundation, "Sleep Apnea," Accessed January 2015, www.sleepfoundation.org/article/sleep-related-problems/obstructive-sleep-apnea-and-sleep.

60. Sleep Disorders Guide, "Sleep Apnea Statistics," Accessed January 2015, www.sleepdisordersguide.com/sleepapnea/sleep-apnea-statistics.html

61. National Sleep Foundation, "Sleep Apnea," 2015.

62. Ibid.

63. Ibid.

64. National Institute of Neurological Disorders and Stroke, "Restless Legs Syndrome Fact Sheet," updated July 25, 2014, www.ninds.nih.gov/disorders/restless_legs/detail_restless_legs.htm

65. Ibid.

66. National Institute of Neurological Disorders and Stroke, "Narcolepsy Fact Sheet," updated January 5, 2015, www.ninds.nih.gov/disorders/narcolepsy/detail_narcolepsy.htm

67. National Sleep Foundation, "Narcolepsy and Sleep," 2014, www.sleepfoundation.org/article/sleep-related-problems/narcolepsy-and-sleep

Pulled Statistics:

Page 100, American College Health Association, American College Health Association— National College Health Assessment II: Reference Group Executive Summary, Spring 2014 (Hanover, MD: American College Health Association, 2014).

Page 102, American College Health Association, American College Health Association— National College Health Assessment II: Reference Group Executive Summary, Spring 2014 (Hanover, MD: American College Health Association, 2014).

Chapter 4: Preventing Violence and Injury

1. Voltaire, "Semiramis," V.1, trans. by J. K. Hoyt, in *The Cyclopaedia of Practical Quotations*, 1896. New York: Funk & Wagnalls Company.

2. World Health Organization (WHO), *Global Status Report on Violence Prevention* (Geneva: World Health Organization, 2014), Available at www.undp.org/content/dam/undp/library/corporate/Reports/UNDP-GVA-violence-2014.pdf

3. Centers for Disease Control and Prevention, "Deaths, Percent of Total Deaths, and Death Rates for the 15 Leading Causes of Death: United States and Each State, 1999–2013," December 31, 2014, Available at www.cdc.gov/nchs/data/dvs/LCWK1_2013.pdf

4. WHO, *Global Status Report on Violence Prevention* 2014.

5. Ibid.

6. Ibid.

7. U.S. Department of Justice, Federal Bureau of Investigation, *Crime in the United States, Preliminary Semiannual Uniform Crime Report for January–June 2013*, May 2014, www.fbi.gov/about-us/cjis/ucr/crime-in-the-u.s/2013/preliminary-semiannual-uniform-crime-report-january-june-2013; J. Rudolph, "Violent Crime up in the U.S. for the First Time in Nearly 2 Decades, Despite FBI Claims," *Huffington Post*, October 17, 2012, www.huffingtonpost.com/2012/10/17/violent-crime-bureau-justice-statistics_n_1974123.html

8. C. Barnett-Ryan, L. Langton, M. Planty, "The Nation's Two Crime Measures," September 18, 2014, *Bureau of Justice Statistics*, www.bjs.gov/index.cfm?ty=pbdetail&iid=5112; Bureau of Justice Statistics, "Reporting Crimes to Police," February 11, 2015, www.bjs.gov/index.cfm?ty=tp&tid=96

9. J. Langton and J. Truman. "Criminal Victimization, 2013 (Revised)," *Bureau of Justice Statistics*, September 18, 2014, www.bjs.gov/index.cfm?ty=tp&tid=96

10. U.S. Department of Justice. Bureau of Justice Statistics. "Criminal Victimization, 2013." 2014 . http://www.bjs.gov/content/pub/pdf/cv13.pdf

11. Ibid.

12. American College Health Association, *American College Health Association—National College Health Assessment II: Reference Group Data Report, Spring 2014* (Hanover, MD: American College Health Association, 2014), Available at www.acha-ncha.org/reports_ACHA-NCHAII.html

13. Ibid.

14. Ibid.

15. National Criminal Justice Reference Service, "Section 6: Statistical Overviews," *NCVRW Resource Guide*, 2014, http://ovc.ncjrs.gov/ncvrw2014/pdf/StatisticalOverviews.pdf.

16. Center for Public Integrity, "Sexual Assault on Campus: A Frustrating Search for Justice," Updated February 2013, www.publicintegrity.org/accountability/education/sexual-assault-campus

17. World Health Organization Violence Prevention Alliance, "The Ecological Framework," 2015, www.who.int/violenceprevention/approach/ecology/en/index.html; World Health Organization, Global Status Report on Violence Prevention, (Geneva: World Health Organization, 2014), Available at www.undp.org/content/dam/undp/library/corporate/Reports/UNDP-GVA-violence-2014.pdf; Centers for Disease Control and Prevention, National Center for Injury Prevention and Control, "Understanding School Violence: Fact Sheet—2015," 2015, www.cdc.gov/violenceprevention/pdf/school_violence_factsheet-a.pdf

18. Substance Abuse and Mental Health Services Administration, "The NSDUH Report: Violent Behaviors and Family Income among Adolescents," August 19, 2010, Newsletter, www.oas.samhsa.gov

19. Centers for Disease Control and Prevention, "Intimate Partner Violence: Risk and Protective Factors," February 11, 2015, www.cdc.gov/violenceprevention/intimatepartnerviolence/riskprotectivefactors.html; D. M. Capaldi et al., "A Systematic Review of Risk Factors for Intimate Partner Violence," *Partner Abuse* 2, no. 2 (2012): 231–80, Available at www.ncbi.nlm.nih.gov

20. World Health Organization Violence Prevention Alliance, "The Ecological Framework," 2015, www.who.int/violenceprevention/approach/ecology/en/index.html; J. H. Derzon, "The Correspondence of Family Features with Problem, Aggressive, Criminal and Violent Behaviors: A Meta-Analysis," *Journal of Experimental Criminology* 6, no. 3 (2010): 263–92, doi: 10.1007/s11292-010-9098-0; L. Kiss et al., "Gender-Based Violence and Socioeconomic Inequalities: Does Living in More Deprived Neighborhoods Increase Women's Risk of Intimate Partner Violence?," *Social Science and Medicine* 74, no. 8 (2012): 1172–79; H. Beydoun et al., "Intimate Partner Violence against Adult Women and Its Association with Major Depressive Disorder, Depressive Symptoms and Postpartum Depression: A Systematic Review and Meta-Analysis," *Social Science & Medicine* 75, no. 6 (2012): 959–75, doi: 10.1016/j.socscimed.2012.04.025

21. M. L. Hunt, A. W. Hughey, and M. G. Burke, "Stress and Violence in the Workplace and on Campus: A Growing Problem for Business, Industry and Academia," *Industry and Higher Education* 26, no. 1 (2012): 43–51; K. Devries et al., "Intimate Partner Violence and Incident Depressive Symptoms and Suicide Attempts: A Systematic Review of Longitudinal Studies," *PLoS Medicine* 10, no. 5 (2013): e1001439.

22. T. Frisell et al., "Violent Crime Runs in Families: A Total Population Study of 12.5 Million Individuals," *Psychological Medicine* 41, no. 1 (2010): 97–105, doi:10.1017S0023329170000462; T. Dishion, "A Developmental Model of Aggression and Violence: Microsocial and Macrosocial Dynamic within an Ecological Framework," in *Handbook of Developmental Psychpathology* (New York: Springer, 2014), 449–65; M. Lee et al., "Exposure to Family Violence and Attachment Styles as Predictors of Dating Violence Perpetuation among Men and Women: A Mediation Model," , *Journal of Interpersonal Violence* 29, no. 1 (2014): 120–43. doi: 10.1177/0886260513504644

23. K. Makin-Byrd and K. L. Bierman, "Individual and Family Predictors of the Perpetration of Dating Violence and Victimization in Late Adolescence," *Journal of Youth Adolescence* 42, no. 4 (2013): 536–50, doi: 10.1007/s10964-012-9810-7; J. H. Derzon, "The Correspondence of Family Features," 2010; C. Cook et al., "Predictors of Bullying and Victimization in Childhood and Adolescence: A Meta-Analytic Investigation," *School Psychology Quarterly* 25, no. 2 (2010): 65–83.

24. R. Puff and J. Segher, *The Everything Guide to Anger Management: Proven Techniques to Understand and Control Anger* (Avon, MA: Adams Media, Inc. A Division of F. and W. Media, 2014).

25. C. J. Ferguson, "Genetic Contributions to Antisocial Personality and Behavior: A Meta-Analytic Review from an Evolutionary Perspective," *The Journal of Social Psychology* 150, no. 2 (2010): 160–80; D. Boisvert and J. Vaske, "Genetic Theories of Criminal Behavior," *The Encyclopedia of Criminology and Criminal Justice* (Boston, MA: Wiley-Blackwell, 2014), 1–6.

26. R. Kendra, K. Bell, and J. Guimond, "The Impact of Child Abuse History, PTSD and Anger Arousal on Dating Violence Perpetrators among College Women," *Journal of Family Violence* 27, no. 3 (2012): 165–75; C. Sousa et al., "Longitudinal Study on the Effects of Child Abuse and Children's Exposure to Domestic Violence, Parent-Child Attachments and Antisocial Behavior in Adolescence," *Journal of Interpersonal Violence* 26, no. 1 (2011): 111–36.

27. W. Gunter and B. Newby, "From Bullied to Deviant: The Victim-Offender-Overlap among Bullying Victims," *Youth Violence and Juvenile Justice* (2014), doi: 10.1177/1541204014521250, (Epub ahead of print.); M. M. Ttofi, D. P. Farrington, and F. Lösel, "School Bullying as a Predictor of Violence Later in Life: A Systematic Review and Meta-Analysis of Prospective Longitudinal Studies," *Aggression and Violent Behavior* 17, no. 5 (2012): 405–18.

28. K. M. Devries et al., "Intimate Partner Violence Victimization and Alcohol Consumption in Women: A Systematic Review and Meta-Analysis," *Addiction* 109 (2014): 379–91, doi: 10.1111/add.12393; A. Abbey, "Alcohol's Role in Sexual Violence Perpetration: Theoretical Explanations, Existing Evidence and Future Directions," *Drugs and Alcohol Review* 30, no. 5 (2012): 481–85; J. M. Boden, D. M. Fergusen, and L. J. Horwood, "Alcohol Misuse and Violent Behavior: Findings from a 30-Year Longitudinal Study," *Drugs and Alcohol Dependence* 122, (2012): 135–41; United Nations Office on Drugs and Crime, "World Drug Report," 2013, www.unodc.org/unodc/secured/wdr/wdr2013/World_Drug_Report_2013.pdf; A. Sanderlund et al. "The Association between Sports Participation, Alcohol Use and Aggression and Violence: A Systematic Review," *Journal of Science and Medicine in Sport* 17, no. 1 (2014): 2–7.

29. P. H. Smith et al., "Intimate Partner Violence and Specific Substance Use Disorders: Findings from the National Epidemiologic Survey on Alcohol and Related Conditions," *Psychology of Addictive Behaviors* 26, no. 2 (2012): 236–45; J. Kuhns et al., "The Prevalence of Alcohol-Involved Homicide Offending: A Meta-Analytic Review," *Homicide Studies* 18, no. 3 (2014): 251–270, doi:10.1177/1088767913493629

30. A. Abbey, "Alcohol's Role in Sexual Violence Perpetration," 2011.

31. Ibid; S. Gervais, et al., "Understanding the Link between Men's Alcohol Use and Sexual Violence Perpetration: The Mediating Role of Sexual Objectification," *Psychology of Violence* 4, no. 2 (2014): 150–69.

32. C. Love et al., "Understanding the Connection between Suicide and Substance Abuse: What the Research Tells Us," SAMHSA Webinar Series, September 11, 2014, http://captus.samhsa.gov/sites/default/files/capt_resource/webcast_suicide_and_substance_abuse_part_1_sept_11_2014_final.pdf; Mary McMurran, ed., *Alcohol-Related Violence Prevention and Treatment* (West Sussex, UK: John Wiley and Sons, 2013); K. Graham et al., "Alcohol-Related Negative Consequences among Drinkers around the World," *Addiction* 106, no. 8 (2011): 1391–1405.

33. American Psychological Association, "Violence in the Media—Psychologists Study TV and Video Game Violence for Potential Harmful Effects," November 2013, www.apa.org/research/action/protect.aspx; V. Pozios et al., "Does Media Violence Lead to the Real Thing?," *New York Times*, August 23, 2013, www.nytimes.com/2013/08/25/opinion/sunday/does-media-violence-lead-to-the-realthing.html; T. Greitemer, "Video Games Do Affect Social Outcomes: A Meta-Analytical Review of the Effects of Violent and Prosocial Video Game Play," *Personality and Social Psychology Bulletin* 40, no. 5 (2014): 578–89

34. W. Gunter and K. Daley, "Causal or Spurious? Using Propensity Score Matching to Detangle the Relationship between Violent Video Games and Violent Behavior," *Computers in Human Behavior* 4, no. 28 (2012): 1348–55.

35. T. Greitemeyer and D. Mugge, "Video Games Do Affect Social Outcomes: A Meta-Analytic Review of the Effects of Violent and Prosocial Video Game Play," *Personality and Social Psychology Bulletin* 40, no. 5 (2014): 578–89; C. J. Ferguson et al, "Not Worth the Fuss After All? Cross-Sectional and Prospective Data on Violent Video Game Influences on Aggression, Visuospatial Cognition and Mathematics Ability in a Sample of Youth," *Journal of Youth and Adolescence* 42, no. 1 (2013): 109–22; J. Perlus et al. "Trends in Bullying, Physical Fighting, and Weapon Carrying among 6th-through 10th-Grade Students from 1998 to 2010: Findings from a National Study," *American Journal of Public Health* 104, no. 6 (2014): 110–6.

36. M. Elson and C. Ferguson, "Twenty-Five Years of Research on Violence in Digital games and Aggression: Empirical Evidence, Perspectives, and a Debate Gone Astray," *European Psychologist* 19, no. 1 (2014): 33–46.

37. C. J. Ferguson et al, "Not Worth the Fuss After All?," 2013.

38. R. A. Ramos et al., "Comfortably Numb or Just Yet Another Movie? Media Violence Exposure Does NOT Reduce Viewer Empathy for Victims of Real Violence among Primarily Hispanic Viewers," *Psychology of Popular Media Culture* 2, no. 1 (2013): 2–10.

39. World Health Organization, "Definitions and Typology of Violence," 2015, www.who.int/violenceprevention/approach/definition/en/

40. Centers for Disease Control and Prevention, "Youth Violence: Definitions," December 2013, www.cdc.gov/violenceprevention/youthviolence/definitions.html; L. L. Dahlberg and E. G. Krug, "Violence: A Global Public Health Problem," in *World Report on Violence and Health* (Geneva: World Health Organization, 2002), 1–21.

41. World Health Organization, "Definitions and Typology of Violence," 2015.

42. Centers for Disease Control and Prevention, "Health, United States, 2013," May 2014, www.cdc.gov/nchs/data/hus/hus13.pdf

43. Centers for Disease Control and Prevention, "Deaths: Preliminary Data for 2013," *National Vital Statistics Reports* 61, no. 6 (2012), Available at www.cdc.gov/nchs/data/nvsr/nvsr61/nvsr61_06.pdf; Centers for Disease Control and Prevention, "Faststats: Assault or Homicide," December 2013, www.cdc.gov/nchs/fastats/homicide.htm

44. U. S. Department of Justice, Federal Bureau of Investigation, "Expanded Homicide Data Table 10," *Crime in the United States 2013*, Available at www.fbi.gov/about-us/cjis/ucr/crime-in-the-u.s/2013/crime-in-the-u.s.-2013/offenses-known-to-law-enforcement/expanded-homicide/expanded_homicide_data_table_10_murder_circumstances_by_relationship_2013.xls

45. A. Cooper and E. Smith, "Homicide in the U.S. Known to Law Enforcement, 2011," *Bureau of Justice Statistics,* December 30, 2013, Available at www.bjs.gov/index.cfm?ty=pbdetail&iid=4863

46. Ibid.

47. Ibid.

48. Ibid.

49. Federal Bureau of Investigation, "Hate Crime Statistics, 2013," February 2015, Available at www.fbi.gov/about-us/cjis/ucr/hate-crime/2013

50. Bureau of Justice Statistics, "Hate Crime Victimization-2004-2012-Statistical Tables," February 2014, www.bjs.gov/index.cfm?ty=pbdetail&iid=4883

51. Ibid.

52. U.S. Department of Justice, "Juvenile Justice Fact Sheet—Highlights of the 2012 National Youth Gang Survey," December 2014, www.ojjdp.gov/pubs/248025.pdf; Federal Bureau of Investigation, "2013 National Gang Threat Assessment-Emerging Trends," February 2015, www.fbi.gov/stats-services/publications/national-gang-report-2013

53. National Gang Center, "National Youth Survey Analysis," February 2015, www.nationalgangcenter.gov/Survey-Analysis

54. FB I, "2013 National Gang Threat Assessment," 2015.

55. D. McDaniel, "Risk and Protective Factors Associated with Gang Affiliation among High-Risk Youth: A Public Health Approach," *Injury Prevention*, January 11, 2012, Available at http://injury-prevention.bmj.com/content/early/2012/01/04/injuryprev-2011-040083.full.pdf+html

56. U.S. Code of Federal Regulations, Title 28CFR0.85.

57. U.S. Department of Homeland Security, "The Internet as a Terrorist Tool for Recruitment and Radicalizaton of Youth-White Paper," April 24, 2009, Available at www.homelandsecurity.org/docs/reports/Internet_Radicalization.pdf

58. P. Lin and J. Gill, "Homicides of Pregnant Women," *Journal of Forensic Medicine and Pathology* (2010), doi: 10-1097/PAF .obo13e3181d3dc3b. (Epub ahead of print.)

59. Violence Policy Center, *American Roulette: Murder-Suicide in the United States*, 4th ed. (Washington, DC: Violence Policy Center, 2012), Available at www.vpc.org

60. S. Catalano, "Intimate Partner Violence: Attributes of Victimization, 1993-2011" *Bureau of Justice Statistics,* November 13, 2013, Available at www.bjs.gov/index.cfm?ty=pbdetail&iid=4801

61. M. C. Black et al., *The National Intimate Partner and Sexual Violence Survey (NISVS): 2010 Summary Report* (Atlanta, GA: National Center for Injury Prevention and Control, Centers for Disease Control and Prevention, 2011), Available at www.cdc.gov

62. L. Walker, *The Battered Woman* (New York: Harper and Row, 1979).

63. L. Walker, *The Battered Woman Syndrome*, 3rd ed. (New York: Springer, 2009).

64. Psychiatric Times, "Battered Woman Syndrome," July 2009, www.psychiatrictimes.com/trauma-and-violence/battered-woman-syndrome

65. Child Welfare Information Gateway, *Definitions of Child Abuse and Neglect* (Washington, DC: U.S. Department of Health and Human Services, Children's Bureau, 2014), Available at www.childwelfare.gov/topics/systemwide/laws-policies/statutes/define/; U. S. Department of Health and Human Services Administration for Children and Families, "Definitions of Child Abuse and Neglect," February 2011, www.childwelfare.gov/systemwide/laws_policies/statutes/define.cfm

66. R. Gilbert and C. Spatz Widom et al. "Burden of Child Maltreatment in 'High Income' Countries," *Lancet* 373, no. 9657 (2009): 68–81; GAO, *Child Maltreatment: Strengthening National Data on Child Fatalities Could Aid in Prevention* (Washington, D.C.: U.S. Government Printing Office, 2011), Available at www.gao.gov/assets/330/320774; Childhelp, National Child Abuse Statistics, "Child Abuse in America–2013," 2013, www.childhelp.org/pages/statistics; National Children's Alliance, "National Statistics on Child Abuse," 2015, www.childhelp.org/child-abuse-statistics

67. Childhelp, "Child Abuse Statistics and Facts," 2015.

68. M. Lachs and J. Berman, " Under the Radar: New York State Elder Abuse Prevalence Study," New York City Department for Aging, May 2011, Available at www.ocfs.state.ny.us/main/reports/Under%20the%20Radar%2005%2012%2011%20final%20report.pdf; Centers for Disease Control and Prevention, "Elder Abuse Prevention," June 2014, www.cdc.gov/Features/ElderAbuse/; National Institute on Aging, "Elder Abuse," February 2015. www.nia.nih.gov/health/publication/elder-abuse

69. J. Grohol, "DSM-5 Changes: PTSD, Trauma and Stress-Related Disorders," *Psych Central-Professional*, May 28, 2013, http://pro.psychcentral.com/dsm-5-changes-ptsd-trauma-stress-related-disorders/004406.html

70. M. Breiding et al., "Prevalence and Characteristics of Sexual Violence, Stalking, and Intimate Partner Violence Victimization—National Intimate Partner and Sexual Violence Survey, United States, 2011," *Morbidity and Mortality Weekly Report* 63, no. SS08 (September 5, 2014), 1–18, Available at www.cdc.gov/mmwr/preview/mmwrhtml/ss6308a1.htm?s_cid=ss6308a1_e

71. Ibid.

72. Ibid.

73. Ibid; C. MaCaskill, "Sexual Violence on Campus: How Too Many Institutions of Higher Education Are Failing to Protect Students," July 9, 2014, www.mccaskill.senate.gov/SurveyReportwithAppendix.pdf; White House Task Force to Protect Students from Sexual Assault, *Not Alone: First Report of White House Task Force to Protect Students from Sexual Assault,* April 2014, www.whitehouse.gov/sites/default/files/docs/report_0.pdf

74. J. Carr, *American College Health Association Campus Violence White Paper* (Baltimore: American College Health Association, 2005), Available at www.acha.org

75. National Criminal Justice Reference Service, "School and Campus Crime," *Resource Guide*, 2013, http://ovc.ncjrs.gov

76. Centers for Disease Control and Prevention, National Center for Injury Prevention and Control, "Understanding Sexual Violence Fact Sheet," 2014, www.cdc.gov

77. Jeanne Clery Act Information, "The Campus Sexual Violence Elimination Act," 2014, www.cleryact.info/campus-save-act.html

78. White House Task Force to Protect Students from Sexual Assault, *Not Alone: First Report of White House Task Force to Protect Students from Sexual Assault,* April 2014, www.whitehouse.gov/sites/default/files/docs/report_0.pdf

79. SB-967, "Student Safety: Sexual Assault," 2013–2014, https://leginfo.legislature.ca.gov/faces/billNavClient.xhtml?bill_id=201320140SB967

80. B. Chappell, "California Enacts 'Yes means Yes' Law, Defining Sexual Consent,"September 29, 2014, www.npr.org/blogs/thetwo-way/2014/09/29/352482932/california-enacts-yes-means-yes-law-defining-sexual-consent

81. R. Bergen and E. Barnhill, National Online Resource Center on Violence Against Women, "Marital Rape: New Research and Directions," National Resource Center on Domestic Violence, 2011.

82. D. Finkelhor and K. Yllö, *License to Rape: Sexual Abuse of Wives* (New York: The Free Press, 1985).

83. Ibid.

84. National Online Resource Center, Violence Against Women, "Marital Rape: New Research and Directions," 2011, www.vawnet.org/applied-research-papers/print-document.php?doc_id=248

85. Association of Title IX Administrators, "The Challenge of Title IX Responses to Campus Relationship and Intimate Partner Violence: The 2015 White Paper, 2015," 2015, Available at www.atixa.org/wordpress/wp-content/uploads/2012/01/Challenge-of-TIX-with-Author-Photos.pdf

86. U.S. Equal Employment Opportunity Commission, "Sexual Harassment," February 2015, www.eeoc.gov/laws/types/sexual_harassment.cfm

87. U.S. Department of Education, "U.S. Department of Education Releases List of Higher Education Institutions with Open Title IX Sexual Violence Investigations," May 1, 2014, www.ed.gov/news/press-releases/us-department-education-releases-list-higher-education-institutions-open-title-ix-sexual-violence-investigations

88. Centers for Disease Control, "Sexual Violence, Stalking, and Intimate Partner Violence Widespread in the US," NISVS 2010 Summary Report, Press Release, December 2011.

89. Centers for Disease Control and Prevention, "Sexual Violence, Stalking, and Intimate Partner Violence Widespread in the US," 2011; National Criminal Justice Reference Service (NCVRW), "Crime Victimization in the United States: Statistical Overviews," in *NCVRW Resource Guide-2012*, June 2014, www.ncjrs.gov/ovc_archives/ncvrw/2012/pdf/StatisticalOverviews.pdf

90. M. Breiding et al., "Prevalence and Characteristics of Sexual Violence, Stalking, and Intimate Partner Violence Victimization," 2014.

91. Centers for Disease Control and Prevention, "Sexual Violence, Stalking, and Intimate Partner Violence Widespread in the US," 2011; NCVRW, "Crime Victimization in the United States," 2014.

92. M. Stoltenborgh et al., "The Current Prevalence of Child Sexual Abuse Worldwide: A Systematic Review and Meta-Analysis," *International Journal of Public Health* 58, no. 3 (2013): 469–83; L. P. Chen et al., "Sexual Abuse and Lifetime Diagnosis of Psychiatric Disorders: Systematic Review and Meta-Analysis," *Mayo Clinic Proceedings* 85, no. 7 (2010): 618–29; Childhelp, "Child Abuse Statistics and Facts," 2015; U.S. Department of Health and Human Services, Children's Bureau, "Child Maltreatment," 2013, www.acf.hhs.gov/sites/default/files/cb/cm2012.pdf

93. U.S. Department of Justice, "Sexual Assault of Young Children as Reported to Law Enforcement: Victim, Incident, and Offender Characteristics," *Bureau of Justice Statics*, March 2015, www.bjs.gov/content/pub/pdf/saycrle.pdf

94. Childhelp, "Child Abuse Statistics and Facts," 2015, www.childhelp.org/pages/statistics; L. P. Chen et al., "Sexual Abuse and Lifetime Diagnosis of Psychiatric Disorders," 2010; M. Stoltenborgh et al., "The Current Prevalence of Child Sexual Abuse Worldwide, 2013; T. Hilberg, C. Hamilton-Giachrtsis, and L. Dixon, "Review of Meta-Analyses on the Association between Child Sexual Abuse and Adult Mental Health Difficulties: A Systematic Approach," *Trauma, Violence, Abuse* 12, no. 1 (2011): 38–49.

95. Childhelp, "Child Abuse in America–2012," 2014.

96. K. Kochanek et. al., "Mortality in the United States, 2013," *NCHS Data Brief* 178, December 2014, www.cdc.gov/nchs/data/databriefs/db178.htm#what

97. Centers for Disease Control and Prevention, "10 Leading Causes of Death by Age Group, United States–2012," November 2014, Available at www.cdc.gov/injury/wisqars/pdf/leading_causes_of_death_by_age_group_2012-a.pdf

98. Centers for Disease Control and Prevention, "Wide-Ranging Online Data for Epidemiologic Research (WONDER)," May 2013, http://wonder.cdc.gov/mortsql.html

99. NHTSA, "The Fatality Analysis Reporting System (FARS) and the National Automotove Sampling System (NASS) General Estimates System (GES)," *Data Webinar*, January 15, 2015 www.nrd.nhtsa.dot.gov/Pubs/13WPPP.pdf; National Highway Traffic Safety Administration, "Traffic Safety Facts: 2012 Data," 2014.

100. NHTSA, "The Fatality Analysis Reporting System (FARS) and the National Automotive Sampling System (NASS)," 2015.

101. Ibid.

102. Ibid.

103. National Highway Traffic Safety Administration, "Traffic Safety Facts, 2013 Data: Alcohol-Impaired Driving," December 2014, www-nrd.nhtsa.dot.gov/Pubs/812102.pdf

104. National Institute on Drug Abuse, "Drug Facts: Drugged Driving," Revised December 2014, www.drugabuse.gov/publications/drugfacts/drugged-driving

105. S. Salomonsen-Sautel et al., "Trends in Fatal Motor Vehicle Crashes Before and After Marijuana Commercialized in Colorado," *Drug and Alcohol Dependence* 140 (2014): 137–44

106. Centers for Disease Control and Prevention, "Drowsy Driving: Asleep at the Wheel," 2014, www.cdc.gov/features/dsDrowsyDriving/index.html

107. Centers for Disease Control and Prevention, "Distracted Driving," October, 2014, www.cdc.gov/motorvehiclesafety/distracted_driving/.

108. NHTSA, "The Fatality Analysis Reporting System (FARS) and the National Automotive Sampling System (NASS)," 2015.; National Highway Traffic Safety Administration, "What Is Distracted Driving? Key Facts and Statistics," February 2015, www.distraction.gov/get-the-facts/facts-and-statistics.html

109. Centers for Disease Control and Prevention, "Distracted Driving," 2014.

110. National Highway Traffic Safety Administration, "What Is Distracted Driving?," 2015.

111. Governors Highway Safety Association, "Distracted Driving Laws," March 2015, www.ghsa.org/html/stateinfo/laws/cellphone_laws.html

112. Centers for Disease Control and Prevention, "Policy Impact: Seat Belts," Updated January 2014, www.cdc.gov/Motorvehiclesafety/seatbeltbrief

113. National Highway Traffic Safety Administration, "Traffic Safety Facts: 2012 Data," March 2014, www-nrd.nhtsa.dot.gov/Pubs/811892.pdf

114. NHTSA, "The Fatality Analysis Reporting System (FARS) and the National Automotove Sampling System (NASS)," 2015.

115. National Highway Traffic Safety Administration, "Traffic Safety Facts 2012 Data: Bicyclists and Other Cyclists," April 2014, www-nrd.nhtsa.dot.gov/Pubs/812018.pdf

116. Ibid.

117. Ibid.

118. Centers for Disease Control and Prevention, "Unintentional Drowning: Get the Facts," October 24, 2014, www.cdc.gov/HomeandRecreationalSafety/Water-Safety/waterinjuries-factsheet.html

119. Ibid.

120. Ibid.

121. Ibid.

122. U. S. Coast Guard, "Coast Guard News: U.S. Coast Guard Releases 2013 Recreational Boating Statistics Report," May 2014, http://coastguardnews.com/u-s-coast-guard-releases-2013-recreational-boating-statistics-report/2014/05/14/?utm_source=feedburner&utm_medium=feed&utm_campaign=Feed%3A+CoastGuardNews+(Coast+Guard+News)

123. Ibid.

124. Ibid.

125. U. S. Coast Guard, "Boating Safety Resource Center: BUI Initiatives," April 2014, www.uscgboating.org/recreational-boaters/boating-under-the-influence.php

126. American Boating Association, "Boating Safety—It Could Mean Your Life," 2013, www.americanboating.org/safety.asp

127. Centers for Disease Control and Prevention, "National Vital Statistics System Mortality Data," March 4, 2015, www.cdc.gov/nchs/deaths.htm

128. Centers for Disease Control and Prevention, "Prescription Drug Overdose," October 2014, www.cdc.gov/homeandrecreationalsafety/overdose/index.html

129. J. B. Mowry et al., "2012 Annual Report of the American Association of Poison Control Centers' National Poison Data System (NPDS): 30th Annual Report," *Clinical Toxicology* 51, no. 10 (2013): 949–1229, doi: 10.3109/15563650.2013.863906

130. American Association of Poison Control Centers, "Prevention," February 2015, www.aapcc.org/prevention

131. Centers for Disease Control and Prevention, "Falls among Older Adults: An Overview," December 2014, www.cdc.gov/homeandrecreationalsafety/falls/adultfalls.html

132. U.S. Fire Administration, "U.S. Fire Deaths, Fire Death Rates, and Risks of Dying in a Fire," November 4, 2014, www.usfa.fema.gov/data/statistics/fire_death_rates.html

133. U.S. Fire Administration, "Campus Fire Safety: Safety Tips for Students and Parents," March 2014, www.usfa.fema.gov/citizens/college

134. Ibid.

135. Ibid.

Pulled Statistics:

Page 118, CDC, "The National Intimate Partner and Sexual Violence Survey (NISVS): 2010 Summary Report," February 26, 2014, www.cdc.gov/

Page 120, White House Task Force to Protect Students from Sexual Assault, "Not Alone: First Report of White House Task Force to Protect Students from Sexual Assault, "April 2014, www.whitehouse.gov/sites/default/files/docs/report_0

Page 127, American College Health Association, American College Health Association—National College Health Assessment II: Reference Group Executive Summary Spring 2014 (Hanover, MD: American College Health Association, 2014).

Chapter 5: Connecting and Communicating in the Modern World

1. J. T. Cacioppo, *Rewarding Social Connections Promote Successful Aging*, American Association for the Advancement of Science Annual Meeting, Chicago, Illinois, 2014.

2. Y. Luo et al., "Loneliness, Health, and Mortality in Old Age: A National Longitudinal Study," *Social Science and Medicine* 74, no. 6 (2012): 907–14.

3. J. T. Cacioppo and B. Patrick, *Loneliness: Human Nature and the Need for Social Connection.* (New York: W. W. Norton, 2008).

4. Ibid.

5. M. T. Frías, A. Brassard, and P. R. Shaver,"Childhood Sexual Abuse and Attachment Insecurities as Predictors of Women's Own and Perceived-Partner Extradyadic Involvement," *Child Abuse and Neglect* (2014), http://dx.doi.org.proxy.lib.uni.edu/10.1016/j.chiabu.2014.02.009; A. Lowell, K. Renk, and A. H. Adgate, "The Role of Attachment in the Relationship between Child Maltreatment and Later Emotional and Behavioral Functioning," *Child Abuse and Neglect* (2014), http://dx.doi.org.proxy.lib.uni.edu/10.1016/j.chiabu.2014.02.006

6. R. Sternberg, "A Triangular Theory of Love," *Psychological Review* 93 (1986): 119–35.

7. R. Sternberg, *Cupid's Arrow: The Course of Love through Time* (Boston: Cambridge University Press, 1998).

8. H. Fisher, *Why We Love* (New York: Henry Holt, 2004); H. Fisher et al., "Defining the Brain System of Lust, Romantic Attraction, and Attachment," *Archives of Sexual Behavior* 31, no. 5 (2002): 413–19.

9. Ibid.

10. L. Festinger, S. Schachter, and K. Back, *Social Pressures in Informal Groups: A Study of Human Factors in Housing* (Stanford, CA: Stanford University Press, 1950); E. J. Finkel and R. F. Baumeister, "Attraction and Rejection," in *Advanced Social Psychology: The State of the Science*, eds. R. F. Baumeister and E. J. Finkel (New York: Oxford University Press, 2010), 419–59.

11. S. Levay and J. Baldwin, *Human Sexuality*, 4th ed. (Sunderland, MA: Sinauer Associates, 2012).

12. L. Lee et al., "If I'm Not Hot, Are You Hot or Not? Physical-Attractiveness Evaluations and Dating Preferences as a Function of One's Own Attractiveness," *Psychological Science* 19, no. 7 (2008): 669–77.

13. J. Holt-Lunstad, T. Smith, and J. Layton, "Social Relationships and Mortality Risk: A Meta-Analytic Review," *PLoS Medicine* 7, no. 7 (2010); J. L. Kohn and S. L. Averett, "The Effect of Relationship Status on Health with Dynamic Health and Persistent Relationships," *Journal of Health Economics* 36 (2014): 69–83.

14. J. Holt-Lunstad, T. Smith, and J. Layton, "Social Relationships and Mortality Risk: A Meta-Analytic Review," *PLoS Medicine* 7, no. 7 (2010): e1000316; M. Ferris, "Social Connectedness and Health," (St. Paul, MN: Wilder Foundation, 2012).

15. J. Holt-Lunstad, T. Smith, and J. Layton, "Social Relationships and Mortality Risk: A Meta-Analytic Review," *PLoS Medicine* 7, no. 7 (2010): e1000316.

16. E. Robinson, J. Thomas, P. Aveyard, and S. Higgs, "What Everyone Else is Eating: A Systematic Review and Meta-Analysis of the Effect of Informational Eating Norms on Eating Behavior," *Journal of the Academy of Nutrition and Dietetics* 114, no. 3 (2014) 414–29; N. A. Christakis and J. H. Fowler, "Social Contagion Theory: Examining Dynamic Social Networks and Human Behavior," *Statistics in Medicine* 32, no. 4 (2013): 556–77.

17. S. Cohen and T. A. Wills, "Stress, Social Support, and the Buffering Hypothesis," *Psychological Bulletin* 98 (1985): 310–57.

18. S. Schnall, K. D. Harber, J. K. Stefanucci, and D. R. Proffitt, "Social Support and the Perception of Geographical Slant," *Journal of Experimental Social Psychology*, 44, no. 5 (2008): 1246–255.

19. K. Hampton, L. S. Goulet, L. Rainie, and K. Purcell, "Social Networking Sites and Our Lives," *Pew Internet and American Life Project,* June 16, 2011, Available at www.pewinternet.org/files/old-media//Files/Reports/2011/PIP%20-%20Social%20networking%20sites%20and%20our%20lives.pdf

20. L. F. Berkman, I. Kawachi, and M. Glymour, eds. *Social Epidemiology* (Oxford University Press, 2014).

21. J. T. Cacioppo and B. Patrick, *Loneliness: Human Nature and the Need for Social Connection.* (New York: W. W. Norton, 2008).

22. K. Hampton, L. S. Goulet, L. Rainie, et al., "Social Networking Sites and Our Lives," *Pew Internet and American Life Project,* 2011.

23. C. R. Rogers, "Interpersonal Relationship: The Core of Guidance," in *Person to Person: The Problem of Being Human,* eds. C. R. Rogers and B. Stevens (Lafayette, CA: Real People Press, 1967).

24. B. Hurn and B. Tomalin, *Cross-Cultural Communication: Theory and Practice* (London: Pagrave-Macmillan, 2013).

25. Ibid.

26. Ibid.

27. J. Wood, *Interpersonal Communication: Everyday Encounters,* 7th ed. (Belmont, CA: Cengage, 2012).

28. Ibid.

29. R. E. Jack et al., "Facial Expressions of Emotion are not Culturally Universal," *Proceedings of the National Academy of Sciences* 109, no. 19 (2012): 7241–244.

30. K. Hampton, L. S. Goulet, L. Rainie, and K. Purcell, "Social Networking Sites and our Lives," Pew Internet and American Life Project.

31. Ibid.

32. Ibid.

33. Ibid.

34. Ibid.

35. Ibid.

36. Ibid.

37. Ibid.

38. E. C. Tandoc, P. Ferrucci, and M. Duffy, "Facebook Use, Envy, and Depression among College Students: Is Facebooking Depressing?," *Computers in Human Behavior* 43, (2015): 139–46.

39. M. Meeker and L. Wu, "2013 Internet Trends," *KPCB,* May 19, 2013, Available at www.kpcb.com/blog/2013-internet-trends

40. J. A. Roberts, L. Yaya, and C. Manolis, "The Invisible Addiction: Cell-phone Activities and Addiction among Male and Female College Students," *Journal of Behavioral Addiction* 3, no. 4 (2014): 254–65.

41. Ibid.

42. K. M. Hertlein and K. Ancheta, "Advantages and Disadvantages of Technology in Relationships: Findings from an Open-Ended Survey," *The Qualitative Report* 19, no. 22 (2014): 1–11.

43. Y. T. Uhls et al., "Five Days at Outdoor Education Camp without Screens Improves Preteen Skills with Nonverbal Emotion Cues," *Computers in Human Behavior* 39, (2014): 387–92.

44. N. Carr, *The Shallows: What the Internet Is Doing to Our Brains* (New York: W. W. Norton, 2011).

45. T. Worley, "Exploring the Association between Relational Uncertainty, Jealousy about Partner's Friendships, and Jealousy Expression in Dating Relationships," *Communication Studies* 65, no. 4 (2014): 370–88; B. Sagarin et al., "Sex Differences in Jealousy: A Meta-Analytic Examination," *Evolution and Human Behavior* 33, no. 6 (2012): 595–614.

46. United States Department of Labor, Bureau of Labor Statistics, "American Time Use Survey Summary–2013 Results," June 2014, www.bls.gov/news.release/atus.t01.htm

47. The Gottman Institute, "Research FAQs," www.gottman.com/research/research-faqs

48. G. F. Kelly, *Sexuality Today,* 11th ed. (New York, NY: McGraw-Hill, 2014).

49. F. Newport and J. Wilke, "Most in U.S. Want Marriage, but Its Importance Has Dropped," *Gallup,* August 2, 2013, www.gallup.com/poll/163802/marriage-importance-dropped.aspx

50. D. B. Elliot, K. Krivickas, and M. W. Brault, "Historical Marriage Trends from 1890–2010: A Focus on Race Differences," Annual Meeting of the Population Association of America, 2012, www.census.gov/hhes/socdemo/marriage/data/acs/ElliottetalPAA2012paper.pdf

51. G. Livingston, "Four-in-Ten Couples are Saying 'I Do' Again," *Pew Research Center,* November 14, 2014, www.pewsocialtrends.org/2014/11/14/four-in-ten-couples-are-saying-i-do-again/

52. U.S. Census Bureau, "Families and Living Arrangements: 2014, Table MS-2 Estimated Median Age at First Marriage, by Sex: 1890 to the Present," www.census.gov/hhes/families/data/marital.html

53. M. Banschick, "The High Failure Rate of Second and Third Marriages," *Psychology Today,* February 6, 2012, www.psychologytoday.com/blog/the-intelligent-divorce/201202/the-high-failure-rate-second-and-third-marriages

54. K. Heller, "The Myth of the High Rate of Divorce," *Psych Central,* April 2, 2014, http://psychcentral.com/lib/2012/the-myth-of-the-high-rate-of-divorce

55. R. M. Kreider and R. Ellis, "Number, Timing, and Duration of Marriages and Divorces: 2009," *Current Population Reports,* P70-125 (Washington, DC: U.S. Census Bureau, 2011), Available at www.census.gov/prod/2011pubs/p70–125.pdf

56. Ibid.

57. A. J. Cherlin, "Americans Prefer Serial Monogamy to Open Relationships," *New York Times* Blog, May 21, 2013, http://www.nytimes.com/roomfordebate/2012/01/20/the-gingrich-question-cheating-vs-open-marriage/americans-prefer-serial-monogamy-to-open-relationships

58. I. Siegler et al., "Consistency and Timing of Marital Transitions and Survival During Midlife: The Role of Personality and Health Risk Behaviors," *Annals of Behavioral Medicine* 45, no. 3 (2013): 338–47, doi: 10.1007/s12160-012-9457-3; A. A. Aizer et al., "Marital Status and Survival in Patients with Cancer," *Journal of Clinical Oncology* 31, no. 31 (2013): 3869–3876, doi: 10.1200/JCO.2013.49.6489

59. C. C. Miller, "Study Finds More Reasons to Get and Stay Married," *New York Times,* January 8, 2015, www.nytimes.com/2015/01/08/upshot/study-finds-more-reasons-to-get-and-stay-married.html?rref=upshot&abt=0002&abg=0&_r=2

60. K. Williams, "Has the Future of Marriage Arrived? A Contemporary Examination of Gender, Marriage, and Psychological Well-Being." *Journal of Health and Social Behavior* 44.4 (2003): 470–87.

61. U.S. Department of Health and Human Services, Vital and Health Statistics, "Health Behaviors of Adults: United States, 2008–2010," DHHS Pub 10, No. 257 (2013): 7–78, Available at www.cdc.gov/nchs/data/series/sr_10/sr10_257.pdf

62. Ibid.

63. Ibid.

64. U.S. Department of Health and Human Services, Division of Vital Statistics, "First Premarital Cohabitation in the United States: 2006–2010 National Survey of Family Growth," *National Health Statistics Report* 64 (2013), Available at www.cdc.gov/nchs/data/nhsr/nhsr064.pdf

65. Ibid.

66. A. Kuperberg, "Age at Co-Residence, Premarital Cohabitation and Marriage Dissolution: 1985–2009," *Journal of Marriage and Family,* 76 no. 2 (2014): 352–69.

67. U.S. Department of Health and Human Services, "First Premarital Cohabitation in the United States," 2013.

68. U.S. Census Bureau, "Characteristics of Same-Sex Households: 2013," 2013, www.census.gov/hhes/samesex/

69. Obergefell v. Hodges, 576 U.S. (2015).

70. Ibid

71. Ibid.

72. A. Blinder and T. Lewin, "Clerk in Kentucky Chooses Jail Over Deal on Same-Sex Marriage," September 3, 2015, http://www.nytimes.com/2015/09/04/us/kim-davis-same-sex-marriage.html?_r=0; Krishnadev Calamur, "In Some States Defiance of Supreme Court's Same-Sex Ruling," June 29, 2015, http://www.npr.org/sections/thetwo-way/2015/06/29/418600672/in-some-states-defiance-over-supreme-courts-same-sex-marriage-ruling.

73. U.S. Census Bureau, "Marital Status: 2007–2011 American Community Survey, 5-Year Estimates, Table S1201," http://factfinder2 .census

Pulled Statistics:

Page 147, A. Smith and M. Duggan, "Online Dating and Relationships," Pew Research (2013), www.pewinternet.org/2013/10/21/online-dating- relationships/

Page 150, K. Parker, W. Wang, and M. Rohol, "Record Share of Americans Have Never Married," Pew Research (2014), www.pewsocialtrends.org/files/2014/09/2014-09-24_Never-Married-Americans.pdf

Focus On: Understanding Your Sexuality

1. I. A. Hughes et al., "Consensus Statement on Management of Intersex Disorders," *Journal of Pediatric Urology* 2, no. 3 (2006): 148–62; Intersex Society of North America, "How Common Is Intersex?," 2008, www.isna.org.

2. G. M. Herek and K. A. McLemore, "Sexual Prejudice," *Annual Review of Psychology* 64 (2013): 309–33.

3. Federal Bureau of Investigation, "Hate Crime Statistics, 2013," (Fall 2014), www.fbi.gov/about-us/cjis/ucr/hate-crime/2013/topic-pages/incidents-and-offenses/incidentsandoffenses_final.pdf

4. M. Rosario and E. Schrimshaw, "Theories and Etiologies of Sexual Orientation," *APA Handbook of Sexuality and Psychology* 1 (2014): 555–96.

5. S. M. Cabrera et al., "Age of Thelarche and Menarche in Contemporary U.S. Females: A Cross-Sectional Analysis," *Journal of Pediatric Endocrinology and Metabolism* 27, 1–2 (2014): 47–51.

6. S. Levay and J. Baldwin, *Human Sexuality,* 4th ed. (Sunderland, MA: Sinauer Associates, 2012).

7. Womenshealth.gov, "Premenstrual Symptoms Fact Sheet," December 23, 2014, http://womenshealth.gov/publications/our-publications/fact-sheet/premenstrual-syndrome.html#e

8. Ibid.

9. Ibid.

10. Mayo Clinic Staff, "Diseases and Conditions: Menstrual Cramps," May 8, 2014, www.mayoclinic.org/diseases-conditions/menstrual-cramps/basics/definition/con-20025447

11. National Institute on Aging, "Menopause", January 22, 2015, Available at www.nia.nih.gov/health/publication/menopause

12. National Institutes of Health, "WHI Follow-Up Study Confirms Risk of Long-Term Combination

Hormone Therapy Outweigh Benefits for Postmenopausal Women," News Release, March 4, 2008, www.public.nhlbi.nih.gov/newsroom/home/; National Heart, Lung, and Blood Institute (NHLBI), "WHI Study Data Confirm Short-Term Health Disease Risks of Combination Hormone Therapy for Postmenopausal Women," News Release, February 15, 2010, www.nih.gov/news/health/feb2010/nhlbi-15.htm

13. M. Beck, "Benefits of Hormone-Replacement Therapy Outweigh Risks, Reviews of Studies Show," Health blog, *The Wall Street Journal*, May 22, 2012, http://blogs.wsj.com/health/2012/05/22/benefits-of-hormone-replacement-therapy-outweigh-risks-reviews-of-studies-show

14. M. Owings, S. Uddin, and S. Williams, "Trends in Circumcision for Male Newborns in U.S. Hospitals: 1979–2010," August 2013, www.cdc.gov/nchs/data/hestat/circumcision_2013/circumcision_2013.pdf

15. American Academy of Pediatrics, "2012 Technical Report, Male Circumcision," *Pediatrics* 130, no. 3 (2012): e756–e785, doi: 10.1542/peds.2012-1990

16. Ibid.

17. G. F. Kelly, *Sexuality Today*, 11th ed. (New York, NY: McGraw-Hill, 2014).

18. Ibid.

19. American College Health Association, *American College Health Association–National College Health Assessment II (ACHA-NCHA II) Reference Group Data Report, Spring 2014* (Hanover, MD: American College Health Association, 2014), Available at www.acha-ncha.org/docs/ACHA-NCHA-II_ReferenceGroup_DataReport_Spring2014.pdf

20. S. Caron, *The Sex Lives of College Students: Two Decades of Attitudes and Behaviors,* (Orono, ME: Maine College Press, 2014).

21. American College Health Association, *American College Health Association–National College Health Assessment II: Reference Group Data Report, Spring 2014*, 2014..

22. Ibid.

23. Ibid.

24. C. Harte and C. Meston. "Recreational Use of Erectile Dysfunction Medications and Its Adverse Effects on Erectile Function in Young, Healthy Men: The Mediating Role of Confidence in Erectile Ability." *Journal of Sexual Medicine*. 2012. 9(7):(1852–59)

25. G. Prestage et al., "Australian Gay and Bisexual Men's Use of Erectile Dysfunction Medications During Recent Sexual Encounters," *The Journal of Sexual Medicine* 11, no. 3, (2014): 809–19; D. J. Snipes and E. G. Benotsh, "High-Risk Cocktails and High-Risk Sex: Examining the Relation between Alcohol Mixed with Energy Drink Consumption, Sexual Behavior, and Drug Use in College Students," *Addictive Behaviors* 38, no. 1 (2013): 1418–23.

26. J. Bliss, "Police, Experts: Alcohol Most Common in Sexual Assaults," *USA Today*, October 28, 2013, www.usatoday.com/story/news/nation/2013/10/28/alcohol-most-common-drug-in-sexual-assaults/3285139

Pulled Statistics:

Page 164, Data from American College Health Association, American College Health Association—National College Health Assessment II (ACHA-NCHA II): Reference Group Data Report Spring 2014 (Hanover, MD: American College Health Association, 2014).

Chapter 6: Considering Your Reproductive Choices

1. American College Health Association, *American College Health Association—National College Health Assessment III (ACHA-NCHA III): Reference Group Data Report, Spring 2014* (Hanover, MD: American College Health Association, 2014), Available at www.achancha.org/docs/ACHA-NCHA-II_ReferenceGroup_DataReport_Spring2014.pdf

2. L. B. Finer and M. R. Zolna, "Shifts in Intended and Unintended Pregnancies in the United States, 2001–2008," *American Journal of Public Health* 104, no. S1 (2014): S44–S48.

3. J. Trussell, "Contraceptive Efficacy," in *Contraceptive Technology*, 20th rev. ed., eds. R. A. Hatcher et al. (New York: Ardent Media, 2011).

4. World Health Organization, "Nonoxynol-9 Ineffective in Preventing HIV Infection," Press Release, June 28, 2002, www.who.int/mediacentre/news/releases/who55/en/

5. J. Trussell, "Contraceptive Efficacy," 2011.

6. Ibid.

7. Ibid.

8. Mayo Clinic Staff, "Tests and Procedures: Spermicide," January 2013, www.mayoclinic.org/tests-procedures/spermicide/basics/risks/prc-20012597; World Health Organization, "Nonoxynol-9 Ineffective in Preventing HIV Infection," 2002.

9. World Health Organization, "Nonoxynol-9 Ineffective in Preventing HIV Infection," 2015, www.who.int/mediacentre/news/notes/release55/en

10. J. Trussell, "Contraceptive Efficacy," 2011.

11. Ibid.

12. Ibid.

13. American College Health Association, *National College Health Assessment III): Reference Group Data Report, Spring 2014*, 2014.

14. J. Trussell, "Contraceptive Efficacy," 2011.

15. Ibid.

16. O. Lidegaard et al., "Thrombotic Stroke and Myocardial Infarction with Hormonal Contraception," *New England Journal of Medicine* 366, no. 24 (2012): 2257–66, doi: 10.1056/NEJMoa1111840

17. J. Trussell, "Contraceptive Efficacy," 2011.

18. E. G. Raymond, "Progestin-Only Pills," in *Contraceptive Technology*, 20th rev. ed., eds. R. A. Hatcher et al. (New York: Ardent Media, 2011).

19. Janssen Pharmaceuticals, "OrthoEvra," October 2012, www.orthoevra.com; Drugs.com, "Xulane," April 2015, www.drugs.com/pro/xulane.html

20. J. Trussell, "Contraceptive Efficacy," 2011.

21. Janssen Pharmaceuticals, "Important Safety Update for U.S. Health Care Professionals ORTHO EVRA," March 2011, www.orthoevra.com/isi-hcp.html

22. J. Trussell, "Contraceptive Efficacy," 2011.

23. Ibid.

24. Pfizer, "Depo-subQ Provera," September 2013, www.depo-subqprovera104.com

25. J. Trussell, "Contraceptive Efficacy," 2011.

26. Merck & Co., Inc., "Nexplanon," Accessed April 2015, www.merck.com/product/usa/pi_circulars/n/nexplanon/nexplanon_pi.pdf

27. J. Jones, W. Mosher, and K. Daniels, "Current Contraceptive Use in the United States, 2006–2010, and Changes in Pattern of Use Since 1995," *National Health Statistics Reports* 60 (2012): 1–25.

28. The American Congress of Obstetricians and Gynecologists, "ACOG Committee Opinion-Adolescents and Long-Acting Reversible Contraception: Implants and Intrauterine Devices," Number 539, October 2012, www.acog.org/Resources_And_Publications/Committee_Opinions/Committee_on_Adolescent_Health_Care/Adolescents_and_Long-Acting_Reversible_Contraception

29. J. Trussell, "Contraceptive Efficacy," 2011.

30. American College Health Association, *National College Health Assessment III: Reference Group Data Report Spring, 2014*, 2014.

31. J. Trussell, "Contraceptive Efficacy," 2011.

32. American College Health Association, *National College Health Assessment III: Reference Group Data Report Spring, 2014*, 2014.

33. J. Trussell, "Contraceptive Efficacy," 2011.

34. Office of Population Research & Association of Reproductive Health Professionals, The Emergency Contraception Website, "Answers to Frequently Asked Questions about Effectiveness," Updated July 2014, http://ec.princeton.edu/questions/eceffect.html

35. American College Health Association, *National College Health Assessment II: Undergraduate Students Reference Group Data Fall 2014*, 2014.

36. K. Daniels, J. Daugherty, and J. Jones, "Current Contraceptive Status among Women Aged 15–44: United States 2011–2013," *National Health Statistics Data Brief*, no. 173 (Hyattsville, MD: National Center for Health Statistics, 2014).

37. J. Trussell, "Contraceptive Efficacy," 2011.

38. Guttmacher Institute, "Fact Sheet: Induced Abortion in the United States," July 2014, www.guttmacher.org/pubs/fb_induced_abortion.html

39. American Psychological Association (APA), Task Force on Mental Health and Abortion, *Report of the Task Force on Mental Health and Abortion* (Washington, DC: American Psychological Association, 2008), Available at www.apa.org/pi/wpo/mental-health-abortion-report.pdf

40. *Roe v. Wade*, 410 U.S. 113 (1973).

41. L. Saad, "Abortion," *Gallup Politics*, Blog, January 22, 2013, www.gallup.com/poll/160058/majority-americans-support-roe-wade-decision.aspx

42. Guttmacher Institute, "In Just the Last Four Years, States Have Enacted 231 Abortion Restrictions," January 2015, https://guttmacher.org/media/inthenews/2015/01/05/index.html

43. APA, *Report of the Task Force*, 2008; J. R. Steinberg, C. E. McCulloch, and N. E. Adler, "Abortion and Mental Health: Findings from the National Comorbidity Survey-Replication," *Obstetrics & Gynecology* 123, no. 2 (2014): 263–70.

44. Ibid.

45. Ibid.

46. Guttmacher Institute, "Fact Sheet: Induced Abortion in the United States," 2014.

47. Ibid.

48. Ibid.

49. Planned Parenthood, "The Abortion Pill (Medication Abortion)," www.plannedparenthood.org/health-topics/abortion/abortion-pill-medication-abortion-4354.asp

50. K. Cleland et al., "Significant Adverse Events and Outcomes After Medical Abortion," *Obstetrics and Gynecology* 121, no. 1 (2013): 166–171.

51. K. Cleland et al., "Significant Adverse Events and Outcomes After Medical Abortion," 2013.

52. M. Lino, *Expenditures on Children by Families, 2013* (Alexandria, VA: U.S. Department of Agriculture, Center for Nutrition Policy and Promotion, 2014), www.cnpp.usda.gov/ExpendituresonChildrenbyFamilies

53. Truven Health Analytics, "The Cost of Having a Baby in the United States," January 2013, http://transform.childbirthconnection.org/wp-content/uploads/2013/01/Cost-of-Having-a-Baby1.pdf

54. T. J. Mathews and B. E. Hamilton, "*First Births to Older Women Continue to Rise*," National Center for Health Statistics Data Brief, No. 152, May 2014, www.cdc.gov/nchs/data/databriefs/db152.pdf

55. J. A. Martin et al., U.S. Department of Health and Human Services, National Center for Health Statistics, "Births: Final Data for 2012," *National Vital Statistics Reports* 62, no. 9 (2013), Available at www.cdc.gov/nchs/data/nvsr/nvsr62/nvsr62_09.pdf#table01

56. American Pregnancy Association, "Miscarriage," Updated June 2014, http://americanpregnancy .org/pregnancycomplications/miscarriage.html

57. Committee on Gynecologic Practice of American College of Obstetricians and Gynecologists; Practice Committee of American Society for Reproductive Medicine, "Age-Related Fertility Decline: A Committee Opinion," *Fertility and Sterility*, 90, Supplement 5 (2008): S154–55.

58. Centers for Disease Control and Prevention (CDC), "Preconception Care and Health Care: Women," January 2015, www.cdc.gov/ preconception/women.html

59. bid.

60. S. M. Schrader and K. L. Marlow, "Assessing the Reproductive Health of Men with Occupational Exposures," *Asian Journal of Andrology* 16, no. 1 (2014): 23–30; CDC, "Preconception Health and Healthcare," September 2014, www.cdc.gov/pre-conception/careformen/exposures.html

61. B. M. D'Onofrio et al., "Paternal Age at Child-bearing and Offspring Psychiatric and Academic Morbidity," *Journal of the American Medical Association Psychiatry*, 71 no. 4 (2014): 432–38; E. Calloway, "Fathers Bequeath More Mutations as They Age," *Nature*, 488 no. 7412 (2012): 439.

62. Planned Parenthood, "Pregnancy Tests," Accessed April 2015, www.plannedparenthood .org/health-topics/pregnancy/pregnancy-test-21227.asp

63. Committee on Obstetric Practice, "Committee Opinion no. 548, American Congress of Obstetricians and Gynecologists: Weight Gain During Pregnancy," *Obstetrics and Gynecology* 121, no. 1 (2013): 210–12, doi: 10.1097/01. AOG.0000425668.87506.4c

64. The American Congress of Obstetricians and Gynecologists, "Tobacco, Alcohol, Drugs, and Pregnancy," December 2013, www.acog.org/~/ media/For%20Patients/faq170.pdf?dmc=1&ts=2 0140516T2242271513

65. National Center for Chronic Disease Prevention and Health Promotion, "Tobacco Use and Pregnancy," *Reproductive Health*, Updated August 2014, www.cdc.gov/Reproductivehealth/Tobac-coUsePregnancy/index.htm; The American Congress of Obstetricians and Gynecologists, "Tobacco, Alcohol, Drugs, and Pregnancy," 2013,

66. CDC, "Facts about Cleft Lip and Cleft Palate," 2014, www.cdc.gov/ncbddd/birthdefects/cleftlip.html

67. B. E. Hamilton et al., "Births: Preliminary Data for 2013," 2014, www.cdc.gov/nchs/data/nvsr/ nvsr63/nvsr63_02.pdf

68. J. Christensen, *CNN News*, "Why So Many C-Sections Have Medical Groups Concerned," May 8, 2014, www.cnn.com/2014/05/08/health/ c-section-report

69. E. Puscheck, "Early Pregnancy Loss," *Medscape Reference: Drugs, Diseases & Procedures*, Updated October 2014, http://reference.medscape.com/ article/266317-overview

70. V. P. Sepilian et al., "Ectopic Pregnancy," *Medscape Reference*, Updated September 2014, http://emedi-cine.medscape.com/article/2041923-overview

71. What to Expect, "Stillbirth," Accessed April 2015, www.whattoexpect.com/pregnancy/pregnancy-health/complications/stillbirth.aspx

72. K. L. Wisner et al., "Onset Timing, Thoughts of Self-harm, and Diagnoses in Postpartum Women with Screen-Positive Depression Findings," *JAMA Psychiatry* 70, no. 5 (2013): 1–9, doi:10.1001/jama-psychiatry.2013.87

73. American Academy of Pediatrics, "Benefits of Breastfeeding for Mom," Updated July 2014, www.healthychildren.org/English/ages-stages/baby/breastfeeding/pages/Benefits-of-Breastfeeding-for-Mom.aspx

74. CDC, "Sudden Unexpected Infant Death and Sudden Infant Death Syndrome," January 2015, www.cdc.gov/sids

75. Ibid.

76. Ibid.

77. CDC, "Infertility FAQs," Reproductive Health, updated June 2013, www.cdc.gov/reproductive-health/Infertility/

78. MayoClinic.com, "Infertility: Causes," July 2014, www.mayoclinic.com/health/infertility/ DS00310/DSECTION=causes

79. U.S. Department of Health and Human Services, "Polycystic Ovary Syndrome (PCOS) Fact Sheet," December 2014, www.womenshealth .gov/publications/our-publications/fact-sheet/ polycystic-ovary-syndrome.html

80. B. Kumbak, E. Oral, and O. Bukulmez, "Female Obesity and Assisted Reproductive Technolo-gies," *Seminars in Reproductive Medicine* 30, no. 6 (2012): 507–16, doi: 10.1055/s-0032-1328879

81. CDC, "Pelvic Inflammatory Disease CDC Fact Sheet," Sexually Transmitted Diseases, Updated July 2014, www.cdc.gov/std/PID/STDFact-PID.htm

82. CDC, "Infertility: FAQs," June 2013, www.cdc .gov/reproductivehealth/Infertility/index.htm#4

83. Ibid.; S. Cabler, A. Agarwal, and S. S. du Plessis, "Obesity and Male Fertility," *Male Infertility* 33 (2012): 349–60.

84. CDC, "Infertility: FAQs," 2013.

85. Ibid.

86. WebMD Medical Reference, "Fertility Drugs," July 2012, www.webmd.com/infertility-and-reproduction/guide/fertility-drugs

87. American Society for Reproductive Medicine, "Fertility Drugs and the Risk for Multiple Births," Accessed March 2015, www.asrm.org/ uploadedFiles/ASRM_Content/Resources/ Patient_Resources/Fact_Sheets_and_Info_Book-lets/fertilitydrugs_multiplebirths.pdf

88. WebMD, "Using a Surrogate Mother, What You Need to Know," September 2013, www.webmd .com/infertility-and-reproduction/guide/using-surrogate-mother.

89. R. M. Kreider and D. A. Loftquist, *Adopted Children and Stepchildren: 2010*, U.S. Census Bureau, April 2014, www.census.gov/content/dam/Cen-sus/library/publications/2014/demo/p20-572.pdf

90. Intercountry Adoption, U.S. Department of State, "FY 2013 Annual Report on Intercountry Adop-tion," Accessed March 2015, http://travel.state.gov/ content/dam/aa/pdfs/fy2013_annual_report.pdf

91. Adoption.com, "Adoption Costs," Accessed March 2015, http://costs.adoption.com

Pulled Statistics:

Page 174, W. D. Mosher and J. Jones, "Use of Con-traception in the United States: 1982–2008," *Vital and Health Statistics* 23, no. 29 (2010), www.cdc .gov/nchs/data/nhsr/nhsr062.pdf

Page 189, Gallup, "U.S. Still Split on Abortion: 47% Pro-Choice, 46% Pro-Life," 2014, www.gallup.com/ poll/170249/split-abortion-pro-choice-pro-life.aspx

Chapter 7: Recognizing and Avoiding Addiction and Drug Abuse

1. J. Grant et al., "Introduction to Behavioral Addic-tions," *American Journal of Behavioral Addictions* 36, no. 5 (2010): 233–41; National Institute on Drug Abuse, National Institutes of Health (NIH), U.S. Department of Health and Human Services, *Drugs, Brains, and Behavior: The Science of Addiction*, NIH Publication no. 07-5605 (Bethesda, MD: National Institute on Drug Abuse, Revised 2010), Available at www.drugabuse.gov

2. American Society of Addiction Medicine, "Defi-nition of Addiction," April 2011, www.asam .org/for-the-public/definition-of-addiction

3. D. E. Smith, "Editor's Note: The Process Addic-tions and the New ASAM Definition of Addic-tion," *Journal of Psychoactive Drugs* 44, no. 1 (2012); National Institute on Drug Abuse, NI H, *Drugs, Brains, and Behavior*, 2010.

4. National Council on Problem Gambling, "Problem Gambling: Have the Conversation in March," February 19, 2015, www.ncpgambling .org/wp-content/uploads/2014/04/PGAM-Press-Release-General-FINAL.pdf

5. American Psychiatric Association, *Diagnostic and Statistical Manual of Mental Disorders*, 5th ed. (Arlington, VA: American Psychiatric Publishing, 2013), p. 585.

6. M. N. Potenza, "Neurobiolgoy of Gambling Behaviors," *Current Opinion in Neurobiology* 23, no.4 (2013): 660–67.

7. Ibid.

8. National Center for Responsible Gambling, "Col-lege Students: Facts and Stats," www.collegegam-bling.org/just-facts/gambling-college-campuses

9. Ibid.

10. H. Hatfield, "Shopping Spree or Addiction?," *WebMD*, 2014, www.webmd.com/mental-health/ features/shopping-spree-addiction; M. Lejoyeux and A. Weinstein, "Compulsive Buying," *The American Journal of Drug and Alcohol Issues* 36, no.5 (2010): 248–53.

11. H. Hatfield, "Shopping Spree or Addiction?,"2014; M. Lejoyeux and A. Weinstein, "Compulsive Buying," 2010.

12. B. Cook and H. A. Hausenblas, "The Role of Exercise Dependence for the Relationship between Exercise Behavior and Eating Pathology: Mediator or Moderator?" *Journal of Health Psychology* 13, no. 4 (2008): 495–502.

13. K. Berczik et al., "Exercise Addiction: Symptoms, Diagnosis, Epidemiology and Etiology," *Substance Use and Misuse* 47 (2012): 403–17.

14. A. Alexander, "Internet Addiction Statistics 2012," April 24, 2012, http://ansonalex.com/ infographics/internet-addiction-statistics-2012-infographic

15. J. Anthony et al., "Problematic Internet Use and Other Risky Behaviors in College Students: An Application of Problem-Behavior Theory," *Ameri-can Psychological Association* 27 no. 1 (2012): 133–41.

16. American College Health Association, *American College Health Association—National College Health Assessment II: Reference Group Data Report Spring 2014* (Hanover, MD: American College Health Association, 2014).

17. Substance Abuse and Mental Health Services Administration, *Results from the 2013 National Survey on Drug Use and Health: Summary of National Findings*, NSDUH Series H-48, HHS Publication No. (SMA) 14-4863 (Rockville, MD: Substance Abuse and Mental Health Services Administration, 2014).

18. L. D. Johnston et al., *Monitoring the Future National Results on Drug Use: 2015 Overview, Key Findings on Adolescent Drug Use* (Ann Arbor: Institute for Social Research, The University of Michigan, 2015).

19. Ibid.

20. National Institute of Drug Abuse, "Drug Facts: Nationwide Trends," NIDA, January 2014, www.drugabuse.gov/publications/drugfacts/ nationwide-trends

21. National Drug Intelligence Center, "National Drug Threat Assessment 2011," 2011, www .justice.gov

22. L. D. Johnston et al., *Monitoring the Future National Results on Drug Use*, 2015.

23. Erowid, The DXM Vault, 2011, www.erowid.org
24. Substance Abuse and Mental Health Services Administration, *Results from the 2013 National Survey*, 2014.
25. Ibid.
26. Ibid.
27. L. D. Johnston et al., *Monitoring the Future National Results on Drug Use*, 2013, http://www.monitoringthefuture.org/pubs/monographs/mtf-overview2013.pdf.
28. American College Health Association, *American College Health Association–National College Health Assessment*, 2014.
29. Ibid.
30. Ibid.
31. Ibid.
32. L. M. Garnier-Dykstra et al., "Nonmedical Use of Prescription Stimulants during College: Four-Year Trends in Exposure Opportunity, Use, Motives, and Sources," *Journal of American College Health* 60, no. 3 (2012): 226–34.
33. Substance Abuse and Mental Health Services Administration, *Results from the 2013 National Survey*, 2014.
34. Ibid
35. Ibid.
36. L. D. Johnston et al., *Monitoring the Future National Survey Results on Drug Use*, 2013.
37. A. Arria, et al., "Drug Use Patterns and Continuous Enrollment in College: Results from a Longitudinal Study," *Journal of Studies on Alcohol and Drugs* 74, (2013): 71–83.
38. A. Arria et al., "Drug Use Patterns in Young Adulthood and Post-College Employment," *Drug and Alcohol Dependence* 127, no. 1–3 (2013): 23–30.
39. Substance Abuse and Mental Health Services Administration, *Results from the 2013 National Survey*, 2014.
40. Addiction Center, "Drinking and Drug Abuse is Higher among Greeks," February 15, 2015, www.addictioncenter.com/college/drinking-drug-abuse-greek-life/
41. Ibid.
42. National Center on Addiction and Substance Abuse at Columbia University, "Wasting the Best and the Brightest: Substance Abuse at America's Colleges and Universities," May 28, 2007, , www.casacolumbia.org
43. Substance Abuse and Mental Health Services Administration, *Results from the 2013 National Survey*, 2014.
44. L. D. Johnston et al., *Monitoring the Future National Results on Drug Use*, 2014, http://www.monitoringthefuture.org/pubs/monographs/mtf-overview2014.pdf.
45. CPDD Community Website, "Methamphetamine Abuse and Parkinson's Disease," July 31, 2011, www.cpddblog.com
46. NIH, National Institute on Drug Abuse, "Methamphetamine: What are the long term effects of Methamphetamine Abuse?" September 2013. www.drugabuse.gov/publications/research-reports/methamphetamine/what-are-long-term-effects-methamphetamine-abuse
47. N. Volkow, "Bath Salts: Emerging and Dangerous Products," *National Institute on Drug Abuse*, February 2011, www.drugabuse.gov/about-nida/directors-page/messages-director/2011/02/bath-salts-emerging-dangerous-products
48. S. Melton, "Bath Salts: An 'Ivory Wave' Epidemic?" *Medscape*, August 26, 2011, wwwmedscape.com/viewarticle/748344
49. Ibid.
50. D. C. Mitchell et al., "Beverage Caffeine Intakes in the U.S.," *Food and Chemical Toxicology*, 63 (2014): 136–42.

51. Ibid.
52. Ibid.
53. Harvard Health Letter, "What Is It about Coffee," January 2012, www.health.harvard.edu
54. National Institute on Drug Abuse, "DrugFacts: Khat," April 2013, www.drugabuse.gov/publications/drugfacts/khat
55. Ibid.
56. Ibid.
57. Substance Abuse and Mental Health Services Administration, *Results from the 2013 National Survey*, 2014.
58. Ibid.
59. National Institute on Drug Abuse, "Drug Facts: Marijuana," January 2014, www.drugabuse.gov/publications/drugfacts/marijuana
60. M. Asbridge et al., "Acute Cannabis Consumption and Motor Vehicle Collision Risk: Systematic Review of Observational Studies and Meta-analysis," *British Medical Journal* 344 (2012): 1–9, doi:10.1136/bmj.e536
61. National Institute on Drug Abuse, "Drug Facts: Marijuana," 2014.
62. Ibid.
63. S. Lev-Ran et al., "The Association between Cannabis Use and Depression: A Systematic Review and Meta-Analysis of Longitudinal Studies," *Psychological Medicine* 44 (2014), doi: 10.1017/S0033291713001438; L. R. Pacek et al., "The Bidirectional Relationships between Alcohol, Cannabis, Co-occurring Alcohol and Cannabis Use Disorders with Major Depressive Disorder: Results from a National Sample," *Journal of Affective Disorders* 148, no. 2 (2013):188–95, doi: 10.1016/j.jad.2012.11.059
64. L. R. Pacek et al., "The Bidirectional Relationships between Use Disorders with Major Depressive Disorder," 2013.
65. L. Degenhardt et al., "The Persistence of the Association between Adolescent Cannabis Use and Common Mental Disorders into Young Adulthood," *Addiction* 108, no. 1 (2013): 124–33.
66. J. Copeland, "Changes in Cannabis Use among Young People: Impact on Mental Health," *Current Opinion in Psychiatry* 26, no. 4 (2013): 325–29.
67. National Institute on Drug Abuse, Marijuana: Facts for Teens," October 2013, www.drugabuse.gov/publications/marijuana-facts-teens; Science Daily, "Marijuana Use Prior to Pregnancy Doubles Risk of Premature Birth," July 17, 2012, www.sciencedaily.com
68. National Institute on Drug Abuse (NIDA), "Drug Facts: Spice," December 2012, www.drugabuse.gov/publications/drugfacts/spice-synthetic-marijuana
69. Ibid.; L. D. Johnston et al., *Monitoring the Future National Survey Results on Drug Use, 1975–2012: Volume I, Secondary School Students*, 2013.
70. NIDA, "Spice," March 2015
71. Ibid.
72. Ibid.
73. National Institutes of Health, National Institute on Drug Abuse, "Drug Facts: Spice," 2012.
74. The Partnership at Drugfree.org, "GHB," www.drugfree.org/drug-guide/ghb
75. Substance Abuse and Mental Health Services Administration, "Results from the 2012 National Survey," 2013, http://archive.samhsa.gov/data/NSDUH/2012SummNatFindDetTables/Index.aspx.
76. National Institutes on Drug Abuse, "Heroin: What is the Scope of Heroin Use in the United States?" November, 2014, www.drugabuse.gov/publications/research-reports/heroin/scope-heroin-use-in-united-states
77. Ibid.
78. T. Cicero, "The Changing Face of Heroin Use in the United States: A Retrospective Analysis of the Past 50 Years," *JAMA* 71, no. 7 (2014): 821–26.

79. Substance Abuse and Mental Health Services Administration, "Results from the 2012 National Survey," 2013.
80. L. D. Johnston et al., *Monitoring the Future National Survey Results on Drug Use*, 2014.
81. National Institute on Drug Abuse, "NIDA InfoFacts: MDMA (Ecstasy)," September 2013, www.drugabuse.gov/infofacts/ecstasy.html
82. The Partnership at DrugFree.org, "Experts: People Who Think They Are Taking "Molly" Don't Know What They Are Getting," June 24, 2013, www.drugfree.org/join-together/drugs/experts-people-who-think-they-are-taking-molly-dont-know-what-theyre-getting
83. National Institute on Drug Abuse, "DrugFacts: Salvia," April 2013, www.drugabuse.gov/publications/drugfacts/salvia
84. Ibid.
85. Ibid.
86. Ibid.
87. The National Collegiate Athletic Association, "NCAA National Study of Substance Use Habits of College Student Athletes—Final Report 2014," August 2014, www.ncaa.org/sites/default/files/Substance%20Use%20Final%20Report_FINAL.pdf
88. H. G. Pope et al., "The Lifetime Prevalence of Anabolic-Androgenic Steroid Use and Dependence in Americans: Current Best Estimates," *American Journal on Addictions* (2013), doi: 10.1111/j.1521-0391.2013.12118.x
89. Ibid.
90. Substance Abuse and Mental Health Services Administration, "Results from the 2013 National Survey," 2014.
91. Office of National Drug Control Policy, "How Illicit Drug Use Affects Business and the Economy," *Executive Office of the President*, www.whitehouse.gov/ondcp/ondcp-fact-sheets/how-illicit-drug-use-affects-business-and-the-economy
92. Ibid.

Pulled Statistics:

Page 212, American College Health Association. *American College Health Association—National College Health Assessment II: Reference Group Executive Summary, Spring 2014* (Hanover, MD: American College Health Association, 2014).

Page 219, Substance Abuse and Mental Health Services Administration, Results from the 2013 National Survey on Drug Use and Health: Summary of National Findings , NSDUH Series H-48, HHS Publication No. (SMA) 14-4863 (Rockville, MD: Substance Abuse and Mental Health Services Administration, 2014).

Chapter 8: Drinking Alcohol Responsibly and Ending Tobacco Use

1. M. Stahre et al., "Contribution of Excessive Alcohol Consumption to Death and Years of Potential Life Lost in the United States," *Prevention of Chronic Disease* 11 (2014): 130293, www.cdc.gov/pcd/issues/2014/13_0293.htm
2. U.S. Department of Health and Human Services, *The Health Consequences of Smoking—50 Years of Progress: A Report of the Surgeon General* (Atlanta, GA: U.S. Centers for Disease Control and Prevention, Office on Smoking and Health, 2014), Available at www.surgeongeneral.gov/library/reports/50-years-of-progress/exec-summary.pdf; Centers for Disease Control and Prevention, "Current Cigarette Smoking among Adults—United States 2005–2013," *Morbidity and Mortality Weekly* 63, no. 47 (2014):1108–1112.

3. T. Naimi et al., "Confounding and Studies of 'Moderate' Alcohol Consumption: The Case of Drinking Frequency and Implications for Low Risk Drinking Guidelines," *Addiction* 108, no. 9 (2013): 1534–543; J. Marrone et al., "Moderate Alcohol Intake Lowers Biochemical Markers of Bone Turnover in Postmenopausal Women," *Journal of the North American Menopause Society* 19, no. 9 (2012): 974–79; C. Stockley, "Is It Merely a Myth That Alcoholic Beverages Such as Red Wine Can Be Cardioprotective?," *Society of Chemical Industry* 92 (2012): 1815–821, doi: 10.1002/jsfa.5696; A. Klatsky, "Alcohol and Cardiovascular Health," *Physiology and Behavior* 100, no. 1 (2010): 76–81, doi: 10.1016/j.physbeh.2009

4. National Center for Health Statistics, "Summary Health Statistics for U.S. Adults: National Health Interview Survey, 2012," *Vital and Health Statistics* 10, no. 260 (2014): 34.

5. Ibid.

6. D. J. Rohsenow et al., "Hangover Sensitivity after Controlled Alcohol Administration as Predictor of Post-College Drinking," *Journal of Abnormal Psychology* 121, no. 1 (2012): 270–75, doi: 10.1037/a0024706

7. K. Jackson et al., "Role of Tobacco Smoking in Hangover Symptoms among University Students," *Journal of Studies on Alcohol and Drugs* 74 (2013): 41–9.

8. M. A. White et al., "Hospitalizations for Alcohol and Drug Overdoses in Young Adults Ages 18–24 in the United States, 1999–2008: Results from the Nationwide Inpatient Sample," *Journal of Studies on Alcohol and Drugs* 72, no. 5 (2011): 774–876.

9. National Institute on Alcohol Abuse and Alcoholism, "Drinking Can Put a Chill on Your Summer Fun," 2012, http://pubs.niaaa.nih .gov; Centers for Disease Control and Prevention, "Unintentional Drowning: Get the Facts," November 2012, www.cdc.gov

10. Centers for Disease Control and Prevention, "Injury Prevention and Control: Home and Recreational Safety: Fire Deaths and Injuries: Fact Sheet," October 2011, www.cdc.gov

11. U.S. Department of Health and Human Services (HHS) Office of the Surgeon General and National Action Alliance for Suicide Prevention, "2012 National Strategy for Suicide Prevention: Goals and Objectives for Action," September 2012, www.surgeongeneral.gov

12. Ibid.

13. American College Health Association, *American College Health Association—National College Health Assessment II: Reference Group Executive Summary Spring 2014* (Hanover, MD: American College Health Association, 2014), Available at www.acha-ncha.org/reports_ACHA-NCHAII .html

14. N. Barnett, et al., "Description and Predictors of Positive and Negative Alcohol-Related Consequences in the First Year of College," *Journal of Studies on Alcohol and Drugs* 75, no.1 (2014): 103–14; M. Bersamin et al., "Young Adults and Casual Sex: The Relevance of College Settings," *Journal of Sex Research* 49, no. 2–3 (2012): 274–81.

15. S. Lawyer et al., "Forcible, Drug-Facilitated, and Incapacitate Rape and Sexual Assault among Undergraduate Women," *Journal of American College Health* 58, no. 5 (2010): 453–60, doi: 10.1080/07448480903540515

16. C. Stappenbeck, "A Longitudinal Investigation of Heavy Drinking and Physical Dating Violence in Men and Women," *Addictive Behaviors* 35, no. 5 (2010): 479–85, doi: 10.1016/j. addbeh.2009.12.027

17. Centers for Disease Control and Prevention, "Ten Leading Causes of Death by Age Group," August 2013, www.cdc.gov/injury/wisqars/leading-causes.html

18. Centers for Disease Control and Prevention, "Vital Signs: Drinking and Driving, a Threat to Everyone—October 2011," October 2013, www .cdc.gov/vitalsigns/drinkinganddriving

19. Ibid.; National Highway Traffic Safety Administration, "Traffic Safety Facts: 2012 Data Alcohol-Impaired Driving," December 2013, www-nrd. nhtsa.dot.gov/Pubs/811870.pdf

20. American College Health Association, *National College Health Assessment II: Reference Group Data Report, Spring 2014,* 2014.

21. Insurance Institute for Highway Safety, "Alcohol-Impaired Driving—2013," www.iihs.org/iihs/topics/t/alcohol-impaired-driving/fatalityfacts/alcohol-impaired-driving/2013

22. Ibid.

23. Ibid.

24. M. Silveri, "Adolescent Brain Development and Underage Drinking in the United States: Identifying Risks of Alcohol Use in College Populations," *Harvard Review of Psychiatry* 20, no. 4 (2012): 189–200.

25. Ibid.

26. S. J. Nielsen et al., "Calories Consumed from Alcoholic Beverages by U.S. Adults, 2007–2010," *NCHS Data Brief*, no. 110 (2012), Available at www.cdc.gov

27. L. Arriola et al., "Alcohol Intake and the Risk of Coronary Heart Disease in Spanish EPIC Cohort Study," *Heart* 96, no. 10 (2010): 124–30; T. Wilson et al., "Should Moderate Alcohol Consumption Be Promoted?," in *Nutrition and Health: Nutrition Guide for Physicians* (New York: Humana Press, 2010): 107–14; The American Heart Association, "Alcohol and Cardiovascular Disease," 2011, www.heart.org

28. Ibid.

29. The American Heart Association, "Alcohol and Heart Health," 2015, www.heart.org

30. J. Abraham et al., "Alcohol Metabolism in Human Cells Causes DNA Damage and Activates the Fanconi Anemia—Breast Cancer Susceptibility (FA-BRCA) DNA Damage Response Network," *Alcoholism: Clinical & Experimental Research* 35, no.12 (2011), doi: 10.1111/j.1530-0277.2011.01563.x

31. W. Y. Chen et al., "Moderate Alcohol Consumption during Adult Life, Drinking Patterns, and Breast Cancer Risk," *Journal of the American Medical Association* 306, no. 17 (2011): 1884–890, doi:10.1001/jama.2011.1590

32. C. S. Berkey et al., "Prospective Study of Adolescent Alcohol Consumption and Risk of Benign Breast Disease in Young Women," *Pediatrics* 125, no. 5 (2010): e1081–87.

33. SAMHSA, "18 Percent of Pregnant Women Drink Alcohol During Early Pregnancy," *The NSDUH Report*, September 9, 2013, www .samhsa.gov/data/sites/default/files/spot123-pregnancy-alcohol-2013/spot123-pregnancy-alcohol-2013.pdf; Y. Liu et al., "Alcohol Intake between Menarche and First Pregnancy: Prospective Study of Breast Cancer Risk," *Journal of the National Cancer Institute* 105, no. 20 (2013): 1571–78.

34. Centers for Disease Control and Prevention, "Fetal Alcohol Spectrum Disorders (FASDs): Alcohol Use During Pregnancy," April 17, 2014, www.cdc.gov/ncbddd/fasd/alcohol-use.html

35. Centers for Disease Control and Prevention, "Fetal Alcohol Spectrum Disorders (FASDs:) Data and Statistics," Updated January 28, 2015, www .cdc.gov/ncbddd/fasd/data.html

36. Ibid.

37. Fetal Alcohol Spectrum Disorders (FASD) Center for Excellence, "What Is FASD?," March 2014, www.Fasdcenter.samhsa.gov

38. American College Health Association, *National College Health Assessment II: Reference Group Executive Summary Spring 2014*, 2014.

39. Substance Abuse and Mental Health Services Administration, "Results from the 2013 National Survey on Drug Use and Health: Summary of National Findings 2013," September 2014, www. samhsa.gov

40. U.S. Department of Health and Human Services, National Institute on Alcohol Abuse and Alcoholism, "Moderate and Binge Drinking," 2012, www.niaaa.nih.gov/alcohol-health/overview-alcohol-consumption/moderate-binge-drinking

41. A. White and R. Hingson, "The Burden of Alcohol Use: Excessive Alcohol Consumption and Related Consequences among College Students," *Alcohol Research: Current Reviews*, 35, no. 2 (2014), Available at http://pubs.niaaa.nih .gov/publications/arcr352/201-218.htm

42. C. Neighbors et al., "Event Specific Drinking among College Students," *Psychology of Addictive Behaviors* 25, no. 4 (2011): 702–707, doi: 10.1037/a0024051

43. M. A. Lewis et al., "Use of Protective Behavioral Strategies and Their Association to 21st Birthday Alcohol Consumption and Related Negative Consequences: A Between and Within Person Evaluation," *Psychology of Addictive Behaviors* 26, no. 2 (2012), 179–86, doi: 10.1037/a0023797

44. National Institute on Alcohol Abuse and Alcoholism, "Fall Semester: A Time for Parents to Revisit Discussions about College Drinking," June 2012, www.collegedrinkingprevention .gov

45. American College Health Association, *National College Health Assessment II: Reference Group Executive Summary Spring 2014*, 2014.

46. C. Foster et al., "National College Health Assessment Measuring Negative Consequences among College Students, "*American Journal of Public Health Research* 2, no.1 (2014): 1–5

47. American College Health Association, *National College Health Assessment II: Reference Group Executive Summary Spring 2014*, 2014.

48. S. Onyper et al., "Class Start Times, Sleep and Academic Performance in College: A Path Analysis," *Chronobiology* 29, no. 3 (2012): 318–35; S. Kenney et al., "Global Sleep Quality as a Moderator of Alcohol Consumption and Consequences in College Students," *Addictive Behaviors* 37, no. 4 (2012): 507–12.

49. R. Hingson et al., "Magnitude of Alcohol-Related Mortality and Morbidity among U.S. College Students Ages 18–24," 2009.

50. Ibid.

51. J. W. LaBrie et al., "Are They All the Same? An Exploratory, Categorical Analysis of Drinking Game Types," *Addictive Behaviors* 38, no. 5 (2013): 2133–39; N. P. Barnett et al., "Predictors and Consequences of Pregaming Using Day and Week-Level Measures," *Psychology of Addictive Behaviors* 27, no. 4 (2013): 921.

52. B. Zamboanga et al., "Knowing Where They're Going: Destination-Specific Pregaming Behaviors in a Multiethnic Sample of College Students," *Journal of Clinical Psychology* 69, no. 4 (2013): 383–96.

53. N. P. Barnett et al., "Predictors and Consequences of Pregaming, ," 2013.

54. J. Alfonso et al., "Do Drinking Games Matter? An Examination by Game Type and Gender in a Mandated Student Sample," *The American Journal of Drug and Alcohol Abuse* 39, no. 5 (2013): 312–19; J. W. LaBrie et al., "Are They All the Same?," 2013.

55. N. P. Barnett et al., "Predictors; and Consequences of Pregaming," 2013.

56. R. Hingson et al., "Magnitude of Alcohol-Related Mortality and Morbidity among U.S. College Students Ages 18–24," 2009.

57. Ibid.

58. A. Barry et al., "Drunkorexia: Understanding the Co-occurrence of Alcohol Consumption and Eating/Exercise Weight Management Behaviors," *Journal of American College Health Association* 60, no. 3 (2012): 236–43, doi: 10.1080/07448481.2011.587487

59. M. Eisenberg and C. Fitz, "'Drunkorexia': Exploring the Who and Why of a Disturbing Trend in College Students' Eating and Drinking Behaviors," *American Journal of College Health* 62, no. 8 (2014):570–77.

60. Ibid.

61. Ibid.

62. Ibid.

63. G. DiFulvio et al., "Effectiveness of the Brief Alcohol and Screening Intervention for College Students (BASICS) Program for Mandated Students," *Journal of American College Health* 60, no. 4 (2012): 269–80.

64. Medline Plus, "Alcoholism and Alcohol Abuse," February 2014, www.nlm.nih.gov/medlineplus/ency/article/000944.htm

65. Center of Behavioral Health Statistics and Quality, "Nearly Half of College Student Treatment Admissions Were for Primary Alcohol Abuse," *Data Spotlight* (2012), www.samhsa.gov

66. K. Beck et al., "Social Contexts of Drinking and Subsequent Alcohol Use Disorder Among College Students," *American Journal of Alcohol Abuse* 39, no.1 (2012): 38–43.

67. A. Arria, "College Student Success: The Impact of Health Concerns and Substance Abuse," Lecture presented at NASPA Alcohol and Mental Health Conference (Fort Worth, TX: January 19, 2013).

68. M. Waldron et al., "Parental Separation and Early Substance Involvement: Results from Children of Alcoholic and Cannabis Twins," *Drug and Alcohol Dependence* 134 (2014): 78–84.

69. A. Levin, "Determining Alcoholism Proves Complicated Endeavor," *Psychiatric News* 47, no. 24 (2012): 20, doi: 10.1176/appi.pn.2012.12b13

70. D. Stacey, "RASGRF2 Regulates Alcohol-Induced Reinforcement by Influencing Mesolimbic Dopamine Neuron Activity and Dopamine Release," *Proceedings of the National Academy of Sciences* 109, no. 51 (2012): 21128–33, doi: 10.1073/pnas.1211844110

71. J. Niels Rosenquist et al., "The Spread of Alcohol Consumption Behavior in a Large Social Network," *Annals of Internal Medicine* 152, no. 7 (2010): 426–33.

72. Centers for Disease Control and Prevention, Fact Sheet, "Excessive Alcohol Use and Risks to Women's Health," November 19, 2014, www.cdc.gov/alcohol/fact-sheets/womens-health.htm

73. Centers for Disease Control and Prevention, "The High Cost of Excessive Drinking to States," February 5, 2015, www.cdc.gov/features/CostsOfDrinking

74. Ibid.

75. Underage Drinking Enforcement Training Center, Underage Drinking Costs, "Underage Drinking," September 2011, www.udetc.org/UnderageDrinkingCosts.as

76. Ibid.

77. Ibid.

78. Substance Abuse and Mental Health Services Administration, "The NSDUH Report—Alcohol Treatment: Need, Utilization, and Barriers," April 2009, www.samhsa.gov

79. A. Laudet et al., "Collegiate Recovery Community Programs: What Do We Know and What Do We Need to Know?," *Journal of Social Work Practice in the Addictions* 14 (2014): 84–100; A. Laudet, et al., "Characteristics of Students Participating in Collegiate Recovery Programs: A National Survey," *Journal of Substance Abuse Treatment* 51 (2014): 38–46.

80. J. Liang and R. Olsen, "Alcohol Use Disorders and Current Pharmacological Therapies: The Role of GABA Receptors," *Acta Pharmacologica Sinica* 35, no. 8 (2014): 981–93.

81. U.S. Department of Health and Human Services, *The Health Consequences of Smoking—50 Years of Progress*, 2014.

82. CDC, "Fast Facts: Tobacco," April 2015, www.cdc.gov/tobacco/data_statistics/fact_sheets/fast_facts/index.htm

83. Substance Abuse and Mental Health Services Administration, "Results from the 2012 National Survey on Drug Use and Health: Summary of National Findings," U.S. Department of Health and Human Services Series H-46, No. (SMA) 13-4795 (Rockville, MD: Substance Abuse and Mental Health Services Administration, 2013), Available at www.samhsa.gov/data/NSDUH/2012SummNatFindDetTables/NationalFindings/NSDUHresults2012.pdf

84. Centers for Disease Control and Prevention, "50th Anniversary of the First Surgeon General's Report on Smoking and Health," January 2014, www.cdc.gov/mmwr/preview/mmwr.html/mm6302a1.htm?s_cid=mm6302a1_w

85. Campaign for Tobacco-Free Kids, "Toll of Tobacco in the United States of America,"February 2014, www.tobaccofreekids.org/research/factsheets/pdf/0072.pdf?utm_source=factsheets_finder&utm_medium=link&utm_campaign=analytics

86. American Lung Association, "General Smoking Facts," June 2011, www.lung.org

87. Tobacco Free Providence, "Sweet Deceit Survey Results," January 2012, www.tobaccofreeprovidence.org

88. American Cancer Society, "Cancer Facts & Figures 2015," April 2015, www.cancer.org/acs/groups/content/@editorial/documents/document/acspc-044552.pdf

89. U.S. Department of Health and Human Services, *The Health Consequences of Smoking—50 Years of Progress*, 2014.

90. Campaign for Tobacco-Free Kids, "Toll of Tobacco in the United States of America," 2014.

91. Campaign for Tobacco-Free Kids, "State Cigarette Excise Tax Rates & Rankings," December 2013, www.tobaccofreekids.org/research/factsheets/pdf/0097.pdf

92. American College Health Association, *American College Health Association–National College Health Assessment II: Reference Group Data Report, Spring 2014*, 2014.

93. Ibid.

94. Substance Abuse and Mental Health Services Administration, "Results from the 2012 National Survey on Drug Use and Health: Summary of National Findings," 2013.

95. Y. Choi et al., "I Smoke but I Am Not a Smoker": Phantom Smokers and the Discrepancy between Self-identity and Behavior," *Journal of American College Health* 59, no. 2 (2011): 117–25.

96. E. Sutfin et al., "Tobacco Use by College Students: A Comparison of Daily and Nondaily Smokers," *American Journal of Health Behavior* 36, no. 2 (2012): 218–29, doi: 10.5993/AJHB.36.2.7

97. U.S. Department of Health and Human Services, *The Health Consequences of Smoking—50 Years of Progress*, 2014.

98. Tobacco-Free Kids, "1998 State Tobacco Settlement 15 Years Later," February 2014, www.tobaccofreekids.org/what_we_do/state_local/tobacco_settlement

99. 111th Congress of the United States of America, *Family Smoking Prevention and Tobacco Control Act of 2009*, HR 1256, www.govtrack.us

100. U.S. Department of Health and Human Services, *The Health Consequences of Smoking—50 Years of Progress*, 2014; U.S. Department of Health and Human Services, "How Tobacco Smoke Causes Disease: The Biology and Behavioral Basis for Smoking Attributable Disease: A Report of the Surgeon General," 2010, Available at www.ncbi.nlm.nih.gov

101. American Cancer Society, "Child and Teen Tobacco Use," March 6, 2015, www.cancer.org/acs/groups/cid/documents/webcontent/002963-pdf.pdf

102. National Institute on Drug Abuse Research Report Series, "Tobacco Addiction," *NIH Publication no. 12-4342*, 2012, Available at www.drugabuse.gov

103. American Cancer Society, "Who Smokes Cigars?" February 19, 2014, www.cancer.org/cancer/cancercauses/tobaccocancer/cigarsmoking/cigar-smoking-who-smokes-cigars

104. K. Sterling et al., "Factors Associated with Small Cigar Use Among College Students," *American Journal of Health Behavior* 37, no. 3 (2013): 325–33.

105. Centers for Disease Control and Prevention, "Smoking and Tobacco Use: Bidis and Kreteks," Updated July 2013, www.cdc.gov/tobacco/data_statistics/fact_sheets/tobacco_industry/bidis_kreteks

106. Centers for Disease Control and Prevention, "Smoking and Tobacco Use: Bidis and Kreteks," June 2011, www.cdc.gov

107. American Cancer Society, "Questions about Smoking, Tobacco, and Health: What about More Exotic Forms of Smoking Tobacco, Such as Clove Cigarettes, Bidis, and Hookahs?," January 2013, www.cancer.org

108. American Cancer Society, "Questions about Smoking, Tobacco, and Health: What about More Exotic Forms of Smoking Tobacco, Such as Clove Cigarettes, Bidis, and Hookahs?," February 2014, www.cancer.org/cancer/cancercauses/tobaccocancer/questionsaboutsmokingtobaccoandhealth/questions-about-smoking-tobacco-and-health-other-forms-of-smoking

109. Centers for Disease Control and Prevention, "Youth and Tobacco Use," February 2014, www.cdc.gov/tobacco/data_statistics/fact_sheets/youth_data/tobacco_use

110. Campaign for Tobacco Free Kids, "Toll of Tobacco in the United States of America," 2014.

111. National Cancer Institute, "Lung Cancer Prevention," February 2014, www.cancer.gov/cancertopics/pdq/prevention/lung/HealthProfessional/page2

112. American Cancer Society, "Cancer Facts & Figures 2015," www.cancer.org/acs/groups/

content/@editorial/documents/document/acspc-044552.pdf

113. Ibid.

114. American Cancer Society, "What Are Oral Cavity and Oropharyngeal Cancers?," February 2014, www.cancer.org/cancer/oralcavityandoropharyngealcancer/detailedguide/oral-cavity-and-oropharyngeal-cancer-what-is-oral-cavity-cancer

115. American Cancer Society, "Cancer Facts & Figures 2015," 2015.

116. Ibid.

117. American Heart Association, *Heart Disease and Stroke Statistics—2015 Update* (Dallas, TX: American Heart Association, 2015), Available at http://circ.ahajournals.org/content/early/2014/12/18/CIR.0000000000000152.full.pdf

118. Ibid.

119. Ibid.

120. Ibid.

121. American Heart Association, "Stroke Risk Factors," October 2012, www.strokeassociation.org/STROKEORG/AboutStroke/UnderstandingRisk/Understanding-Risk_UCM_308539_SubHomePage.jsp; CDC, "Health Effects of Cigarette Smoking," February 2014, www.cdc.gov/tobacco/data_statistics/fact_sheets/health_effects/effects_cig_smoking

122. U.S. Department of Health and Human Services, *The Health Consequences of Smoking—50 Years of Progress: A Report of the Surgeon General,* 2014.

123. Johns Hopkins Health Alerts, "Emphysema: Symptoms and Remedies," March 2012, www.johnshopkinshealthalerts.com

124. C. B. Harte et al., "Association between Cigarette Smoking and Erectile Tumescence: The Mediating Role of Heart Rate Variability," *International Journal of Impotence Research* (2013*)*: doi: 10.1038/ijir.2012.43

125. Centers for Disease Control and Prevention, "Tobacco Use and Pregnancy," Modified January 2014, www.cdc.gov/reproductivehealth/TobaccoUsePregnancy

126. Ibid.

127. Centers for Disease Control and Prevention, "Current Cigarette Smoking among Adults—United States 2005–2013," *Morbidity and Mortality Weekly* 63, no. 47 (2014): 1108–12; M. Thun et al., "50-Year Trends in Smoking-Related Mortality in the United States," *The New England Journal of Medicine* 368 (2013): 351–64, doi: 10.1056/NEJMsa1211127; American Cancer Society, "Women and Smoking: An Epidemic of Smoking-Related Cancer and Disease in Women," Revised February 2014, www.cancer.org/Cancer/CancerCauses/TobaccoCancer/WomenandSmoking/women-and-smoking-intro

128. American Academy of Periodontology, "Gum Disease Risk Factors, www.perio.org/consumer/risk-factors

129. I. Moreno-Gonzalez, et al., "Smoking Exacerbates Amyloid Pathology in a Mouse Model of Alzheimer's Disease," *Nature Communications* 4 (2013), www.nature.com/ncomms/journal/v4/n2/abs/ncomms2494.html; J. Cataldo et al., "Cigarette Smoking Is a Risk Factor of Alzheimer's Disease: An Analysis Controlling for Tobacco Industry Affiliation," *Journal of Alzheimer's Disease* 19, no. 2 (2010): 465–80, doi: 10.3233/JAD-2010-1240

130. Centers for Disease Control and Prevention, "Smoking and Tobacco Use Facts: Secondhand Smoke," April 2014, www.cdc.gov/tobacco/data_statistics/fact_sheets/secondhand_smoke/general_facts

131. Ibid

132. Ibid.

133. Ibid.

134. Ibid.

135. National Cancer Institute, "Secondhand Smoke and Cancer," January 2011, www.cancer.gov/cancertopics/factsheet/Tobacco/ETS

136. U.S. Department of Health and Human Services, *The Health Consequences of Involuntary Exposure to Tobacco Smoke,* November 2011; Centers for Disease Control and Prevention, "Smoking and Tobacco Use Fact Sheet," February 2014, www.cancer.org/docroot/ped/content/ped_10_2x_secondhand_smoke-clean_indoor_air.asp

137. Centers for Disease Control and Prevention, "Tobacco Use: Smoking Cessation," February 2014, www.cdc.gov/tobacco/data_statistics/fact_sheets/cessation/quitting/index.htm#quitting

138. American Lung Association, "Benefits of Quitting," March 2012, www.lungusa.org

139. N. Hopper, "What a Pack of Cigarettes Costs Now, State by State," *The Awl,* August 1, 2014, www.theawl.com/2014/08/how-much-a-pack-of-cigarettes-costs-state-by-state

140. American Cancer Society, "Guide to Quitting Smoking: A Word about Quitting Success Rates," February 2014, www.cancer.org/Healthy/StayAwayfromTobacco/GuidetoQuittingSmoking/guide-to-quitting-smoking-success-rates

141. Everyday Health, "A Guide to Using the Nicotine Patch," May 2011, www.everydayhealth.com

142. U.S. Food and Drug Administration, "Public Health Advisory: FDA Requires New Boxed Warnings for the Smoking Cessation Drugs Chantix and Zyban," July 2009, http://www.fda.go

Pulled Statistics:

Page 232, National Institute on Alcohol Abuse and Alcoholism, "Drinking Facts and Statistics," 2014, www.niaaa.nih.gov/alcohol-health/overview-alcohol-consumption/alcohol-facts-and-statistics.

Page 238, www.niaaa.nih.gov/alcohol-health/overview-alcohol-consumption/alcohol-facts-and-statistics

Chapter 9: Nutrition: Eating for a Healthier You

1. L. L. Wilkinson et al., "Attachment Anxiety, Disinhibited Eating and Body Mass Index in Adulthood," *Appetite* 57, no. 2 (2011): 543.

2. U.S. Department of Agriculture, "Part D: Section 6: Sodium, Potassium, and Water," *Report of the Dietary Guidelines Advisory Committee on the Dietary Guidelines for Americans, 2010* (Washington, DC.: U.S. Department of Agriculture, Agricultural Research Service, 2010).

3. S. C. Killer, A. K. Blannin, and A. E. Jeukendrup, "No Evidence of Dehydration with Moderate Daily Coffee Intake: A Counterbalanced Cross-Over Study in a Free-Living Population," *PLoS ONE* 9, no. 1 (2014): e84154, doi:10.1371/journal.pone.0084154

4. American College of Sports Medicine (ACSM), "Selecting and Effectively Using Hydration for Fitness," 2011, www.acsm.org/docs/brochures/selecting-and-effectively-using-hydration-for-fitness.pdf

5. U.S. Department of Agriculture, *What We Eat in America,* NHANES 2009–2010, 2010

6. Food and Nutrition Board, Institute of Medicine, *Dietary Reference Intakes for Energy, Carbohydrate, Fiber, Fat, Fatty Acids, Cholesterol, Protein, and Amino Acids (Macronutrients),* (Washington, DC: National Academies Press, 2005), Available at www.nap.edu/openbook.php?isbn=0309085373

7. S. M. Phillips and L. J. C. van Loon, "Dietary Protein for Athletes: From Requirements to Optimum Adaptation," *Journal of Sports Science* 29, no. S1 (2011): S29–S38.

8. Institute of Medicine of the National Academies, "Dietary, Functional, and Total Fiber," *Dietary Reference Intakes for Energy, Carbohydrate, Fiber, Fat, Fatty Acids, Cholesterol, Protein, and Amino Acids* (Washington, DC: The National Academies Press, 2005), 339–421, Available at www.nap.edu/openbook.php?isbn=0309085373

9. Ibid.

10. Ibid.

11. C. E. Ramsden et al., "Use of Dietary Linoleic Acid for Secondary Prevention of Coronary Heart Disease and Death: Evaluation of Recovered Data from the Sydney Diet Heart Study and Updated Meta-Analysis," *British Medical Journal* 346 (2013): e8707, doi: http://dx.doi.org/10.1136/bmj.e8707; L. Gillingham, S. Harris-Janz, and P. Jones, "Dietary Monounsaturated Fatty Acids Are Protective against Metabolic Syndrome and Cardiovascular Disease Risk Factors," *Lipids* 46, no. 3 (2011): 209–28, doi: 10.1007/s11745-010-3524-y

12. W. Willet, "Dietary Fats and Coronary Heart Disease," *Journal of Internal Medicine,* no. 1 (2012): 13–24; N. Bendson et al., "Consumption of Industrial and Ruminant Trans Fatty Acids and Risk of CHD: A Systemic Review and Meta-Analysis of Cohort Studies," *European Journal of Clinical Nutrition* 65 (2011): 773–83.

13. U.S. Food and Drug Administration, "FDA Targets Trans Fats in Processed Foods," FDA Consumer Updates, December 2013, www.fda.gov/ForConsumers/ConsumerUpdates/ucm372915.htm

14. Ibid.

15. H. J. Silver et al., "Consuming a Balanced High Fat Diet for 16 Weeks Improves Body Composition, Inflammation and Vascular Function Parameters in Obese Premenopausal Women," *Metabolism* (January 17, 2014), doi: 10.1016/j.metabol.2014.01.004; Z. Shadman, "Association of High Carbohydrate versus High Fat Diet with Glycated Hemoglobin in High Calorie Consuming Type 2 Diabetics," *Journal of Diabetes and Metabolic Disorders* 12, no. 1 (2013): 27.

16. Food and Nutrition Board, Institute of Medicine, *Dietary Reference Intakes for Energy, Carbohydrate, Fiber, Fat, Fatty Acids, Cholesterol, Protein, and Amino Acids (Macronutrients)* (Washington, DC: National Academies Press, 2005), Available at www.nap.edu/openbook.php?isbn=0309085373.

17. National Institutes of Health Office of Dietary Supplements, "Dietary Supplement Fact Sheet: Vitamin D," June 2011, http://ods.od.nih.gov/factsheets/VitaminD-HealthProfessional

18. Institute of Medicine Committee to Review Dietary Reference Intakes for Vitamin D and Calcium, *Dietary Reference Intakes for Calcium and Vitamin D,* eds. A. Ross, C. Taylor, A. Yaktine, H. Del Valle (Washington, DC: National Academies Press, 2011), Available at www.iom.edu/Reports/2010/Dietary-Reference-Intakes-for-Calcium-and-Vitamin-D.aspx

19. Ibid.

20. U.S. Department of Agriculture, *What We Eat in America*, 2010.

21. Ibid.; C. Ayala et al., "Application of Lower Sodium Intake Recommendations to Adults—United States, 1999-2006," *Morbidity and Mortality Weekly* (*MMWR*) 58, no. 11 (2009): 281-83.

22. American Heart Association, "Sodium (Salt)," February 2014, www.heart.org/HEARTORG/GettingHealthy/NutritionCenter/HealthyDietGoals/Sodium-Salt-or-Sodium-Chloride_UCM_303290_Article.jsp

23. R. L. Bailey et al., "Estimation of Total Usual Calcium and Vitamin D Intakes in the United States," *Journal of Nutrition* 140, no. 4 (2010): 817–22, doi: 10.3945/jn.109.118539

24. S. A. McNaughton et al., "An Energy-Dense, Nutrient-Poor Dietary Pattern Is Inversely Associated with Bone Health in Women," *Journal of Nutrition* 141, no. 8 (2011): 1516–23, doi: 10.3945/jn.111.138271

25. World Health Organization, "Miconutrient Deficiencies: Iron Deficiency Anemia," 2014, www.who.int/nutrition/topics/ida/en/index.html

26. U.S. Centers for Disease Control and Prevention (CDC), "Iron and Iron Deficiency," *Nutrition for Everyone*, February 23, 2011, www.cdc.gov/nutrition/everyone/basics/vitamins/iron.html

27. C. Geissler and M. Singh, "Iron, Meat, and Health," *Nutrients* 3, no. 3 (2011): 283–316, doi: 10.3390/nu3030283

28. Academy of Nutrition and Dietetics, "Position of the Academy of Nutrition and Dietetics: Functional Foods" *Journal of the Academy of Nutrition and Dietetics*, 113 (2013): 1096–1103.

29. Ibid.

30. Ibid.

31. M. E. Obrenovich, et al., "Antioxidants in Health, Disease, and Aging," *CNS & Neurological Disorders Drug Targets* 10, no. 2 (2011): 192–207; V. Ergin, R. E. Hariry, and C. Karasu, "Carbonyl Stress in Aging Process: Role of Vitamins and Phytochemicals as Redox Regulators," *Aging and Disease* 4, no. 5 (2013): 276–94, doi: 10.14336/AD.2013.0400276

32. E. A. Klein et al., "Vitamin E and the Risk of Prostate Cancer: The Selenium and Vitamin E Cancer Prevention Trial (SELECT)," *Journal of the American Medical Association* 306, no. 14 (2011): 1549–56, doi: 10.1001/jama.2011.1437

33. U.S. Department of Agriculture, Economic Research Service, "Loss-Adjusted Food Availability Documentation: Overview: Calories," November 2, 2012, www.ers.usda.gov

34. D. Grotto and E. Zied, "The Standard American Diet and Its Relationship to the Health Status of Americans," *Nutrition in Clinical Practice* 25, no. 6 (2010): 603–12, doi: 10.1177/0884533610386234

35. U.S. Department of Agriculture and U.S. Department of Health and Human Services, *Dietary Guidelines for Americans, 2010,* 7th ed. (Washington, DC: U.S. Government Printing Office, 2010), Available at www.cnpp.usda.gov/publications/dietaryguidelines/2010/policydoc/policydoc.pdf

36. Ibid.

37. Ibid.

38. U.S. Department of Agriculture, "Empty Calories: How Do I Count the Empty Calories I Eat?," June 4, 2011, www.choosemyplate.gov/foodgroups/emptycalories_count_table.html

39. U.S. Food and Drug Administration, "Nutrition Facts Label: Proposed Changes Aim to Better Inform Food Choices," February 2014, www.fda.gov/ForConsumers/ConsumerUpdates/ucm387114.htm

40. U.S. Food and Drug Administration, "Label Claims for Conventional Foods and Dietary Supplements," December 2013, www.fda.gov/Food/IngredientsPackagingLabeling/LabelingNutrition/ucm111447.htm

41. The Vegetarian Resource Group, "How Often Do Americans Eat Vegetarian Meals? And How Many Adults in the U.S. Are Vegan?" May 18, 2012, www.vrg.org/journal/vj2011issue4/vj2011issue4poll.php

42. F. Newport, "In U.S. 5% Consider Themselves Vegetarians," *Gallup*, July 26, 2012, www.gallup.com/poll/156215/Consider-Themselves-Vegetarians.aspxw

43. Y. Yokoyama et al., "Vegetarian Diets and Blood Pressure: A Meta-Analysis," *Journal of the American Medical Association Internal Medicine*, February 2014, doi:10.1001/jamainternmed.2013.14547

44. C. G. Lee et al., "Vegetarianism as a Protective Factor for Colorectal Adenoma and Advanced Adenoma in Asians," *Digestive Diseases and Science* (2013), doi: 10.1007/s10620-013-2974-5

45. Office of Dietary Supplements, "Frequently Asked Questions," July 2013, http://ods.od.nih.gov/Health_Information/ODS_Frequently_Asked_Questions.aspx#; V. A. Moyer, "Vitamin, Mineral, and Multivitamin Supplements for the Primary Prevention of Cardiovascular Disease and Cancer: U.S. Preventive Services Task Force Recommendation Statement," *Annals of Internal Medicine* 160. no. 8 (2014): 558–64, doi:10.7326/M14-0198

46. R. Chowdhury et al., "Association between Fish Consumption, Long Chain Omega 3 Fatty Acids, and Risk of Cerebrovascular Disease: Systematic Review and Meta-Analysis," *British Medical Journal* 345 (2012): e6698, www.ncbi.nlm.nih.gov/pmc/articles/PMC3484317

47. Office of Dietary Supplements, "Vitamin A Fact Sheet for Consumers," June 2013, http://ods.od.nih.gov/factsheets/VitaminA-QuickFacts/; Office of Dietary Supplements, "Vitamin E Fact Sheet for Consumers," June 2013, http://ods.odnih.gov/factsheets/list-all/VitaminE-QuickFacts/; Office of Dietary Supplements, "Vitamin D Fact Sheet for Consumers," June 2013, http://ods.od.nih.gov/factsheets/VitaminD-QuickFacts

48. Academy of Nutrition and Dietetics, "It's About Eating Right: Dietary Supplements," January 2013, www.eatright.org/public/content.aspx?id=7918

49. U.S. Department of Health and Human Services, "Food Safety Modernization Act (FSMA)," November 2013, www.fda.gov/Food/GuidanceRegulation/FSMA/ucm304065.htm

50. The Organic Trade Association, "Eight in Ten U.S. Parents Report They Purchase Organic Products," April 2013, www.ota.com/news/press-releases/17124

51. USDA Economic Research Service, "Organic Market Overview," April 7, 2014, www.ers.usda.gov/topics/natural-resources-environment/organic-agriculture/organic-market-overview.aspx

52. K. Brandt et al., "Agroecosystem Management and Nutritional Quality of Plant Foods: The Case of Organic Fruits and Vegetables," *Critical Reviews in Plant Sciences* 30, no. 1–2 (2011): 177–97; C. Smith-Spangler et al., "Are Organic Foods Safer or Healthier Than Conventional Alternatives? A Systematic Review," *Annals of Internal Medicine* 157, no. 5 (2012): 348–66, doi:10.7326/0003-4819-157-5-201209040-00009

53. U.S. Environmental Protection Agency, "Pesticides and Foods: Health Problems Pesticides May Pose," May 2012, www.epa.gov/pesticides/food/risks.htm

54. U.S. Department of Agriculture, Pesticide Data Program: 21st Annual Summary, Calendar Year 2011, Agricultural Marketing Service, February 2013, www.ams.usda.gov/AMSv1.0/getfile?dDocName=stelprdc5102692

55. CDC, "Estimates of Food-Borne Illnesses in the United States," January 2014, www.cdc.gov/foodborneburden/index.html

56. CDC, "Trends in Foodborne Illness in the United States, 2012,"April 2013, www.cdc.gov/features/dsfoodnet2012

57. CDC, "Listeria (Listeriosis)," March 16, 2015, www.cdc.gov/listeria

58. Ibid.

59. Ibid.

60. Ibid.

61. R. Johnson, "The U.S. Trade Situation for Fruit and Vegetable Products," Congressional Research Service, January 2014, www.fas.org/sgp/crs/misc/RL34468.pdf

62. S. Clark et al., "Frequency of US Emergency Department Visits for Food-related Acute Allergic Reactions," *Journal of Allergy Clinical Immunology* 127, no. 3, (2011): 682–83, doi: 10.1016/j.jaci.2010.10.040

63. National Institute of Allergy and Infectious Diseases, "Food Allergy," August 2013, www.niaid.nih.gov/topics/foodallergy/Pages/default.aspx

64. R. S. Gupta et al., "The Prevalence, Severity, and Distribution of Childhood Food Allergy in the United States," *Journal of Pediatrics* 128, no. 1 (2011): e9–e17, doi: 10.1542/peds.2011-0204

65. National Institute of Allergy and Infectious Diseases, "Food Allergy," August 2013, www.niaid.nih.gov/topics/foodallergy/Pages/default.aspx

66. U.S. Food and Drug Administration, "Food Allergies: What You Need to Know," April 2013, www.fda.gov/food/resourcesforyou/consumers/ucm079311.htm

67. A. Rubio-Tapia et al., "The Prevalence of Celiac Disease in the United States," *American Journal of Gastroenterology* 107 (2012):1 538–44

68. Panel, NIAID-Sponsored Expert, "Guidelines for the Diagnosis and Management of Food Allergy in the United States: Report of the NIAID-sponsored Expert Panel," *Journal of Allergy and Clinical Immunology* 126, no. 6 (2010): S1–S58.

69. J. N. Keith et al., "The Prevalence of Self-Reported Lactose Intolerance and the Consumption of Dairy Foods among African American Adults Less than Expected," *Journal of the National Medical Association* 103 (2011): 36–45.

70. G. Pinholster, "AAAS Board of Directors: Legally Mandating GM Food Labels Could 'Mislead and Falsely Alarm Consumers,'" American Association for the Advancement of Science News, October 2012, www.aaas.org/news/aaas-board-directors-legally-mandating-gm-food-labels-could-mislead-and-falsely-alarm; World Health Organization, "20 Questions on Genetically Modified Foods," Accessed March 2014, www.who.int/foodsafety/publications/biotech/20questions/en

Pulled Statistics:

Page 276, C. Ogden, B. Kit, M. Carroll, S. Park, "Consumption of Sugar Drinks in the United States, 2005–2008," *NCHS Data Brief*, no. 71. (Hyattsville, MD: National Center for Health Statistics, 2011), www.cdc.gov/nchs/data/databriefs/db71.htm.

Page 281, K. Heidal, S. Colby, G. Mirabella, et al., "Cost and Calorie Analysis of Fast Food Consumption in College Students," *Food and Nutrition Sciences* 3, no. 7, (2012): 942–46, doi:10.4236/fns.2012.37124

Chapter 10: Reaching and Maintaining a Healthy Weight

1. M. Ng et al., " Global, Regional, and National Prevalence of Overweight and Obesity in Children and Adults during 1980–2013: A Systematic Analysis for the Global Burden of Disease Study 2013," *Lancet* 384, no. 9945 (2014): 766–81; C. L. Ogden et al., "Prevalence of Childhood and Adult Obesity in the United States, 2011–2012," *Journal of the American Medical Association* 311, no. 8 (2014): 806–14, doi:10.1001/jama.2014.732; C. L. Ogden et al., "Prevalence of Obesity among Adults: United States, 2011-2012," *National Center for Health Statistics Data Brief* 131 (2013), www.cdc.gov/nchs/data/databriefs/db131.htm

2. Centers for Disease Control and Prevention (CDC), "Health, United States, 2013." Figure 10. Overweight and Obesity among Adults Aged 20 and Over by Sex, United States, 1988-1994, then, 2009-2012, May 2014, www.cdc.gov/nchs/data/hus/hus13.pdf

3. C. L. Ogden et al., "Prevalence of Obesity among Adults: United States, 2011–2012," *NCHS Data Brief* no 131 (Hyattsville, MD: National Center for Health Statistics, 2013).

4. D. Mozaffarian et al., "Heart Disease and Stroke Statistics—2015 Update: A Report From the American Heart Association," *Circulation* 131, no . 4 (2015): 434–41.

5. Ibid.

6. Ibid.

7. Ibid.

8. Ibid.

9. World Health Organization (WHO), "Obesity and Overweight Fact Sheet," January 2015, www.who.int/mediacentre/factsheets/fs311/en

10. Ibid.; International Obesity Taskforce, "Obesity–The Global Epidemic," 2014, www.iaso .org/iotf/obesity/obesitytheglobalepidemic; M. Ng et al., "Global, Regional, and National Prevalence of Overweight and Obesity in Children and Adults, 2014.

11. K. M. Flegal et al., "Association of All-Cause Mortality with Overweight and Obesity Using Standard Body Mass Index Categories: A Systematic Review and Meta-Analysis," *Journal of the American Medical Association* 309, no. 1 (2013): 71–82.

12. American Heart Association, "With a Very Heavy Heart: Obesity and Cardiovascular Disease," February 2014, www.heart.org/idc/groups/heart-public/@wcm/@adv/documents/downloadable/ucm_461353.pdf

13. American Diabetes Association, "Statistics about Diabetes and Pre-diabetes," February 19, 2015, www.diabetes.org/diabetes-basics/statistics

14. C. L. Himes and S. L. Reynolds. "Effect of Obesity on Falls, Injury, and Disability," *Journal of the American Geriatrics Society* 60, no. 1 (2012): 124–29; L. A. Schaap, A. Koster, and M. Visser, "Adiposity, Muscle Mass, and Muscle Strength in Relation to Functional Decline in Older Persons," *Epidemiologic Reviews* 35, no. 1 (2013): 1.

15. D. Spruijt-Metz, "Etiology, Treatment, and Prevention of Obesity in Childhood and Adolescence: A Decade in Review," *Journal of Research on Adolescence* 21 (2011): 129–52, doi: 10.1111/j.1532-7795.2010.00719.x; S. A. Affenito et al., "Behavioral Determinants of Obesity: Research Findings and Policy Implications," *Journal of Obesity* 2012 (2012), www.hindawi .com/journals/jobes/2012/150732

16. K. Silventoinen et al., "The Genetic and Environmental Influences on Childhood Obesity: A Systematic Review of Twin and Adoption Studies," *International Journal of Obesity* 34, no. 1 (2010): 29–40; D. Cummings and M. Schwartz, "Genetics and Pathophysiology of Human Obesity," *Annual Review of Medicine* 54 (2003): 453–71.

17. T. Tanaka, J. S. Ngwa, and F. J. van Rooij, "Genome-Wide Meta-Analysis of Observational Studies Shows Common Genetic Variants Associated with Macronutrient Intake," *American Journal of Clinical Nutrition* 97, no. 6 (2013): 1395–402; M. M. Hetherington and J. E. Cecil, "Gene-Environment Interactions in Obesity," *Forum Nutrition* 63 (2010): 195–203; M. Graff, J. S. Ngwa, and T. Workalemahu, "Genome-Wide Analysis of BMI in Adolescents and Young Adults Reveals Additional Insights into the Effects of the Genetic Loci over the Life Course," *Human Molecular Genetics* 22, no. 17 (2013): 3597–607.

18. D. Withers, et al., "A Link between FTO, Ghrelin and Impaired Brain Food-cue Responsivity," *The Journal of Clinical Investigation* 123, no. 8 (2013): 3339–351, doi: 10.1172/JC144403

19. M. Graff, J. S. Ngwa and T. Workalemahu, "Genome-Wide Analysis of BMI in Adolescents and Young Adults Reveals Additional Insights," 2013.

20. T. O. Kilpelainen et al., "Physical Activity Attenuates the Influence of *FTO* Variants on Obesity Risk: A Meta-Analysis of 218,166 Adults and 19,268 Children," *PLoS Medicine* 8, no.11 (2012): e1001116, doi:10.1371/journal.pmed.1001116; A. S. Richardson et al., "Moderate to Vigorous Physical Activity Interactions with Genetic Variants and Body Mass Index in a Large US Ethnically Diverse Cohort," *Pediatric Obesity* 9, no. 2 (2013): e35–46, doi: 10.1111/j.2047-6310.2013.00152

21. J. C. Wells, "The Evolution of Human Adiposity and Obesity: Where Did It All Go Wrong?," *Disease Models and Mechanisms* 5, no. 5 (2012): 595–607, doi:10.1242/dmm.009613; J. R. Speakman et al., " Evolutionary Perspectives on the Obesity Epidemic: Adaptive, Maladaptive, and Neutral Viewpoints," *Annual Review of Nutrition* 33 (2013): 289–317.

22. A. Tremblay et al., "Adaptive Thermogenesis Can Make a Difference in the Ability of Obese Individuals to Lose Body Weight," *International Journal of Obesity* 37 (2013): 759–64.

23. J. Buss et al., "Associations of Ghrelin with Eating Behaviors, Stress, Metabolic Factors, and Telomere Length among Overweight and Obese Women: Preliminary Evidence of Attenuated Ghrelin Effects in Obesity," *Appetite* 76, no. 1 (2014): 84–94; B. Biondi, "Thyroid and Obesity: An Intriguing Relationship," *Journal of Clinical Endocrinology and Metabolism* 95, no. 8 (2010): 3614–17; T. Reinehr, "Obesity and Thyroid Function," *Molecular and Cellular Endocrinology* 316, no. 2 (2010): 165–71.

24. D. E. Cummings et al., "Plasma Ghrelin Levels After Diet-Induced Weight Loss or Gastric Bypass Surgery," *New England Journal of Medicine* 346, no. 21 (2002): 1623–30.

25. M. Khatib et al., "Effect of Ghrelin on Regulation of Growth Hormone Release: A Review," *The Health Agenda* 2, no. 1 (2014), Available at www .healthagenda.net/wp-content/uploads/2013/11/Effect-of-ghrelin-on-regulation-of-growth-hormone-release-A-review.pdf; C. DeVriese et al., "Focus on the Short- and Long-Term Effects of Ghrelin on Energy Homeostasis," *Nutrition* 26, no. 6 (2010): 579–84; T. Castaneda et al., "Ghrelin in the Regulation of Body Weight and Metabolism," *Frontiers in Neuroendocrinology* 31, no. 1 (2010): 44–60.

26. P. Marzullo et al. "Investigations of Thyroid Hormones and Antibodies in Obesity: Leptin Levels Are Associated with Thyroid Autoimmunity Independent of Bioanthropometric, Hormonal and Weight-Related Determinants," *The Journal of Clinical Endocrinology and Metabolism* 95, no. 8 (2010): 3965–72; H. Feng et al., "Review: The Role of Leptin in Obesity and the Potential for Leptin Replacement Therapy," *Endocrine* 44 (2013): 33–39.

27. L. K. Mahan and S. Escott-Stump, *Krause's Food, Nutrition, and Diet Therapy,* 13th ed. (New York: W. B. Saunders, 2012).

28. USDA Economic Research Service, "Food Availability (per capita) Data System," March 2014, www.ers.usda.gov/data-products/food-availability

29. E. Ford and W. Dietz, "Trends in Energy Intake among Adults in the United States: Findings from NHANES," *American Journal of Clinical Nutrition*, April 2013, http://bit.ly/XUJ7Dq

30. Centers for Disease Control and Prevention, "Facts about Physical Activity," May 2014, http://www.cdc.gov/physicalactivity/data/facts.htm

31. M. Wang, L. Pbert, and S. Lemon, "Influence of Family, Friend and Co-worker Social Support and Social Undermining on Weight Gain Prevention among Adults," *Obesity* 22, no. 9 (2014): 1973–80; T. Lehey, J. LaRose, J. Fave, and R. Wing, "Social Influences Are Associated with BMI and Weight Loss Intentions in Young Adults," *Obesity* 19, no. 6 (2011): 1157–62.

32. C. Gillespie et al., "The Growing Concern of Poverty in the United States: An Exploration of Food Prices and Poverty on Obesity Rates for Low-Income Citizens," *Undergraduate Economic Review* 8, no. 1 (2012): 1–38.

33. J. F. Sallis et al., "Role of Built Environments in Physical Activity, Obesity and Cardiovascular Disease," *Circulation* 125, no. 5 (2012): 729–37; J. Kolodziejczyk et al., "Influence of Specific Individual and Environmental Variables on the Relationship between Body Mass Index and Health-related Quality of Life in Overweight and Obese Adolescents," *Quality of Life Research* 24, no. 1 (2015): 251–61.

34. CDC, "About BMI for Adults," February 2015, www.cdc.gov/healthyweight/assessing/bmi/adult_bmi/index.html

35. J. I. Mechanick et al., "Clinical Practice Guidelines for the Perioperative Nutritional, Metabolic and Nonsurgical Support of the Bariatric Surgery Patient—2013 Update," *Endocrine Practice* 19, no. 2 (2013): e1–36, www.aace.com/files/publish-ahead-of-print-final-version.pdf

36. C. L. Ogden, M. D. Carroll, B. K. Kit, K. M. Flegal, "Prevalence of childhood and adult obesity in the United States, 2011–2012," *JAMA*, 2014, 311(8):806–814

37. American Heart Association, "Body Composition Tests," April 2013, www.heart.org/HEARTORG/GettingHealthy/NutritionCenter/Body-Composition-Tests_UCM_305883_Article.jsp; S. J. Mooney, A. Baecker, and A. G. Rundel, "Comparison of Anthropometric and Body Composition Measures as Predictors of Components of the Metabolic Syndrome in the Clinical Setting," *Obesity Research and Clinical Practice* 7, no. 1 (2013): e55–e66.

38. C. L. Ogden et al., "Prevalence of Childhood and Adult Obesity in the United States," 2014; National Center for Health Statistics, "Health, United States, 2011: With Special Features on Socioeconomic Status and Health," Hyattsville, MD; U.S. Department of Health and Human Services, 2012, Available at www.cdc.gov/nchs/data/hus/hus11.pdf

39. R. Puhl, "Weight Stigmatization toward Youth: A Significant Problem in Need of Societal Solutions," *Childhood Obesity* 7, no. 5 (2011): 359–63; S. A. Mustillo, K. Budd, and K. Hendrix, "Obesity, Labeling, and Psychological Distress in Late-Childhood and Adolescent Black and White Girls: The Distal Effects of Stigma," *Social Psychology Quarterly* 76, no. 3 (2013): 268–89.

40. L. Goh et al., "Anthropometric Measurements of General and Central Obesity and the Prediction of Cardiovascular Disease Risk in Women: A Cross-sectional Study," BMJ Open 4, (2014): e004138, doi:10.1136/bmjopen-2013-004138; M. Bombelli et al., "Impact of Body Mass Index and Waist Circumference on the Long Term Risk of Diabetes Mellitus, Hypertension and Cardiac Organ Damage," *Hypertension* 58, no. 6 (2011): 1029–35; S. Czernichow et al., "Body Mass Index, Waist Circumference and Waist-Hip Ratio: Which is the Better Discriminator of Cardiovascular Disease Mortality Risk? Evidence from an Individual-Participant Meta-Analysis of 82,864 Participants from Nine Cohort Studies," *Obesity Reviews* 12, no. 9 (2011): 1467–78.

41. National Heart, Lung, and Blood Institute, "Classification of Overweight and Obesity by BMI, Waist Circumference and Associated Disease Risks," 2012, www.nhlbi.nih.gov/health/public/heart/obesity/lose_wt/bmi_dis.htm

42. University of Maryland Medical Center, Rush University, "Waist to Hip Ratio Calculator," March 2014, www.healthcalculators.org/calculators/waist_hip.asp

43. P. Brambilla et al., "Waist Circumference-to-Height Ratio Predicts Adiposity Better than Body Mass Index in Children and Adolescents," *International Journal of Obesity* 37, no. 7 (2013): 943–46.

44. L. Gray, N. Cooper, A. Dunkley et al., "A Systematic Review and Mixed Treatment Comparison of Pharmacological Interventions for the Treatment of Obesity," *Obesity Reviews* 13, no. 6 (2012): 483–98.

45. ConsumerSearch, "Diet Pills: Reviews," 2012, www.consumersearch.com/diet-pills

46. U.S. Food and Drug Administration, "Fen-Phen Safety Update Information," December 2014, www.fda.gov

47. C. E. Weber et al., "Obesity and Trends in Malpractice Claims for Physicians and Surgeons," *Surgery* 154, no. 2 (2013): 299–304.

48. Mayo Clinic, "Gastric Bypass Surgery," April 7, 2014, www.mayoclinic.com/health/gastric-bypass/MY00825

49. John's Hopkins Health Library, "BPD/DS Weight-Loss Surgery," March 2014, www.hopkinsmedicine.org/healthlibrary/test_procedures/gastroenterology/bpdds_weight-loss_surgery_135,64

50. F. Rubino et al., "Metabolic Surgery to Treat Type 2 Diabetes: Clinical Outcomes and Mechanisms of Action," *Annual Review of Medicine* 61 (2010): 393–411; S. Brethauer et al., "Can Diabetes Be Surgically Cured? Long-Term Metabolic Effects of Bariatric Surgery in Obese Patients with Type 2 Diabetes Mellitus," *Annals of Surgery* 258, no. 4 (2013): 628–37.

Pulled Statistics:

Page 298, C. D. Fryar and R. B. Ervin, "Caloric Intake from Fast Food among Adults: United States, 2007–2010," *NCHS Data Brief*, No. 114. (2013), www.cdc.gov

Page 308, Centers for Disease Control and Prevention, "Adult Obesity Facts: Obesity Affects Some Groups More than Others," September 2014, www.cdc.gov/obesity/data/adult.html

Focus On: Enhancing Your Body Image

1. University of the West of England, "30% of Women Would Trade at Least One Year of Their Life to Achieve Their Ideal Body Weight and Shape," March 2011, http://info.uwe.ac.uk/news/UWENews/news.aspx?id=1949

2. M. Bucchianeri et al., "Body Dissatisfaction from Adolescence to Young Adulthood: Findings from a 10-year Longitudinal Study," *Body Image* 10, no. 1 (2013): 1–7.

3. University of Minnesota Health Talk, "Social Media May Inspire Unhealthy Body Image," May 2013, www.healthtalk.umn.edu/2013/05/15/thigh-gap-and-social-media

4. Ibid.

5. Centers for Disease Control and Prevention, "FASTSTATS: Obesity and Overweight," April 29, 2015, www.cdc.gov/nchs/fastats/obesity-overweight.htm

6. J. B. Webb et al., "Do You See What I See?: An Exploration of Inter-Ethnic Ideal Body Size Comparisons among College Women," *Body Image* 10, no. 3 (2013): 369–79.

7. V. Swami et al., "The Attractive Female Body Weight and Female Body Dissatisfaction in 26 Countries across 10 World Regions: Results of the International Body Project I," *Personality and Social Psychology Bulletin* 36, no. 3 (2010): 309–25.

8. Mayo Clinic Staff, "Body Dysmorphic Disorder," May 2013, www.mayoclinic.com/health/body-dysmorphic-disorder/DS00559

9. J. D. Feusner et al., "Abnormalities of Object Visual Processing in Body Dysmorphic Disorder," *Psychological Medicine* 41, no. 11 (2011): 2385–97, doi: 10.1017/S0033291711000572

10. Body Image Health, "The Model for Healthy Body Image and Weight," March 2014, http://bodyimagehealth.org/model-for-healthy-body-image

11. I. Ahmed et al., "Body Dysmorphic Disorder," *Medscape Reference*, January 2014, http://emedicine.medscape.com/article/291182-overview

12. Mayo Clinic Staff, "Body Dysmorphic Disorder," 2013; KidsHealth, "Body Dysmorphic Disorder," May 2013, http://kidshealth.org/parent/emotions/feelings/bdd.html

13. I. Ahmed et al., "Body Dysmorphic Disorder," 2014.

14. J. Reel, *Eating Disorders: An Encyclopedia of Causes, Treatment and Prevention*, (New York: Greenwood Publishing, 2013); A. Taheri et al., "The Relationship between Social Physique Anxiety and Anthropometric Characteristics of the Non-athletic Female Students," *Annals of Biological Research* 3, no. 6 (2012): 2727–29; A. Sicilia et al., "Exercise Motivation and Social Physique Anxiety in Adolescents," *Psychologica Belgica* 54, no. 1 (2014): 111–29, doi: http://dx.doi.org/10.5334/pb.ai

15. American Psychiatric Association, *Diagnostic and Statistical Manual of Mental Disorders*, 5th ed. (Washington, DC: American Psychiatric Association, 2013).

16. National Eating Disorders Association, "Get the Facts on Eating Disorders," May 2015, www.nationaleatingdisorders.org/get-facts-eating-disorders

17. D. A. Gagne et al., "Eating Disorder Symptoms and Weight and Shape Concerns in a Large Web-Based Convenience Sample of Women Ages 50 and Above: Results of the Gender and Body Image (GABI) Study," *International Journal of Eating Disorders* 45, no. 7 (2012): 832–44, doi: 10.1002/eat.22030

18. American College Health Association, *National College Health Assessment II: Undergraduates Reference Group Executive Summary Spring 2014* (Hanover, MD: American College Health Association, 2014), Available at www.acha-ncha.org/reports_ACHA-NCHAII.html

19. L. M. Gottschlich, "Female Athlete Triad," *Medscape Reference, Drugs, Diseases & Procedures*, January 25, 2012, http://emedicine.medscape.com/article/89260-overview#a0156

20. Alliance for Eating Disorder Awareness, "What Are Eating Disorders?," 2013, www.allianceforeatingdisorders.com/portal/what-are-eating-disorders#.Uycs4_Pn9lY

21. Ibid.

22. National Eating Disorders Association, "Anorexia Nervosa," April 2014, www.nationaleatingdisorders.org/anorexia-nervosa

23. S. A. Swanson et al., "Prevalence and Correlates of Eating Disorders in Adolescents: Results from the National Comorbidity Survey Replication Adolescent Supplement," *Archives of General Psychiatry* 68, no. 7 (2011): 714–23, doi: 10.1001/archgenpsychiatry.2011.22

24. P. Crocker et al., "Body-Related State Shame and Guilt in Women: Do Causal Attributions Mediate the Influence of Physical Self-concept and Shame and Guilt Proneness," *Body Image* 11, no. 1 (2013): 19–26; A. R. Smith, T. E. Joiner, and D. R. Dodd, "Examining Implicit Attitudes toward Emaciation and Thinness in Anorexia Nervosa," *International Journal of Eating Disorders* 47, no. 2 (2013): 138–47; R. N. Carey, N. Donaghue, and P. Broderick, "Concern among Australian Adolescent Girls: The Role of Body Comparisons with Models and Peers," *Body Image* 11, no. 1 (2014): 81–84.

25. A.D.A.M. Medical Encyclopedia, U.S. National Library of Medicine, "Anorexia Nervosa," February 13, 2012, www.ncbi.nlm.nih.gov; B. Suchan et al., "Reduced Connectivity between the Left Fusiform Body Area and the Extrastriate Body Area in Anorexia Nervosa Is Associated with Body Image Distortion," *Behavioural Brain Research* 241 (2013): 80–85, doi: 10.1016/j.bbr.2012.12.002; G. Frank et al., "Anorexia Nervosa and Obesity Are Associated with Opposite Brain Reward Response," *Neuropsychopharmacology* 37, no. 9 (2012): 2031–46, doi: 10.1038/npp.2012.51

26. R. Kessler et al., "The Prevalence and Correlates of Binge Eating Disorder in the World Health Organization World Mental Health Surveys," *Biological Psychiatry* 73, no. 9 (2013): 904–14, doi: 10.1016/j.biopsych.2012.11.020

27. National Institute of Mental Health, "Eating Disorders," January 2013, www.nimh.nih.gov/health/topics/eating-disorders/index.shtml

28. T. A. Oberndorfer et al., "Altered Insula Response to Sweet Taste Processing After Recovery from Anorexia and Bulimia Nervosa," American Journal of Psychiatry 170, no. 10 (2013): 1143–51.

29. Mayo Clinic, "Binge-Eating Disorder," April 2012, www.mayoclinic.com/health/binge-eating-disorder/DS00608

30. R. Kessler et al., "The Prevalence and Correlates of Binge Eating Disorder," 2013.

31. National Eating Disorder Association, "Other Specified Feeding or Eating Disorder," March 2014, www.nationaleatingdisorders.org/other-specified-feeding-or-eating-disorder

32. K. N. Franco, Cleveland Clinic Center for Continuing Education, "Eating Disorders," 2011, www.clevelandclinicmeded.com/medicalpubs/diseasemanagement/psychiatry-psychology/

eating-disorders; Mirasol Eating Disorder Recovery Centers, "Eating Disorder Statistics," March 2014, www.mirasol.net/eating-disorders/information/eating-disorder-statistics.php

33. M. Smith, L. Robinson, and J. Segal, "Helping Someone with an Eating Disorder," *Helpguide.org*, February 2014, www.helpguide.org/mental/eating_disorder_self_help.htm; C. Biggs, "On the Outside: Helping a Friend through an Eating Disorder," *Act: Every Action Counts*, February 28, 2013, http://act.mtv.com/posts/neda-week-helping-a-friend-through-an-eating-disorder

34. National Eating Disorder Association, "Find Help and Support," March 2014, www.nationaleating-disorders.org/find-help-support

35. H. Goodwin, E. Haycraft, and C. Meyer, "The Relationship between Compulsive Exercise and Emotion Regulation in Adolescents," *British Journal of Health Psychology* 17, no. 4 (2012): 699–710.

36. J. J. Waldron, "When Building Muscle Turns into Muscle Dysmorphia," Association for Sport Applied Psychology, March 2014, www.appliedsportpsych.org/resource-center/health-fitness-resources/when-building-muscle-turns-into-muscle-dysmorphia

37. M. Silverman, "What is Muscle Dysmorphia?" Massachusetts General Hospital, February 18, 2011, https://mghocd.org/what-is-muscle-dysmorphia; J. J. Waldron, "When Building Muscle Turns into Muscle Dysmorphia," 2014.

38. L. M. Gottschlich et al., "Female Athlete Triad," 2014.

Pulled Statistics:

Page 318, C. Ross, "Why Do Women Hate Their Bodies?" World of Psychology, Blog, Psych Central, June 2, 2012, http://psychcentral.com/blog/archives/2012/06/02/why-dowomen-hate-their-bodies

Chapter 11: Improving Your Personal Fitness

1. Centers for Disease Control and Prevention (CDC), "Behavioral Risk Factor Surveillance System Prevalence and Trends Data," March 2014, http://apps.nccd.cdc.gov/BRFSS/display .asp?yr=2012&state=US&qkey=8041&grp=0&SUBMIT3=Go

2. Ibid.

3. Ibid.

4. C. E. Garber et al., "American College of Sports Medicine Position Stand: Quantity and Quality of Exercise for Developing and Maintaining Cardiorespiratory, Musculoskeletal and Neuromotor Fitness in Apparently Healthy Adults: Guidance for Prescribing Exercise," *Medicine and Science in Sports and Exercise* 33, no. 7 (2011): 1334–59, doi:10.1249/MSS.0b013e318213fefb

5. American College Health Association, *American College Health Association-National College Health Assessment II (ACHA-NCHA II): Reference Group Executive Summary, Spring 2014* (Hanover, MD: American College Health Association, 2014), Available at www.acha-ncha.org/docs/ACHA-NCHAII_ReferenceGroup_ExecutiveSummary_Spring2014.pdf

6. Lee et al., "Impact of Physical Inactivity on the World's Major Non-communicable Diseases," *Lancet* 380, no. 9838 (2012): 219–29.

7. S. Plowman and D. Smith, *Exercise Physiology for Health, Fitness, and Performance*, 3rd ed. (Philadelphia, PA: Lippincott Williams & Wilkins, 2011).

8. 8S. Grover et al., "Estimating the Benefits of Patient and Physician Adherence to Cardiovascular Prevention Guidelines: The MyHealth-Checkup Survey," *Canadian Journal of Cardiology* 27, no. 2 (2011): 159–66, doi: 10.1016/j.cjca.2011.01.007

9. American Heart Association, "About Cholesterol," Updated July 31, 2014, www.heart.org

10. L. Montesi et al., "Physical Activity for the Prevention and Treatment of Metabolic Disorders," *Internal and Emergency Medicine* 8, no. 8 (2013): 655–66.

11. Ibid.

12. D. C. Lee et al., "Changes in Fitness and Fatness on the Development of Cardiovascular Disease Risk Factors Hypertension, Metabolic Syndrome, and Hypercholesterolemia," *Journal of the American College of Cardiology* 59, no. 7 (2012): 665–72, doi: 10.1016/j.jacc.2011.11.013

13. M. Uusitupa, J. Tuomilehto, and P. Puska, "Are We Really Active in the Prevention of Obesity and Type 2 Diabetes at the Community Level?," *Nutrition and Metabolism in Cardiovascular Diseases* 21, no. 5 (2011): 380–89, doi: 10.1016/j.numecd.2010.12.007

14. National Diabetes Information Clearinghouse, U.S. Department of Health and Human Services, *Diabetes Prevention Program (DPP)*, (Bethesda, MD: National Diabetes Information Clearinghouse, 2008), NIH Publication no. 09–5099, Available at http://diabetes.niddk.nih.gov

15. J. Erdrich, X. Zhang, E. Giovannucci, and W. Willet, "Proportion of Colon Cancer Attributable to Lifestyle in a Cohort of US Women," *Cancer, Causes & Control* (2015), doi: 10.1007/s10552-015-0619-z (Epub ahead of print); M. Harvie, A. Howell, and D. Evans, "Can Diet and Lifestyle Prevent Breast Cancer: What is the Evidence?" *ASCO Educational Book* 35, (2015): e66–73, doi: 10.14694/EdBook_AM.2015.35.e66

16. World Cancer Research Fund/American Institute for Cancer Research, *Policy and Action for Cancer Prevention. Food, Nutrition, and Physical Activity: A Global Perspective* (Washington, DC: American Institute for Cancer Research, 2009), Available at www.dietandcancerreport.org

17. Ibid.; F. Canches-Gomas et al., "Physical Inactivity and Low Fitness Deserve More Attention to Alter Cancer Risk and Prognosis," *Cancer Prevention Research* 8 (2015): 105–110; D. Schmid and M. Leitzman, "Association between Physical Activity and Mortality among Breast Cancer and Colorectal Cancer Survivors: A Systematic Review and Meta-analysis," *Annals of Oncology* 25, no. 7 (2014): 1293–1311, doi: 10.1093/annonc/mdu012; D. Brenner et al., "Physical Activity After Breast Cancer: Effect on Survival and Patient-reported Outcomes," *Current Breast Cancer Reports* 6 (2014): 193–204.

18. C. Denlinger, et al. "Survivorship: Health Lifestyles," *Journal of National Comprehensive Cancer Network* 12, no. 9 (2014): 122–27; D. Brenner et al. "Physical Activity After Breast Cancer," 2014.

19. M. Nilsson et al., "Increased Physical Activity Is Associated with Enhanced Development of Peak Bone Mass in Men: A Five Year Longitudinal Study," *Journal of Bone and Mineral Research* 27, no. 5 (2012): 1206–14, doi: 10.1002/jbmr.1549; M. Callréus et al., "Self-Reported Recreational Exercise Combining Regularity and Impact Is Necessary to Maximize Bone Mineral Density in Young Adult Women: A Population-Based Study of 1,061 Women 25 Years of Age," *Osteoporosis International* 23, no. 10 (2012): 2517–26, doi: 10.1007/s00198-011-1886-5

20. R. Rizzoli, C. A. Abraham, and M. L. Brandi, "Nutrition and Bone Health: Turning Knowledge and Beliefs in Healthy Behavior," *Current Medical Research & Opinion* 30, no. 1 (2014): 131–41.

21. V. A. Catenacci et al., "Physical Activity Patterns Using Accelerometry in the National Weight Control Registry," *Obesity* 19, no. 6 (2011): 1163–70, doi: 10.1038/oby.2010.264

22. T. L. Gillum et al., "A Review of Sex Differences in Immune Function After Aerobic Exercise," *Exercise Immunology Review* 17 (2011): 104–20.

23. MedLine Plus, National Institutes of Health, "Exercise and Immunity," Updated May 15, 2012, www.nlm.nih.gov

24. N. P. Walsh et al., "Position Statement. Part Two: Maintaining Immune Health," *Exercise and Immunology Review* 17 (2011): 64–103.

25. M. W. Kakanis et al., "The Open Window of Susceptibility to Infection After Acute Exercise in Healthy Young Male Elite Athletes," *Exercise Immunology Review* 16 (2010): 119–37.

26. C. Huang et al., "Cardiovascular Reactivity, Stress, and Physical Activity," *Frontiers in Physiology* 4 (2013): 1–13, doi:10.3389/fphys.201300314

27. S. Covell et al. "Physical Activity Level and Future Risks of Mild Cognitive Impairment or Dementia: A Critically Appraised Topic," *Neurologist* 19, no. 3 (2015): 89–91; T. M. Burkhalter and C. H. Hillman, "A Narrative Review of Physical Activity, Nutrition, and Obesity to Cognitive and Scholastic Performance across the Human Lifespan," *Advances in Nutrition: An International Review Journal* 2, no. 2 (2011): 201S –206S; C. Hogan, "Exercise Holds Immediate Benefits for Affect and Cognition in Younger and Older Adults," *Psychology of Aging* 28, no. 2 (2013): 587–94.

28. M. Daly, D. McMinn, and J. Allan, "A Bidirectional Relationship between Physical Activity and Executive Function in Older Adults," *Frontiers in Human Neuroscience* 8 (2014): 1–9.

29. J. Hu et al., "Exercise Improves Cognitive Function in Aging Patients," *International Journal of Clinical and Experimental Medicine* 7, no. 10 (2014): 3144–49.

30. M. Beckett et al., "A Meta-analysis of Prospective Studies in the Role of Physical Activity and the Prevention of Alzheimer's Disease in Older Adults," *BMC Geriatrics* 15, no. 9 (2015), doi:10.10.1186/s12877-015-0007-2

31. J. Woodcock, O. Franco, N. Orsini, and I. Roberts, "Non-Vigorous Physical Activity and All-Cause Mortality: Systematic Review and Meta-Analysis of Cohort Studies," *International Journal of Epidemiology* 40, no. 1 (2011): 121–38.

32. J. Berry et al., "Lifetime Risks for Cardiovascular Disease Mortality by Cardiorespiratory Fitness Levels Measured at Ages 45, 55, and 65 Years in Men: The Cooper Center Longitudinal Study," *Journal of the American College of Cardiology* 57, no. 15 (2011): 1604–10, doi: 10.1016/j.jacc.2010.10.056

33. D. Dunlop et al., "Sedentary Time in US Older Adults Associated with Disability in Activities of Daily Living Independent of Physical Activity," *Journal of Physical Activity and Health* 12, no. 1(2015): 93–101.

34. American College of Sports Medicine, *ACSM's Guidelines for Exercise Testing and Prescription*, 9th ed. (Baltimore, MD: Lippincott Williams & Wilkins, 2014).

35. C. E. Garber et al., "American College of Sports Medicine Position Stand: Quantity and Quality of Exercise for Developing and Maintaining Cardiorespiratory, Musculoskeletal and Neuromotor Fitness in Apparently Healthy Adults: Guidance for Prescribing Exercise," *Medicine and Science in Sports and Exercise* 43, no. 7 (2011): 1334–59.

36. Ibid.

37. Ibid.

38. American College of Sports Medicine, *ACSM's Resource Manual for Guidelines for Exercise Testing and Prescription* (Philadelphia, PA: Lippincott Williams & Wilkins, 2014).

39. W. Micheo, L. Baerga, and G. Miranda, "Basic Principles Regarding Strength, Flexibility, Flexibility, and Stability Exercises," *Physical Medicine & Rehabilitation* 4, no. 11 (2012): 805–11, doi: 10.1016/j.pmrj.2012.09.583

40. Ibid.

41. M. Pahor et al., "Effect of Structured Physical Activity on Prevention of Major Mobility Disability in Older Adults: The LIFE Study Randomized Clinical Trial," *JAMA* 311, no. 23 (2014): 2387–96, doi:10.1001/jama.2014.5616

42. American College of Sports Medicine, *Guidelines for Exercise Testing and Prescription*, 2014.

43. Ibid.

44. D. G. Behm and A. Chaouachi, "A Review of the Acute Effects of Static and Dynamic Stretching on Performance," *European Journal of Applied Physiology* 111, no. 11 (2011): 2633–51, doi: 10.1007/s00421-011-1879-2

45. K. C. Huxel Bliven and B. E. Anderson, "Core Stability Training for Injury Prevention," *Sports Health: A Multidisciplinary Approach* 5, no.6 (2013): 514–22.

46. Ibid.

47. D. G. Behm and J. C. Colao Sanchez, "Instability Resistance Training Across the Exercise Continuum," *Sports Health: A Multidisciplinary Approach* 5, no. 6 (2013): 500–3.

48. Ibid.

49. M. N. Sawka et al., "American College of Sports Medicine Position Stand: Exercise and Fluid Replacement," *Medicine and Science in Sports and Exercise* 39, no. 2 (2007): 377–90.

50. Ibid.

51. K. Pritchett and R. Pritchett, "Chocolate Milk: Post-Exercise Recovery Beverage for Endurance Sports," *Medicine and Sports Science* 59 (2011): 127–34.

52. K. B. Fields et al., "Prevention of Running Injuries," *Current Sports Medicine Reports* 9, no. 3 (2010): 176–82, doi: 10.1249/JSR.0b013e3181de7ec5

53. American Academy of Ophthalmology, "Eye Health in Sports and Recreation," March 2014, www.aao.org/eyesmart/injuries/eyewear.cfm

54. Ibid.

55. Bicycle Helmet Safety Institute, "Helmet-Related Statistics from Many Sources," January 2014, www.helmets.org/stats.htm

56. American College Health Association, *National College Health Assessment II: Reference Group Data Report, Spring 2013*, 2013.

57. Bicycle Helmet Safety Institute, "Helmet-Related Statistics from Many Sources," 2014.

58. N. G. Nelson et al., "Exertional Heat-Related Injuries Treated in Emergency Departments in the U.S., 1997–2006," *American Journal of Preventive Medicine* 40, no. 1 (2011): 54–60, doi: 10.1016/j.amepre.2010.09.031

59. E. E. Turk, "Hypothermia," *Forensic Science Medical Pathology* 6, no. 2 (2010): 106–115, doi: 10.1007/s12024-010-9142-4

60. Ibid.

61. American Council on Exercise, "Exercising in the Cold," Fit Facts, Blog, 2010, www.acefitness.org

Pulled Statistics:

Page 330, Centers for Disease Control and Prevention–Division of Nutrition, Physical Activity and Obesity, "How Much Physical Activity Do Adults Need?" *Physical Activity for Everyone*, June 2015, www.cdc.gov/physicalactivity/basics/adults/index.htm

Page 334, Centers for Disease Control and Prevention (CDC), "Nutrition, Physical Activity and Obesity: Data, Trends, and Maps," June 30, 2015, www.cdc.gov/nccdphp/DNPAO/index.html

Chapter 12: Reducing Your Risk of Cardiovascular Disease and Cancer

1. M. Naghavi et al., "Global, Regional, and National Age–Sex Specific All-Cause and Cause-Specific Mortality for 240 Causes of Death, 1990–2013: A Systematic Analysis for the Global Burden of Disease Study 2013," *The Lancet* 117, no. 171 (2015): 385.

2. Ibid.

3. World Health Organization, "10 Facts on the State of Global Health," April 2015, www.who.int/features/factfiles/global_burden/facts/en/index3.html

4. American Cancer Society, *Cancer Facts and Figures 2015* (Atlanta, GA: American Cancer Society, 2015), Available at www.cancer.org/acs/groups/content/@editorial/documents/document/acspc-044552.pdf

5. Ibid.

6. Ibid.

7. D. Mozaffarian et al., "Heart Disease and Stroke Statistics, 2015 Update," *Circulation* 131 (2015): e29–2322.

8. Ibid.

9. Ibid.

10. Ibid.

11. Ibid.

12. Ibid.

13. Ibid.

14. American Heart Association, "Cardiovascular Health," April 2015, www.heart.org/idc/groups/heart-public/@wcm/@sop/@smd/documents/downloadable/ucm_462014.pdf; D. M. Lloyd-Jones et al., "Defining and Setting National Goals for Cardiovascular Health Promotion and Disease Reduction: The AHA's Strategic Impact Goal through 2020 and Beyond," *Circulation* 121 (2010): e14–e31.

15. American Heart Association, "Cardiovascular Health," 2015; D. Mozaffarian et al., "Heart Disease and Stroke Statistics," 2015.

16. D. Mozaffarian et al., "Heart Disease and Stroke Statistics," 2015.

17. H. Ning et al., "Status of Cardiovascular Health in US Children Up to 11 Years of Age. The National Health and Nutrition Examination Surveys 2003–2010." *Circulation: Cardiovascular Quality and Outcomes* 8, no. 2 (2015): 164–171, doi: 10.1161/CIRCOUTCOMES.114.001274); L. Hayman and S. Camhi. "Ideal Cardiovascular Health in Adolescence is Associated with Reduced Risks of Hypertension, Metabolic Syndrome and High Cholesterol," *Evidence Based Nursing* 16, no. 1 (2013): 24–5, doi:10.1136/eb-2012-100887

18. American Heart Association, "Why Blood Pressure Matters," August 2014, www.heart.org/HEARTORG/Conditions/HighBloodPressure/WhyBloodPressureMatters/Why-Blood-Pressure-Matters_UCM_002051_Article.jsp

19. D. Mozaffarian et al., "Heart Disease and Stroke Statistics," 2015.

20. Ibid.

21. Ibid.

22. Ibid.

23. L. Rutten-Jacobs et al., "Cardiovascular Disease Is the Main Cause of Long-Term Excess Mortality after Ischemic Stroke in Young Adults," *Hypertension* 65, no. 3 (2015): 670–75.

24. D. Mozaffarian et al., "Heart Disease and Stroke Statistics," 2015.

25. Centers for Disease Control and Prevention, "High Blood Pressure Facts," February 19, 2015, www.cdc.gov/bloodpressure/facts.htm

26. C. Rosendorf et al., "Treatment of Hypertension in Patients with Coronary Artery Disease: A Scientific Statement from the American Heart Association, American College of Cardiology, and American Society of Hypertension," *Journal of the American College of Cardiology* 65, no. 18, (2015): 1998–2038; P. James et al., "2014 Evidence-Based Guideline for the Management of High Blood Pressure in Adults: Report From the Panel Members Appointed to the Eighth Joint National Committee (JNC 8)," *Journal of American Medical Association,* 311, no. 5 (2014): 507–20, doi:10.1001/jama213.284427

27. D. Mozaffarian et al., "Heart Disease and Stroke Statistics," 2015; American Heart Association, About Peripheral Artery Disease, August 2014, www.heart.org/HEARTORG/Conditions/More/PeripheralArteryDisease/About-Peripheral-Artery-Disease-PAD_UCM_301301_Article.jsp

28. Ibid.

29. D. Mozaffarian et al., "Heart Disease and Stroke Statistics," 2015.

30. American Heart Association, "Angina in Women Can Be Different than Men," April 2015, www.heart.org/HEARTORG/Conditions/HeartAttack/WarningSignsofaHeartAttack/Angina-in-Women-Can-Be-Different-Than-Men_UCM_448902_Article.jsp

31. D. Mozaffarian et al., "Heart Disease and Stroke Statistics," 2015; American Heart Association, "Angina (Chest Pain)," April 2015, www.heart.org/HEARTORG/Conditions/HeartAttack/SymptomsDiagnosisofHeartAttack/Angina-Chest-Pain_UCM_450308_Article .jsp; American Heart Association, "Angina in Women," 2015.

32. D. Mozaffarian et al., "Heart Disease and Stroke Statistics," 2015.

33. Ibid.

34. B. M. Kissel et al., "Age at Stroke: Temporal Trends in Stroke Incidence in a Large, Biracial Population," *Neurology* 79 (2012): 1781–87.

35. Ibid.

36. American Stroke Association, "Stroke Treatments," May 2013, www.strokeassociation.org/STROKEORG/AboutStroke/Treatment/Stroke-Treatments_UCM_310892_Article.jsp

37. C. J. L. Murray et al., "The State of US Health, 1990–2010 Burden of Diseases, Injuries, and Risk Factors," *Journal of the American Medical Association* 310, no. 6 (2013): 591–608.

38. D. Mozaffarian et al., "Heart Disease and Stroke Statistics," 2015; A. Noortie, "Ischaemic Stroke in Young Adults: Risk Factors and Long-term Consequences," *Nature Reviews Neurology* 10, no. 6 (2014):315–25; S. Saydah, "Cardiometabolic Risk Factors among US Adolescents and Young Adults and Risk of Early Mortality," *Pediatrics* 131 (2013): e679–86.

39. L. Nelson et al., "Hypertension and Inflammation in Alzheimer's Disease: Close Partners in Disease Development and Progression!," *Journal of Alzheimer's Disease* 41, no. 2 (2014): 331–33; S. Sharp et al., "Hypertension Is a Potential Risk Factor for Vascular Dementia: Systematic Review," *International Journal of Geriatric Psychiatry* 26, no. 7, (2011): 661–69.

40. H. Beltrain-Sanchez et al., "Prevalence and Trends in Metabolic Syndrome in the Adult U.S. Population, 1999–2010," *Journal of the American*

College of Cardiology 62, no. 8, (2013): 607–703; D. Mozaffarian et al., "Heart Disease and Stroke Statistics," 2015.

41. D. Mozaffarian et al., "Heart Disease and Stroke Statistics," 2015; S. Grundy et al., "Definition of Metabolic Syndrome. Report of the National Heart, Lung, and Blood Institute/American Heart Association Conference on Scientific Issues Related to Definition," *Circulation* 109, no. 2, (2011): 433–38.

42. A. Noortie. "Ischaemic Stroke in Young Adults," 2014; S. Saydah, "Cardiometabolic Risk Factors among US Adolescents and Young Adults and Risk of Early Mortality," 2013.

43. D. Mozaffarian et al., "Heart Disease and Stroke Statistics," 2015.

44. Ibid.

45. National Cancer Institute, "Fact Sheet: Harms of Smoking and Benefits of Quitting," January 2011, www.cancer.gov

46. D. Keene et al., "Effect on Cardiovascular Risk of High Density Lipoprotein Targeted Drug Treatments Niacin, Fibrates, and CETP Inhibitors: Meta-analysis of Randomised Controlled Trials Including 117,411 Patients," *British Medical Journal* 349 (2014): g4379, doi: http://dx.doi.org/10.1136/bmj.g4379; G. Schwarts et al., "Effects of Dalcetrapib in Patients with a Recent Acute Coronary Syndrome," *New England Journal of Medicine* 367 (2012): 2089–99; C. Zheng and M. Aikawa, "High Density Lipoproteins: From Function to Therapy," *American College of Cardiology* 60, no. 23 (2012): 2380–83.

47. D. Mozaffarian et al., "Heart Disease and Stroke Statistics," 2015.

48. National Center For Health Statistics, "Health, United States, 2011: With Special Features on Socioeconomic Status and Health," 2012, www.cdc.gov

49. D. Mozaffarian et al., "Heart Disease and Stroke Statistics," 2015.

50. Ibid.; Y. Chida and A. Steptoe, "Greater Cardiovascular Responses to Laboratory Mental Stress Are Associated with Poor Subsequent Cardiovascular Risk Status: A Meta-Analysis of Prospective Evidence," *Hypertension* 55 (2010): 1026–32.

51. T. Kotchen, A. Cowley and E. Frohlich, "Salt in Health and Disease–A Delicate Balance," *New England Journal of Medicine* 368 (2013): 1229–37.

52. A. Steptoe and M. Kivimaki, "Stress and Cardiovascular Disease: An Update on Current Knowledge," *Annual Review of Public Health* 34 (2013): 337–54, doi: 10.1146/annurev-publhealth-031912-114452; C. Vlachopoulous, P. Xaplanteris, and C. Stefanadis, "Mental Stress, Arterial Stiffness, Central Pressures and Cardiovascular Risk," *Hypertension* 56, no. 3 (2010): e28–e30.

53. A. Steptoe and M. Kivimaki, "Stress and Cardiovascular Disease," 2013; R. C. Thurston, M. Rewak, and L.D. Kubzansky, "An Anxious Heart: Anxiety and the Onset of Cardiovascular Diseases," *Progress in Cardiovascular Diseases* 55, no. 6 (2013):524–37.

54. D. Mozaffarian et al., "Heart Disease and Stroke Statistics," 2015.

55. T Huang and F. Hu, "Gene-Environmental Interactions and Obesity: Recent Developments and Future Directions," *BMC Medical Genomics* 8, Supplement 1 (2015): S2; G. Thanassoulis et al., "A Genetic Risk Score Is Associated with Incident Cardiovascular Disease and Coronary Artery Calcium," *Circulation: Cardiovascular Genetics* 5, no. 1 (2012): 113–21; C. Chow et al., "Parental History

and Myocardial Infarction Risk across the World: The Interheart Study," *Journal of the American College of Cardiology* 57 (2011): 619–27.

56. D. Mozaffarian et al., "Heart Disease and Stroke Statistics," 2015.

57. Ibid.

58. The Emerging Risk Factors Collaboration, "C-Reactive Protein, Fibrinogen and CVD Prediction," *New England Journal of Medicine* 367 (2012): 1310–20.

59. "The PLAC Test: Predicting Heart Attack Risk in People with No Symptoms." *Scientific American-Health After 50*, 27, no. 2 (2015): 1–2.

60. R. Chowdhury et al., "Association of Dietary, Circulating, and Supplement Fatty Acids with Coronary Risk: A Systematic Review and Meta Analysis," *Annals of Internal Medicine* 160, no. 6 (2014): 398–406, doi:10.7326?M13-1788; The ORIGIN Trial Investigators, "n-3 Fatty Acids and Cardiovascular Outcomes in Patients with Dysglycemia," *New England Journal of Medicine* 367 (2012): 309–18, doi: 10.1056/NEJMoa1203859

61. American Heart Association, "Fish and Omega 3 Fatty Acids," May 14, 2014, www.heart.org/HEARTORG/General/Fish-and-Omega-3-Fatty-Acids_UCM_303248_Article.jsp

62. B. Keavney, "C-reactive Protein and the Risk for Cardiovascular Disease," British Medical Journal 342 (2011): d144; The Emerging Risk Factors Collaboration, "C-reactive Protein Concentration and Risk of Coronary Heart Disease, Stroke, and Mortality: An Individual Participant Meta-analysis," The Lancet 375, no. 9709 (2010): 132–140.

63. D. Wald, J. Morris, and N. Wald, "Reconciling the Evidence on Serum Homocysteine and Ischemic Heart Disease: A Meta-Analysis," *PLoS ONE* 6, no. 2: e16473; J. Abraham and L. Cho, "The Homocysteine Hypothesis: Still Relevant to the Prevention and Treatment of Cardiovascular Disease?," *Cleveland Clinic Journal of Medicine* 77, no. 12 (2010): 911–18.

64. American Heart Association, "Homocysteine, Folic Acid, and Cardiovascular Disease," March 18, 2014., www.heart.org

65. FDA, "Can an Aspirin a Day Help Prevent a Heart Attack?," May 5, 2014, www.fda.gov/ForConsumers/ConsumerUpdates/ucm390539.htm; Y. Ikeda et al., "Low-Dose Aspirin for Primary Prevention of Cardiovascular Events in Japanese Patients 60 Years or Older with Atherosclerotic Risk Factors: A Randomized Clinical Trial," *Journal of the American Medical Association* 312, no. 23 (2014): 2510–20; C. M. Rembold, "ACP Journal Club Review: Aspirin Does Not Reduce CHD or Cancer Mortality but Increases Bleeding," *Annals of Internal Medicine* 156, no. 12 (2012): JC6-3.

66. American Heart Association, "Prevention and Treatment of Heart Attack," August 2014, www.heart.org

67. D. Mozaffarian et al., "Heart Disease and Stroke Statistics," 2015.

68. American Cancer Society, *Cancer Facts and Figures*, 2015, www.cancer.org

69. American Cancer Society, "Cancer Treatment and Survivorship–Facts and Figures 2014–2015," 2014, www.cancer.org/acs/groups/content/@research/documents/document/acspc-042801.pdf

70. American Cancer Society, *Cancer Facts and Figures*, 2015.

71. National Cancer Institute, "Fact Sheet: Cancer Staging, 2015," January 6, 2015, www.cancer.gov/cancertopics/diagnosis-staging/staging/staging-fact-sheet

72. American Cancer Society, *Cancer Facts and Figures*, 2015.

73. Ibid.

74. American Cancer Society, *Cancer Facts and Figures*, 2015; Centers for Disease Control and Prevention, Smoking and Cancer, April 2015, www.cdc.gov/tobacco/data_statistics/sgr/50th-anniversary/pdfs/fs_smoking_cancer_508.pdf

75. M. Thun et al., "50 Year Trends in Smoking-Related Mortality in the U.S.," *New England Journal of Medicine* 368, (2013): 351–64.

76. American Cancer Society, *Cancer Facts and Figures*, 2015.

77. C. Eheman et al., "Annual Report to the Nation on the Status of Cancer, 1975–2008, Featuring Cancers Associated with Excess Weight and Lack of Sufficient Physical Activity," *Cancer* 118, no. 9 (2012): 2338–66, doi: 10.1002/cncr.27514/full; American Cancer Society, "Nutrition and Physical Activity Research Highlights," April 2015, www.cancer.org/research/acsresearchupdates/nutrition-and-physical-activity-research-highlights; W. Blot and R Tarone, "Doll and Peto's Quantitative Estimates of Cancer Risks: Holding Generally True for 35 Years," *Journal of the National Cancer Institute* 107, no. 4, (2015): djr044, http://jnci.oxfordjournals.org/content/107/4/djv044.full

78. H. R. Harris et al., "Body Fat Distribution and Risk of Premenopausal Breast Cancer in the Nurses' Health Study II," *Journal of the National Cancer Institute* 103, no. 3 (2011): 373–78.

79. R. Kaaks and T. Kuhn, "Epidemiology: Obesity and Cancer—The Evidence is Fattening Up," *Nature Reviews Endocrinology* 10 (2014): 644–45.

80. K. Bhaskaran et al., "Body-mass Index and Risk of 22 Specific Cancers: A Population-based Cohort Study of 5.24 million UK Adults," *The Lancet* 384 (2014): 755–65; C. Eheman et al., "Annual Report to the Nation on the Status of Cancer," 1975–2008, 2012.

81. American Cancer Society, "Family Cancer Syndromes," June 25, 2014, www.cancer.org/cancer/cancercauses/geneticsandcancer/heredity-and-cancer

82. American Cancer Society, "Breast Cancer Overview: What Causes Breast Cancer?," February 26, 2015, www.cancer.org/Cancer/BreastCancer/DetailedGuide/breast-cancer-what-causes

83. American Cancer Society, "Cancer Facts and Figures for Hispanic/Latinos," 2012–2014, April 2015, www.cancer.org/acs/groups/content/@epidemiologysurveillance/documents/document/acspc-034778.pdf; M. Banegas et al., "The Risk of Developing Invasive Breast Cancer in Hispanic Women," *Cancer* 119, no. 7 (2013): 1373–80.

84. O. Kiraly et al., "Inflammation-Induced Cell Proliferation Potentiates DNA Damage-Induced Mutations in Vivo," *PLoS Genetics* 11, no. 2 (2015): e1004901; S. Sebastian et al., "Colorectal Cancer in Inflammatory Bowel Disease: Results of the 3rd ECCO Pathogenesis Scientific Workshop (I)," *Journal of Crohn's and Colitis* 8, no. 1 (2014): 5–18.

85. National Cancer Institute, "Cell Phones and Cancer Risk," March 2013, www.cancer.gov; S. Joachim et al., "Cellular Telephone Use and Cancer Risk: Update of a Nationwide Danish Cohort," *Journal of the National Cancer Institute* 98, no. 23 (2006): 1707–13.

86. American Cancer Society, "Can Infections Cause Cancer?," September 24, 2014, www.cancer.org/cancer/cancercauses/othercarcinogens/infectiousagents/infectiousagentsandcancer/infectious-agents-and-cancer-intro; American Cancer Society, "Infectious Agents and Cancer," March 2013, www.cancer.org

87. American Cancer Society, "Can Infections Cause Cancer,?" 2014.
88. American Cancer Society, *Cancer Facts and Figures*, 2015.
89. National Cancer Institute, "Cervical Cancer," April 2015, www.cancer.gov
90. American Cancer Society, *Cancer Facts and Figures*, 2015.
91. American Cancer Society, "Lung Cancer Risks for Non-Smokers," October 31, 2014, www.cancer.org/cancer/news/why-lung-cancer-strikes-nonsmokers
92. American Cancer Society, *Cancer Facts and Figures*, 2015.
93. American Cancer Society, "When Smokers Quit, What Are the Benefits Over Time?," February 2014, www.cancer.org/healthy/stayawayfromtobacco/guidetoquittingsmoking/guide-to-quitting-smoking-benefits
94. American Cancer Society, *Cancer Facts and Figures*, 2015.
95. Ibid.
96. Ibid.
97. American Cancer Society, "Statistics Report: 1.5 million Cancer Deaths Avoided in 2 Decades," December 31, 2014, www.cancer.org/cancer/news/news/facts-figures-report-cancer-deaths-avoided-in-2-decades
98. American Cancer Society, *Cancer Facts and Figures*, 2015.
99. Ibid.
100. Ibid.
101. Ibid.
102. Susan G. Komen for the Cure, "Genetic Testing for BRCA1 and BRCA2 Gene," January 2015, ww5.komen.org/BreastCancer/GeneMutationsampGeneticTesting.html
103. I. Lahart et al., "Physical Activity, Risk of Death and Recurrence in Breast Cancer Survivors: A Systematic Review and Meta-analysis of Epidemiological Studies," *Acta Oncologica* 54, no. 5 (2015): 635–54, doi:10.3109/0284186X.2014.998275; Y. Wu et al., "Physical Activity and Risk of Breast Cancer: A Meta-analysis of Prospective Studies," *Breast Cancer Research and Treatment* 137, no. 3 (2013): 869–82; R. Patterson, L. Cadmus, and T. Emond, "Physical Activity, Diet, Adiposity and Female Breast Cancer Prognosis: A Review of Epidemiological Literature," *Maturitas* 66 (2010): 5–15.
104. Y. Wu et al., "Meta-Analysis of Studies on Breast Cancer Risk and Diet in Chinese Women," *International Journal of Clinical and Experimental Medicine* 8, no. 11 (2015): 73–85; D. Aune et al., "Dietary Fiber and Breast Cancer Risks: A Systematic Review and Meta Analysis of Prospective Studies," *Annals of Oncology* 23, no. 6. (2012): 1394–402, doi: 10.1093/annuls/mdr589
105. American Cancer Society, *Cancer Facts and Figures*, 2015.
106. Ibid.
107. FDA, "FDA Approves 1st Non-invasive DNA Screening for Colorectal Cancer," August 11, 2014, www.fda.gov/NewsEvents/Newsroom/PressAnnouncements/ucm409021.htm
108. Ibid.; National Cancer Institute, "Colorectal Cancer Prevention," 2015, www.cancer.gov/cancertopics/pdq/prevention/colorectal/Patient/page3#_139
109. American Cancer Society, *Cancer Facts and Figures*, 2015.
110. Ibid.
111. Ibid.
112. Ibid.
113. Ibid.
114. Ibid.
115. Ibid.
116. Ibid.
117. Ibid.
118. American Cancer Society, "Prostate Cancer," April, 2015, www.cancer.org
119. American Cancer Society, *Cancer Facts and Figures*, 2015.
120. Ibid.
121. Ibid.
122. Ibid.
123. Ibid.
124. Ibid.; American Cancer Society, "Testicular Cancer," 2015, www.cancer.org/acs/groups/cid/documents/webcontent/003142-pdf.pdf
125. National Cancer Institute, "Testicular Cancer," 2013, www.cancer.gov
126. American Cancer Society, "Testicular Cancer," 2015.
127. American Cancer Society, *Cancer Facts and Figures*, 2015.

Pulled Statistics:

Page 356, D. Mozaffarian et al., "Heart Disease and Stroke Statistics, 2015 Update," *Circulation* 131 (2015): e29–2322.

Page 359, D. Mozaffarian et al., "Heart Disease and Stroke Statistics, 2015 Update," *Circulation* 131 (2015): e29–2322.

Page 371, American Cancer Society, *Cancer Facts and Figures 2015* (Atlanta, GA: American Cancer Society, 2015), Available at www.cancer.org/acs/groups/content/@editorial/documents/document/acspc-044552.pdf

Focus On: Minimizing Your Risk for Diabetes

1. E. Selvin et al., "Trends in Prevalence and Control of Diabetes in the United States, 1988–1994 and 1999–2010," *Annals of Internal Medicine* 160, no. 8 (2014): 517–25.
2. Centers for Disease Control and Prevention, "National Diabetes Statistics Report, 2014," May 2015, www.cdc.gov/diabetes/pubs/statsreport14/national-diabetes-report-web .pdf; American Diabetes Association, "Fast Facts," March 2015, http://professional.diabetes.org/admin/UserFiles/0%20-%20Sean/Documents/Fast_Facts_3-2015.pdf; Centers for Disease Control and Prevention, "Early Release of Selected Estimates Based on Data from the National Health Interview Survey–January to June, 2014," May 2015, www .cdc.gov/nchs/data/nhis/earlyrelease/earlyrelease201412.pdf
3. Centers for Disease Control and Prevention, "National Diabetes Statistics Report, 2014," May 2015.
4. Centers for Disease Control and Prevention, "Summary Health Statistics for U.S. Adults: National Health Interview Survey, 2012," *Vital and Health Statistics* 10, no. 260 (2014), available at www.cdc.gov/nchs/products/series/series10.htm
5. T. Dall et al., "The Economic Burden of Elevated Blood Glucose Levels in 2012: Diagnosed and Undiagnosed Diabetes, Gestational Diabetes Mellitus, and Prediabetes," *Diabetes Care* 37, no. 12, (2014): 3172–79.
6. Ibid.
7. American Diabetes Association, "Diabetes Basics: Type 1," May 2014, www.diabetes.org/diabetes-basics/type-1
8. Ibid.
9. Centers for Disease Control and Prevention, "National Diabetes Statistics Report, 2014," May 2015.
10. Ibid.
11. R. Hamman et al., "The SEARCH for Diabetes in Youth Study: Rationale, Findings, and Future Directions," *Diabetes Care* 37, no. 12 (2014): 3336–44, doi: 10.2337/dc14-0574
12. D. J. Pettitt et al., "Prevalence of Diabetes in U.S. Youth in 2009: The SEARCH for Diabetes in Youth Study," *Diabetes Care* 37, no. 2 (2014): 402–08.
13. R. Mihaescu et al., "Genetic Risk Profiling for Prediction of Type 2 Diabetes," *PLoS Currents* 3 (2011): doi: 10.1371/currents.RRN1208, www.ncbi.nlm .nih.gov/pmc/articles/PMC3024707; E. Ntzani, K. Evangelia, and F. Kavvoura, "Genetic Risk Factors for Type 2 Diabetes: Insights from the Emerging Genomic Evidence," *Current Vascular Pharmacology* 10, no. 2 (2012): 147–55; K. Colclough et al., "Clinical Utility Gene Card: Maturity-Onset Diabetes of the Young," *European Journal of Human Genetics* (2014): doi: 10.1038/ejhg.2014.14
14. J. Logue et al., "Association between BMI Measured within a Year After Diagnosis of Type 2 Diabetes and Mortality," *Diabetes Care* 36, no. 4 (2013): 887–93; M. Ashwell, P. Gunn, and S. Gibson, "Waist-to-Height Ratio Is a Better Screening Tool than Waist Circumference and BMI for Adult Cardiometabolic Risk Factors: Systematic Review and Meta-Analysis," *Obesity Reviews* 13, no. 3 (2012): 275–86.
15. M. Schulze et al., "Body Adiposity Index, Body Fat Content and Incidence of Type 2 Diabetes," *Diabetologia* (2012), doi: 10.1007/s00125-012-2499-z
16. L. Bromley et al., "Sleep Restriction Decreases the Physical Activity of Adults at Risk for Type 2 Diabetes," *Sleep* 35, no. 7 (2012): 977–84, doi: 10.5665/sleep.1964
17. R. Hancox and C. Landlus, "Association between Sleep Duration and Haemoglobin A1C in Young Adults," *Journal of Epidemiology and Community Health* 66, no. 10 (2011): 957–61; H. C. Hung et al., "The Association between Self-Reported Sleep Quality and Metabolic Syndrome," *PLoS One* 8, no. 1 (2013): e54304, doi:10.1371/journal.pone.0054304; T. Ohkuma et al., "Impact of Sleep Duration on Obesity and the Glycemic Level in Patients with Type 2 Diabetes," *Diabetes Care* 36, no. 3 (2013): 611–17.
18. M. Cosgrove, L. Sargeant, R. Caleyachetty, and S. Griffin, "Work Related Stress and Type 2 Diabetes: A Systematic Review and Meta-Analysis," *Occupational Medicine* (2012), doi: 10.1093/occmed/kqs002; T. Monk and D. J. Buysse, "Exposure to Shiftwork as a Risk Factor for Diabetes," *Journal of Biological Rhythms* 28, no. 5 (2013): 356–59; M. Novak et al., "Perceived Stress and Incidence of Type 2 Diabetes: A 35 Year Follow up Study of Middle Aged Swedish Men," *Diabetic Medicine* 30, no. 1 (2013): e8-3-16.
19. Centers for Disease Control and Prevention (CDC), "National Diabetes Statistics Report, 2014"; CDC, "Prediabetes: Could It Be You?," 2014, www.cdc.gov/diabetes/pubs/statsreport14/prediabetes-infographic.pdf
20. N. Yahia et al., Assessment of College Students' Awareness and Knowledge about Conditions Relevant to Metabolic Syndrome," *Diabetology & Metabolic Syndrome* 6, no. 1 (2014): 111; J. M. Schilter and L. C. Dalleck, "Fitness and Fatness: Indicators of Metabolic Syndrome and Cardiovascular Disease Risk Factors in College Students?," *Journal of Exercise Physiology Online* 13, no. 4 (2010): 29–39.
21. American Heart Association, "Metabolic Syndrome," May 2014, www.heart.org/HEARTORG/Conditions/More/MetabolicSyndrome/Metabolic-Syndrome_UCM_002080_SubHomePage.jsp

22. National Heart Lung and Blood Institute, "What Is Metabolic Syndrome?," November 2011, www.nhlbi.nih.gov/health/dci/Diseases/ms/ms_whatis.html

23. National Heart, Lung, and Blood Institute, "Who Is at Risk for Metabolic Syndrome?," November 2011, www.nhlbi.nih.gov/health/health-topics/topics/ms/atrisk.html

24. Ibid.

25. CDC, "Prediabetes: Could It Be You?," 2014.

26. Centers for Disease Control and Prevention, "Diabetes in the United States – A Snapshot," June, 2014, http://www.cdc.gov/media/dpk/2014/images/diabetes-report/Infographic1-web.pdf

27. L. S. Geiss et al., "Diabetes Risk Reduction Behaviors among U.S. Adults with Prediabetes," *Journal of Preventive Medicine* 38, no. 4 (2010): 403–09; Centers for Disease Control, "National Diabetes Prevention Program: About the Program," October 2012, www.cdc.gov

28. American Diabetes Association, "What Is Gestational Diabetes?," June 2014, www.diabetes .org/diabetes-basics/gestational/what-is-gestational-diabetes.html

29. Ibid; C. Kim et al., "Gestational Diabetes and the Incidence of Type 2 Diabetes: A Systematic Review," *Diabetes Care* 25, no. 10 (2002): 1862–68; G. Chodick et al., "The Risk of Overt Diabetes Mellitus among Women with Gestational Diabetes: A Population-Based Study," *Diabetic Medicine* 27, no. 7 (2010): 779–85.

30. National Healthy Mothers, Healthy Babies Coalition, "The Lasting Impact of Gestational Diabetes on Mother and Children," May 2015, www .hmhb.org/virtual-library/interviews-with-experts/gestational-diabetes

31. P. M. Catalano et al., "The Hyperglycemia and Adverse Pregnancy Outcome Study: Associations of GDM and Obesity with Pregnancy Outcomes," *Diabetes Care* 35, no. 4 (2012): 780, doi: 10.2337/dc11-1790

32. Centers for Disease Control and Prevention, "National Diabetes Statistics Report, 2014," May 2015; American Diabetes Association, "Living with Diabetes: Complications," May 2014, www .diabetes.org/living-with-diabetes/complications/; K. Weinspach et al., "Level of Information about the Relationship between Diabetes Mellitus and Periodontitis—Results from a Nationwide Diabetes Information Program," *European Journal of Medical Research* 18, no. 1 (2013): 6, doi: 10.1186/2047-783X-18-6

33. National Kidney Foundation, "Fast Facts," February 2015, www.kidney.org/news/newsroom/factsheets/FastFacts.cfm

34. Ibid.

35. Centers for Disease Control and Prevention. "National Diabetes Statistics Report, 2014," May 2015.

36. Ibid.

37. Prevent Blindness America, "Diabetic Retinopathy Prevalence by Age," May 2014, www .visionproblemsus.org/diabetic-retinopathy/diabetic-retinopathy-by-age.html

38. American Diabetes Association, "Diabetes and Oral Health Problems," October 2014, www .diabetes.org/living-with-diabetes/treatment-and-care/oral-health-and-hygiene/diabetes-and-oral-health.html

39. Ibid.

40. K. Behan, "New ADA Guidelines for Diagnosis, Screening of Diabetes," *Advance Laboratory* 20, no. 1 (2011): 22, available at http://laboratory-manager.advanceweb.com

41. American Diabetes Association, "Diagnosing Diabetes and Learning about Prediabetes," March 2014, www.diabetes.org/diabetes-basics/diagnosis

42. Diabetes Prevention Program Research Group, "Reduction in the Incidence of Type 2 Diabetes with Lifestyle Intervention or Metformin," *New England Journal of Medicine* 345 (2002): 393–403.

43. American Diabetes Association, "Healthy Weight Loss," 2013, www.diabetes.org; W. Knowles et al., "10 Year Follow-Up of Diabetes Incidence and Weight Loss in the DPP Outcomes Study," *The Lancet* 374, no. 9702 (2009): 1677–86.

44. Linus Pauling Institute, "Glycemic Index and Glycemic Load," April 2014, http://lpi .oregonstate.edu/infocenter/foods/grains/gigl .html

45. S. Jonnalagadda et al., "Putting the Whole Grain Puzzle Together: Health Benefits Associated with Whole Grains—Summary of American Society for Nutrition 2010 Satellite Symposium," *Journal of Nutrition* 41, no. 5 (2011): 10115–25.

46. R. Post et al., "Dietary Fiber for the Treatment of Type 2 Diabetes Mellitus: A Meta Analysis," *Journal of the American Board of Family Medicine* 25, no. 1 (2012): 16–23; S. Bhupathiraju et al., "Glycemic Index, Glycemic Load and Risk of Type 2 Diabetes: Results from 3 Large US Cohorts and an Updated Meta-Analysis," *Circulation* 129, Supplement 1 (2014): AP140; A. Olubukola, P. English, and J. Pinkney, "Systematic Review and Meta-Analysis of Different Dietary Approaches to the Management of Type 2 Diabetes," *The American Journal of Clinical Nutrition* 97, no. 3 (2013): 505–16.

47. Wallin et al., "Fish Consumption, Dietary Long-Chain N-3 Fatty Acids, and the Risk of Type 2 Diabetes: Systematic Review and Meta Analysis of Prospective Studies," *Diabetes Care* 35, no. 4 (2012): 918–29; L. Djousse et al., "Dietary Omega-3 Fatty Acids and Fish Consumption and Risk of Type 2 Diabetes," *American Journal of Clinical Nutrition* 93, no. 1 (2011): 113–50.

48. Jeppesen, K. Schiller, and M. Schultze, "Omega-3 and Omega-6 Fatty Acids and Type 2 Diabetes," *Current Diabetes Reports* 13, no. 2 (2013): 279–88.

49. American Diabetes Association, "What We Recommend," December 2013, www.diabetes .org/food-and-fitness/fitness/types-of-activity/what-we-recommend.html; National Diabetes Information Clearing House, "Diabetes Prevention Program," September 2013, http://diabetes.niddk.nih.gov/dm/pubs/preventionprogram/index.aspx

50. S. R. Kashyap et al., "Metabolic Effects of Bariatric Surgery in Patients with Moderate Obesity and Type 2 Diabetes," *Diabetes Care* 36, no. 8 (2013): 2175–82.

51. P. R. Schauer et al., "Bariatric Surgery versus Intensive Medical Therapy for Diabetes–3 Year Outcomes," *New England Journal of Medicine* 370 (2014): 2002–13, doi: 10.1056/NEJMoa1401329

52. P. Poirier et al., on behalf of the American Heart Association Obesity Committee of the Council on Nutrition, Physical Activity, and Metabolism, "Bariatric Surgery and Cardiovascular Risk Factors: A Scientific Statement from the American Heart Association," *Circulation* 123, no. 15 (2011): 1683–701, doi: 10.1161/CIR.0b013e3182149099

53. Medtronic, "Medtronic Gains Approval of First Artificial Pancreas Device System with Threshold Suspend Automation," September 2013, http://newsroom.medtronic .com/phoenix.zhtml?c=251324&p=irol-newsArticle&id=1859361

Pulled Statistics:

Page 393, National Kidney Foundation, "Diabetes and Kidney Disease," Accessed May 2015, www.kidney .org/news/newsroom/factsheets/Diabetes-And-CKD

Chapter 13: Protecting against Infectious Diseases and Sexually Transmitted Infections

1. M. Day et al., "Surveillance of Zoonotic Infectious Disease Transmitted by Small Companion Animals," *Emerging Infectious Diseases* (2012), wwwnc.cdc.gov/eid/article/18/12/12-0664_article

2. World Health Organization (WHO), "Factsheet on the World Malaria Report–2014," December 2014, www.who.int/malaria/media/world_malaria_report_2014/en/; Centers for Disease Control and Prevention, "Dengue," March 26, 2015, www.cdc.gov/Dengue/

3. E. Hoberg and D. Brooks, "Evolution in Action: Climate Change, Biodiversity Dynamics and Emerging Infectious Disease," *Philosophical Transactions of the Royal Society of London B: Biological Sciences* 370, no. 1665 (2015), doi: 10.1098/rstb.2013.0553; S. Altizer et al., "Climate Change and Infectious Diseases: From Evidence to a Predictive Framework," *Science* 341, no. 6145 (2013): 514–19; WHO, "Climate Change and Infectious Disease," May 2015, www.who.int/globalchange/publications/climatechangechap6.pdf; J. Remais et al., "Convergence of Non-communicable and Infectious Diseases in Low- and Middle-Income Countries," *International Journal of Epidemiology* 42, no. 1 (2013): 221–27, doi: 10.1093/ije/dys135; Environmental Protection Agency, "Climate Impacts on Human Health," April 2013, www .epa.gov/climatechange/effects/health.html

4. B. T. Kerridge et al., "Conflict and Diarrheal and Related Diseases: A Global Analysis," *Journal of Epidemiology and Global Health* 3, no. 4 (2013): 269–77; K. F. Cann et al., "Extreme Water-Related Weather Events and Waterborne Disease," *Epidemiology and Infection* 141, no. 4 (2013): 671–86.

5. Centers for Disease Control and Prevention (CDC), "Birth–18 years and 'Catch-Up' Immunization Schedules," May 26, 2015, www.cdc .gov/vaccines/schedules/hcp/child-adolescent .html

6. CDC, "Get Smart: Know When Antibiotics Work," April 17, 2015, www.cdc.gov/getsmart/community/about/index.html

7. L. Hicks et al., "U.S. Outpatient Antibiotic Prescribing, 2010," *New England Journal of Medicine* 368, no. 15 (2013): 1468–69.

8. CDC, "Health-Associated Infections," January 12, 2015, www.cdc.gov/HAI/surveillance/; S. Magill et al., "Multistate Point-Prevalence Survey of Health Care–Associated Infections," *New England Journal of Medicine* 370, no. 13 (2014):1198–208.

9. CDC, "Health-Associated Infections," 2015; S. Magill et al., "Multistate Point-Prevalence Survey," 2014.

10. CDC, "General Information about MRSA in the Community," September 2013, www.cdc.gov/mrsa/community/index.html

11. Centers for Disease Control and Prevention-Newsroom, "Nearly Half a Million Americans Suffered from *Clostridium difficile* Infections in a Single Year," February 2015, www.cdc.gov/media/releases/2015/p0225-clostridium-difficile.html

12. CDC, "Group B Streptococcus (Group B Strep) and Pregnancy," January 2011, www.cdc.gov/pregnancy/infections-groupb.html

13. CDC, "Chapter 8: Meningococcal Disease: Manual for the Surveillance of Vaccine Preventable Disease," April 1, 2014, Available at www .cdc.gov/vaccines/pubs/surv-manual/ chpt08-mening.html

14. Ibid.

15. Ibid.

16. WHO, "Tuberculosis Fact Sheet," March 2015, www.who.int/mediacentre/factsheets/fs104/en/

17. CDC, "Tuberculosis (TB): Data and Statistics," April 2014, www.cdc.gov/tb/statistics/

18. Ibid.

19. CDC, "Tuberculosis," April 2015, www.cdc .gov/ tb/

20. CDC, "Tuberculosis (TB): Treatment," August 2012, www.cdc.gov/tb/topic/treatment/default. htm

21. Ibid.

22. CDC, "Common Colds: Protect Yourself and Others," February 2015, www.cdc.gov/features/ rhinoviruses/

23. Ibid.

24. Web MD, "Causes of the Common Cold," January 2015, www.webmd.com/cold-and-flu/cold-guide/common_cold_causes; CDC, "Common Colds: Protect Yourself and Others," February 2015.

25. M. G. Thompson et al., "Updated Estimates of Mortality Associated with Seasonal Influenza through the 200--2007 Influenza Season," *MMWR* 59, no. 33 (2010): 1057–62.

26. CDC, "Seasonal Influenza: Key Facts about Influenza (Flu) and Flu Vaccine," February 2013, www .cdc.gov

27. CDC, "Selecting the Viruses in the Seasonal Influenza (Flu) Vaccine," February 2014, www .cdc.gov/flu/about/season/vaccine-selection .htm

28. J. S. Schiller, B. W. Ward, G. Freeman, "Early Release of Selected Estimates Based on Data from the 2013 National Health Interview Survey," CDC, National Center for Health Statistics, June 2014, www.cdc.gov/nchs/nhis.htm

29. Ibid.

30. CDC, "Viral Hepatitis Surveillance, United States, Disease Burden from Viral Hepatitis A, B, and C in the United States–2013," April 2015, www .cdc.gov/hepatitis/Statistics/index .htm; CDC, "Reported Cases of Acute Hepatitis A, by State, United States, 2007–2011," August 2013, www .cdc.gov/hepatitis/Statistics/2011Surveillance/ Table2.1.htm; World Health Organization, "Global Policy Report on Prevention and Control of Viral Hepatitis in WHO Member States," July 2013, http://www .who.int/hiv/pub/hepatitis/global_report/en/

31. CDC, "Viral Hepatitis Surveillance-United States-2013," 2015; CDC, "Reported Cases of Acute Hepatitis A, by State," 2013, www.cdc .gov/hepatitis/Statistics/2011Surveillance/ Table2.1.htm; WHO, "Global Policy Report on Prevention and Control of Viral Hepatitis," 2013.

32. E. Aspinall et al., "Are Needle and Syringe Programmes Associated with a Reduction in HIV Transmission among People Who Inject Drugs: A Systematic Review and Meta-analysis," *International Journal of Epidemiology*, 43, no. 1 (2014): 235–48, doi: 10.1093/ije/dyt243 (Epub ahead of print December 12, 2013); A. Dutta et al., "Key Harm Reduction Interventions and Their Impact on Reduction of Risky Behavior and HIV Incidence among People Who Inject Drugs in Low-Income and Middle-Income Countries," *Current Opinion HIV AIDS* 7, no. 4 (2012): 362–8, doi: 10.1097/COH.0b013e328354a0b5

33. CDC, "Viral Hepatitis Surveillance, United States, Disease Burden from Viral Hepatitis A, B, and C in the United States-2013," April 2015, www.cdc .gov/hepatitis/Statistics/index.htm

34. CDC, "Viral Hepatitis Statistics and Surveillance–2011," August 2013, www.cdc.gov/ hepatitis/Statistics/2011Surveillance/ Commentary.htm#hepB

35. CDC, "Hepatitis C FAQs for the Public," April 2015, www.cdc.gov/hepatitis/C/cFAQ .htm#cFAQ21; CDC, "Viral Hepatitis Surveillance-United States, Disease Burden from Viral Hepatitis A, B, and C," 2015.

36. CDC, "Hepatitis C FAQs," April 2015.

37. Ibid.

38. Ibid.

39. R. Seither et al., "Vaccination Coverage among Children in Kindergarten–United States 2013-2014 School Year," *MMWR* 63, no. 41 (2014): 913–20; California Department of Public Health, "Vaccine Preventable Disease Surveillance in California- Annual Report-2013," 2014, www. cdph.ca.gov/programs/immunize/Documents/ VPD-DiseaseSummary2013.pdf

40. CDC, "West Nile Virus (WNV) Activity Reported to ArboNET, by State, United States, 2011," April 2012, www.cdc.gov

41. WHO, "Cumulative Number of Confirmed Human Cases of Avian Influenza A (H5N1) Reported to WHO," 2013, www.who.int

42. Ibid.

43. CDC, "Avian Influenza A (H7N9) Virus," April 2013, www.cdc.gov; CDC, "Highly Pathogenic Asian-Origin Avian Influenza A (H5N1) Virus," May 2015, www.cdc.gov/flu/avianflu/h5n1-virus.htm

44. CDC, "The 2009 H1N1 Pandemic," August 2010, www.cdc.gov/h1n1flu/cdcresponse.htm

45. CDC, "2013 Sexually Transmitted Disease Surveillance," March 2015, www.cdc.gov/std/stats13/; CDC, "Fact Sheet-Reported STDs in the United States," December 2014, www.cdc .gov/nchhstp/ newsroom/docs/std-trends-508.pdf

46. CDC, "Fact Sheet–Reported STDs in the United States," December 2014, www.cdc.gov/ nchhstp/newsroom/docs/std-trends-508.pdf

47. CDC, "STDs in Adolescents and Young Adults," December 2014, www.cdc.gov/std/stats13/adol. htm

48. Ibid.

49. Ibid.

50. CDC, "Chlamydia—CDC Fact Sheet, Detailed Version," December 2014, www.cdc.gov/std/chlamydia/STDFact-chlamydia-detailed.htm

51. Ibid.

52. CDC, "CDC Fact Sheet–Reported STDS in the United States–2013 National Data for Chlamydia, Gonorrhea, and Syphilis," December 2014, www .cdc.gov/nchhstp/newsroom/docs/ std-trends-508.pdf

53. Ibid; CDC, "STDS in Adolescents and Young Adults," December 2014, www.cdc.gov/std/ stats13/adol.htm

54. CDC, "CDC Fact Sheet–National Data for Chlamydia, Gonorrhea, and Syphilis," 2014.

55. Ibid.

56. Ibid.

57. CDC, "Genital Herpes–CDC Fact Sheet (Detailed)," December 2014, www.cdc.gov/std/ herpes/stdfact-herpes-detailed.htm

58. Ibid; American Sexual Health Association, "Herpes: Fast Facts," May 2015, www .ashasexualhealth.org/stdsstis/herpes/ fast-facts-and-faqs/

59. CDC, "Genital Herpes–CDC Fact Sheet," 2014.

60. CDC, "Genital HPV Infection–CDC Fact Sheet," February 2015, www.cdc.gov/std/HPV/STDFact-HPV.htm

61. CDC, "What is HPV?," January 22, 2015, www .cdc.gov/hpv/whatishpv.html

62. CDC, "Genital HPV Infection Fact Sheet," 2015; American Sexual Health Association, "HPV: Fast Facts," April 2014, www.ashasexualhealth .org/ stdsstis/hpv/fast-facts/; CDC, "What is HPV?," 2015.

63. National Women's Law Center, "Pap Smears," 2010, http://hrc.nwlc.org; CDC, "Cervical Cancer," March 2013, www.cdc.gov

64. The Henry J. Kaiser Foundation, "The HPV Vaccine: Access and Use in the U.S.," February 26, 2015, http://kff.org/womens-health-policy/fact-sheet/the-hpv-vaccine-access-and-use-in-u/

65. CDC, "What is HPV?," 2015; CDC, "What Should I Know About Screening?," January 2015, www. cdc.gov/cancer/cervical/basic_info/screening. htm; CDC, "Cervical Cancer," May 2015, www. cdc.gov/cancer/cervical

66. CDC, "Human Papillomavirus (HPV) and Oropharyngeal Cancer–Fact Sheet," November 2013, www.cdc.gov/std/hpv/stdFact-HPVan-doralcancer.htm

67. Ibid.

68. CDC, "Trichomoniasis: CDC Fact Sheet," April 2015, www.cdc.gov/std/trichomonas/ stdfact-trichomoniasis.htm

69. Ibid.

70. UNAIDS, "Global HIV/AIDS Fact Sheet–2014," May 2015, www.unaids.org/sites/default/files/ en/media/unaids/contentassets/documents/ factsheet/2014/20140716_FactSheet_en.pdf

71. UNAIDS, "Global HIV/AIDS Fact Sheet–2014," May 2015; Joint United Nations Programme on HIV/AIDS (UNAIDS) and World Health Organization (WHO), *2013 UNAIDS Report on the Global AIDS Epidemic* (Geneva: UNAIDS, 2013), Available at www.unaids.org/en/resources/publications/2013/name,85053,en.asp

72. UNAIDS, "Global HIV/AIDS Fact Sheet–2014," May 2015.

73. CDC, "HIV in the United States: At a Glance," December 2013, www.cdc.gov/hiv/resources/ factsheets/us.htm; Care.org, "HIV&AIDS: Facts," January 2014, www.care.org/work/health/hiv-aids/hiv-aids-facts; Joint UNAIDS and WHO, *2013 UNAIDS Report*, 2013, Available at www.unaids.org/ en/resources/publications/2013/name,85053,en.asp

74. CDC, "HIV in the United States," 2015; CDC, "Today's HIV/AIDS Epidemic," March 2015, www.cdc.gov/nchhstp/newsroom/docs/ hivfactsheets/todaysepidemic-508.pdf

75. CDC, "HIV in the United States," 2015; CDC, "Today's HIV/AIDS Epidemic," 2015.

76. Ibid.

77. CDC, "Today's HIV/AIDS Epidemic," 2015.

78. CDC, "HIV among Women," March 2015, www. cdc.gov/HIV/risk/gender/women/facts/index.html

79. WHO, "Mother to Child Transmission of HIV," April 2014, www.who.int/hiv/topics/mtct/en

80. Pharmaceutical Research and Manufacturers of America, "Medicine in Development: 2014 Report," May 2015, www.phrma.org/sites/ default/files/pdf/2014-meds-in-dev-hiv-aids .pdf

81. Ibid.

82. Ibid.

Pulled Statistics:

Page 414, CDC, "Incidence, Prevalence, and Cost of Sexually Transmitted Infections in the United States," February 2013, www.cdc.gov/std/stats/ sti-estimates-fact-sheet-feb-2013.pdf

Page 423, WHO, "HIV/AIDS," November 2014, www .who.int/mediacentre/factsheets/fs360/en/

Focus On: Reducing Risks for Chronic Diseases and Conditions

1. American Lung Association, "Estimated Prevalence and Incidence of Lung Disease," May 2014, www.lung.org/finding-cures/our-research/trend-reports/estimated-prevalence.pdf; Centers for Disease Control and Prevention, "Leading Causes of Death," February 6, 2015, www .cdc.gov/nchs/fastats/leading-causes-of-death .htm

2. American Lung Association, "Chronic Obstructive Pulmonary Disease (COPD) Fact Sheet," May 2014, www.lung.org/lung-disease/copd/resources/facts-figures/COPD-Fact-Sheet.html

3. Ibid.

4. American Lung Association, "Chronic Obstructive Pulmonary Disease," 2014; Centers for Disease Control and Prevention, "Chronic Obstructive Pulmonary Disease Among Adults—United States, 2011," November 2012, www.cdc .gov

5. American Lung Association, "Chronic Obstructive Pulmonary Disease," 2014; American Lung Association, "Trends in COPD," 2013, www .lung.org/finding-cures/our-research/trend-reports/copd-trend-report.pdf

6. American Lung Association, "Trends in COPD," 2013.

7. Ibid.

8. National Institute of Allergy and Infectious Diseases, "Asthma-Common Fungus Promotes Airway Sensitivity in Asthma," April 10, 2015, www.niaid.nih.gov/topics/asthma/research/Pages/FungalAllergenFeature.aspx

9. Ibid.

10. American Lung Association, "Reduce Asthma Triggers," June 2015, www.lung.org/lung-disease/asthma/taking-control-of-asthma/reduce-asthma-triggers.html

11. American Lung Association, "Reduce Asthma Triggers," 2015; U. Gohil, A. Modan, and P. Gohil, "Aspirin-Induced Asthma–A Review," Global Journal of Pharmacology 4, no. 1 (2010): 19–30.

12. Centers for Disease Control and Prevention, "Most Recent Asthma Data," April 23, 2015, www.cdc.gov/asthma/most_recent_data.htm; Centers for Disease Control and Prevention, "Early Release of Selected Estimates Based on Data From the National Health Interview Survey, January–September 2014," March 2015, www .cdc.gov/nchs/data/nhis/earlyrelease/earlyrelease201503_15.pdf; Centers for Disease Control and Prevention, "Faststats: Asthma," May 14, 2015, www.cdc.gov/nchs/fastats/asthma.htm; American Lung Association, "Estimated Prevalence and Incidence of Lung Disease," May 2014, www.lung.org/finding-cures/our-research/trend-reports/estimated-prevalence.pdf

13. Centers for Disease Control and Prevention, "Early Release of Selected Estimates," 2015.

14. Ibid.; Centers for Disease Control and Prevention, "Faststats: Asthma," 2015.

15. Centers for Disease Control and Prevention, "Faststats: Asthma," 2015.

16. National Institute of Allergy and Infectious Diseases, "Allergic Diseases," May 2015, www .niaid.nih.gov/topics/allergicdiseases/Pages/default.aspx

17. Ibid.; Centers for Disease Control and Prevention, "Allergies and Hay Fever," February 2014, www.cdc.gov/nchs/fastats/allergies.htm

18. National Institute of Allergy and Infectious diseases, "Pollen Allergy," January 2012, www .niaid.nih.gov

19. R. Burch et al., "The Prevalence and Burden of Migraine and Severe Headache in the United States: Updated Statistics from Government Health Surveillance Studies," Headache: The Journal of Head and Face Pain 55, no. 1 (2015): 21–34, doi: 10.1111/head.12482

20. J. Lucado, K. Paez, and A. Elixhauser, "Headaches in U.S. Hospitals and Emergency Departments, 2008," HCUP Statistical Brief, no. 111 (2011), Available at www.hcup-us.ahrq.gov

21. National Headache Foundation, "Press Kits: Categories of Headache," June 2014, www .headaches.org/press/NHF_Press_Kits/Press_Kits_-_Categories_Of_Headache

22. WebMD, "Migraines and Headache Health Center: Tension Headaches," 2013, www .webmd.com

23. Mayo Clinic, "Tension Headache: Basics and Symptoms," July 2013, www.mayoclinic.org/diseases-conditions/tension-headache/basics/definition/con-20014295

24. R. Burch et al., "The Prevalence and Burden of Migraine and Severe Headache in the United States," 2015, doi: 10.1111/head.12482; National Institute of Neurological Disorders and Stroke, "NINDS Migraine Information Page," February 23, 2015, www.ninds.nih.gov/disorders/migraine/migraine.htm; National Headache Foundation, "Migraine," June 2015, www .headaches.org/education/Headache_Topic_Sheets/Migraine

25. R. Burch et al., "The Prevalence and Burden of Migraine and Severe Headache," 2015; National Institute of Neurological Disorders and Stroke, "NINDS Migraine Information Page," 2015.

26. National Headache Foundation, "Migraines," 2015.

27. National Institute of Neurological Disorders and Stroke, NINDS Migraine Information Page," 2015.

28. Ibid.

29. National Headache Foundation, "Cluster Headaches," 2013, www.headaches.org

30. National Institute of Diabetes and Digestive and Kidney Diseases. "Definition and Facts for Irritable Bowel Syndrome," June 2015, www .niddk.nih.gov/health-information/health-topics/digestive-diseases/irritable-bowel-syndrome/Pages/definition-facts.aspx

31. National Institute of Diabetes and Digestive and Kidney Diseases, "Irritable Bowel Syndrome," 2015; H. F. Herlong, Digestive Disorders. The Johns Hopkins White Papers. Baltimore, MD: Johns Hopkins Medicine, 2013.

32. National Institute of Diabetes and Digestive and Kidney Diseases, "Irritable Bowel Syndrome," 2015.

33. Ibid.

34. National Digestive Diseases Information Clearinghouse, "Irritable Bowel Syndrome," 2015; H. F. Herlong, Digestive Disorders, 2013.

35. National Institutes of Diabetes and Digestive and Kidney Diseases. "Crohn's Disease," September 2014, www.niddk.nih.gov/health-information/health-topics/digestive-diseases/crohns-disease

36. Centers for Disease Control and Prevention, "Inflammatory Bowel Disease," May 2014, www .cdc.gov/ibd

37. National Institutes of Diabetes and Digestive and Kidney Diseases, "Crohn's Disease," 2014.; National Digestive Diseases Information Clearinghouse, " Irritable Bowel Syndrom," 2015.

38. Centers for Disease Control and Prevention, "Inflammatory Bowel Disease (IBD)," 2014.

39. H. F. Herlong, Digestive Disorders, 2013.

40. Ibid.

41. "Global Burden of Diseases, Injuries and Risk Factors Study 2013," The Lancet, June 2015, www .thelancet.com/themed/global-burden-of-disease

42. Bone and Joint Initiative-USA, "The Burden of Musculoskeletal Diseases in the United States: Prevalence, Societal and Economic Cost," May 2015, www.boneandjointburden.org/facts-brief

43. Centers for Disease Control, "Data and Statistics, Arthritis," March 11, 2015, www.cdc.gov/arthritis/data_statistics

44. Centers for Disease Control, "Arthritis: National Statistics," February 25, 2015, www .cdc.gov/arthritis/data_statistics/national-statistics.html; Arthritis Foundation, "The Heavy Burden of Arthritis in the U.S.," March 2012, www.arthritis.org/files/images/AF_Connect/Departments/Public_Relations/Arthritis-Prevalence-Fact-Sheet--3-7-12.pdf

45. Centers for Disease Control, "National Arthritis Statistics: Future Burden of Arthritis," February 2015, www.cdc.gov/arthritis/data_statistics/national-statistics .html#FutureArthritisBurden

46. Arthritis Foundation, "Arthritis Facts," June 2015, www.arthritis.org/about-arthritis/understanding-arthritis/arthritis-statistics-facts.php; National Institute of Arthritis and Musculoskeletal and Skin Disease, "Handout on Health: Osteoarthritis," April 2015, www .niams.nih.gov/Health_Info/Osteoarthritis/default.asp

47. National Institute of Arthritis and Musculoskeletal and Skin Disease, "Handout on Health: Osteoarthritis," 2015.

48. Calvo-Munoz, "Prevalence of Low Back Pain in Children and Adolescents: A Meta-analysis," BMC Pediatrics 13, no 1 (2013): 14, doi:10.1186/2431-13-14

49. Ibid.

50. American College Health Association, American College Health Association-National College Health Assessment II: Reference Group Executive Summary, Spring, 2014 (Hanover, MD): American College Health Association.

51. F. Balague et al., "Non-Specific Low Back Pain," The Lancet 379, no. 9814 (2012): 482–91, doi: 10.1016/S0140-6736(11)60610-7; National Information Institute of Neurological Disorders and Stroke, "NINDS Back Pain Information Page," April 2014, www.ninds.nih.gov/disorders/back-pain/backpain.htm

52. F. Balague et al., "Non-Specific Low Back Pain," 2012; National Information Institute of Neurological Disorders and Stroke, "NINDS Back Pain Information Page," 2015; R. Shri et al., "Obesity as a Risk Factor for Sciatica: A Meta-analysis," American Journal of Epidemiology (2014): doi:10.1093/aje/Kwn007

53. National Institute of Neurological Disorders and Stroke, "Low Back Pain Fact Sheet," April 2015, http://www.ninds.nih.gov/disorders/backpain/detail_backpain.htm; M. Mehra et al., "The Burden of Chronic Low Back Pain with and without a Neuropathic Component: A Healthcare Resource Use and Cost Analysis," Journal of Medical Economics 15, no. 2 (2011): 245–52.

54. National Institute of Neurological Disorders, "NINDS Repetitive Motion Disorders Information Page," October 2011, www.ninds.nih.gov

Pulled Statistics:

Page 429, American Lung Association, "Chronic Obstructive Pulmonary Disease (COPD) Fact Sheet," March 2015. www.lung.org

Page 433, National Institute of Diabetes and Digestive and Kidney Diseases, "Definition and Facts for Irritable Bowel Syndrome," September 2014, www.niddk.nih.gov/health-information/health-topics/digestive-diseases/irritable-bowel-syndrome

Chapter 14: Preparing for Aging, Death, and Dying

1. Central Intelligence Agency, *The World Factbook. Country Comparisons: Life Expectancy at Birth,* 2014, www.cia.gov/library/publications/the-world-factbook/rankorder/2102rank.html
2. Administration on Aging, U.S. Department of Health and Human Services, "A Profile of Older Americans: 2014," 2014, www.aoa.acl.gov/Aging_Statistics/Profile/2014/docs/2014-Profile.pdf
3. Federal Interagency Forum on Aging-Related Statistics, "Older Americans 2012: Key Indicators of Well-Being," June 2012, www.agingstats.gov
4. Central Intelligence Agency, *The World Factbook,* 2014.
5. Administration on Aging, "A Profile of Older American," 2014.
6. Ibid.
7. Ibid.
8. Ibid.
9. Genworth, "Compare Long-Term Care Costs Across the United States," February 2015, www.genworth.com/corporate/about-genworth/industry-expertise/cost-of-care.html
10. Administration on Aging, "A Profile of Older Americans," 2014.
11. National Osteoporosis Foundation, "Debunking the Myths," June 2015, http://nof.org/OPmyths
12. Centers for Disease Control and Prevention, "Arthritis-Related Statistics," March 2014, www.cdc.gov/arthritis/data_statistics/arthritis_related_stats.htm
13. J. Weinstein et al., "The Aging Kidney," *NIH-Advanced Chronic Kidney Disease* 17, no. 4 (2011): 302–307; Merck Manual Consumer Version, "Effects of Aging on Urinary Tract," June 2015, www.merckmanuals.com
14. Ibid.
15. National Institute on Deafness and Other Communication Disorders, "Age-Related Hearing Loss," November 2013, www.nidcd.nih.gov/health/hearing/Pages/Age-Related-Hearing-Loss.aspx; F. Lin et al., "Hearing Loss and Cognitive Decline in the Elderly," *Journal of American Medical Association-Internal Medicine* 173, no. 4 (2013): 293–99, doi: 10.1001/jamainternmed.2013.1868
16. J. Solheim et al., "Daily Life Consequences of Hearing Loss in the Elderly," *Disability Rehabilitation* 33, no. 23–24 (2011): 2179–85, doi: 10.3109/09638288.2011.563815; F. Lin et al., "Hearing Loss and Cognitive Decline," 2013.
17. T. E. Howe et al., "Exercise for Improving Balance in Older People," *Cochrane Database of Systematic Reviews* (2012), www.cochrane.org/CD004963/MUSKINJ_exercise-for-improving-balance-in-older-people
18. M. N. Lochlainne et al., "Sexual Activity and Aging," *Journal of American Medical Directors Association* 14, no. 8 (2013): 565–72; R. von Simson et al., "Sexual Health and the Older Adult," *Student BMJ* 20 (2012): e688, doi: 10.1136/sbmj.e688
19. Alzheimer's Association, "2015 Alzheimer's Disease Facts and Figures," 2015, www.alz.org
20. Ibid.
21. L. Hebert et al., "Alzheimer Disease in the United States (2010–2050) Estimated Using the 2010 Census," *Neurology* 80, no. 19 (2013), doi: 10.1212/WNL.0b013e31828726f5
22. Ibid.
23. Ibid.
24. Alzheimer's Association, "What Is Alzheimer's?" 2015, www.alz.org
25. Centers for Disease Control and Prevention, "Making Physical Activity a Part of an Older Adult's Life," November 2011, www.cdc.gov
26. By permission. From *Merriam-Webster's Collegiate® Dictionary,* 11th Edition © 2013 by Merriam-Webster, Inc., Available at www.Merriam-Webster.com
27. President's Commission on the Uniform Determination of Death, *Defining Death: Medical, Ethical and Legal Issues in the Determination of Death* (Washington, DC: U.S. Government Printing Office, 1981).
28. Ad Hoc Committee of the Harvard Medical School to Examine the Definition of Brain Death, "A Definition of Irreversible Coma," *Journal of the American Medical Association* 205 (1968): 377.
29. Elisabeth Kübler-Ross, *On Death and Dying* (New York: Scribner, 2014).
30. Victorian Government Health Information, "Death and Dying," July 2014, www.health.vic.gov
31. Behavioural Neuropathy Clinic, "Grief and the grieving process," 2015, www.adhd.com.au/grief.htm
32. American Bar Association Commission on Law and Aging, *Consumer's Tool Kit for Health Care Advance Planning,* 2d ed., 2012, www.americanbar.org/content/dam/aba/uncategorized/2011/2011_aging_bk_consumer_tool_kit_bk.authcheckdam.pdf
33. Aging with Dignity, "Five Wishes," 2013, www.agingwithdignity.org
34. National Hospice and Palliative Care Organization, "NHPCO Facts and Figures: Hospice Care in America, 2014 Edition," 2014, www.nhpco.org
35. U.S. Department of Health and Human Services, "The Need Is Real," June 2015, www.organdonor.gov/about/data.html

Pulled Statistics

Page 441, Administration on Aging, U.S. Dept. of Health and Human Services, "A Profile of Older Americans: 2014," 2015, www.aoa.gov/Aging_Statistics/Profile/2014/docs/2014_Profile.pdf

Page 445, U.S. Census Bureau, "2010 Census Shows 65 and Older Population Growing Faster than Total U.S. Population," November 2011, www.census.gov

Chapter 15: Promoting Environmental Health

1. World Wildlife Fund, "Living Planet Index," July 2015, wwf.panda.org/about_our_earth/all_publications/living_planet_report/living_planet_index2/
2. P. Gerland et al., "World Population Stabilization Unlikely This Century," *Science* 346, no. 6206 (2014): 231–37; Worldwatch Institute, "U.N. Raises 'Low' Population Projections for 2050," June 2014, www.worldwatch.org/node/6038
3. United Nations, "Global Environment Outlook: Environment for Development (GEO-5): Summary for Policy Makers," 2012, www.uncsd2012.org; United Nations, "UNEP Yearbook: Emerging Issues in our Global Environment, 2014," 2015, www.unep.org/yearbook/2014/
4. World Wildlife Fund, "Living Planet Index," 2015.
5. Ibid.
6. Ibid.
7. Ibid.
8. United Nations, "UNEP Yearbook, 2014," 2015.
9. G. Ceballos et al., "Accelerated Modern Human-induced Species Losses: Entering the Sixth Mass Extinction," *Science Advances* 1, no. 5 (2015): e1400253, doi: 10.1126/sciadv.1400253
10. The IUCN Red List of Threatened Species, "IUCN Red List Status: Mammals," June 2015, www.iucnredlist.org/initiatives/mammals/analysis/red-list-status
11. Ibid., J. Croxall et al., "Seabird Conservation Status, Threats and Priority Actions: A Global Assessment," *Bird Conservation International* 22 (2012): 1–34, doi: 10.1017/S0959270912000020
12. G. Whillemyer et al., "Illegal Killing for Ivory Drives Global Decline in African Elephants," *Proceedings of the National Academy of Sciences* 111, no. 36 (2014): 13117–121; W. Ripple, et al., "Collapse of the World's Largest Herbivores," *Science Advances* 1, no. 4 (2015): e1400103.
13. United Nations Environmental Program, "Towards a Green Economy: Pathways to Sustainable Development and Poverty Eradication," June 2015, www.unep.org/greeneconomy/greeneconomyreport/tabid/29846/default.aspx; V. Christensson et al., "A Century of Fish Biomass Decline in the Ocean," *Marine Ecology Program Series* 512 (2014): 155–166, doi: 10.3354/meps10946
14. United Nations, "UNEP Yearbook, 2014," 2015.
15. U.S. Energy Information Administration, "Independent Statistics and Analysis," 2013, www.eia.gov
16. Central Intelligence Agency, "The World Factbook, Country Comparison: Total Fertility Rate," June 2014, www.cia.gov/library/publications/the-world-factbook/rankorder/2127rank.html; C. Haub and T. Kaneda, "2014 World Population Data Sheet," Population Reference Bureau, World Population, 2014, www.prb.org/Publications/Datasheets/2014/2014-world-population-data-sheet/data-sheet.aspx
17. C. Haub and T. Kaneda, "2014 World Population Data Sheet," 2014.
18. Population Reference Bureau, "The Decline in U.S. Fertility," 2014, www.prb.org/Publications/Datasheets/2014/2014-world-population-data-sheet/us-fertility-decline-factsheet.aspx; Central Intelligence Agency, "The World Factbook: Country Comparison: Total Fertility Rate," 2014.
19. U.S. Environmental Protection Agency, "Air Enforcement," June 2014, www2.epa.gov/enforcement/air-enforcement
20. U.S. Environmental Protection Agency, "Overview of Greenhouse Gases: Emissions and Trends: Carbon Dioxide," April 2014, www.epa.gov/climatechange/ghgemissions/gases/co2.html
21. A. Soos, "Acid Rain Change," *Environmental News Network,* 2013, www.enn.com
22. U.S. Environmental Protection Agency, "Reducing Acid Rain," 2012, www.epa.gov
23. U.S. Environmental Protection Agency, "Acid Rain: Effects of Acid Rain—Surface Waters and Aquatic Animals," 2012, www.epa.gov
24. Ibid.; A. Soos, "Acid Rain Change," 2013.
25. U.S. Environmental Protection Agency, "Acid Rain: Effects of Acid Rain—Human Health," 2012, www.epa.gov
26. U.S. Environmental Protection Agency, "Questions About Your Community: Indoor Air," 2013, www.epa.gov/region1/communities/indoorair.html
27. U.S. Environmental Protection Agency, "An Introduction to Indoor Air Quality," Updated November 2014, www.epa.gov/iaq/ia-intro.html
28. Ibid.
29. U.S. Environmental Protection Agency, "Ozone Layer Depletion: Ozone Science: Brief Questions and Answers on Ozone Depletion," Updated February 2010, www.epa.gov; Environment, Health and Safety Online, "Ozone Depletion and UV Radiation," 2013, www.ehso.com; National Aeronautics and Space Administration, "Ozone Hole Watch," 2013, http://ozonewatch.gsfc.nasa.gov

30. White House, "Remarks by the President on Climate Change-Georgetown University," Press Release, June 2013, www.whitehouse.gov/the-press-office/2013/06/25/remarks-president-climate-change

31. U.S. Global Change Research Group, "Climate Change Impacts in the United States," May 2014, http://nca2014.globalchange.gov/downloads/report; NASA, "Global Climate Change. Evidence of Change: How Do We Know?," June 2014, http://climate.nasa.gov/evidence; U.S. Environmental Protection Agency, "Climate Change Facts: Answers to Common Questions," 2014; J. C. L. Olivier et al., "Trends in Global CO_2 Emissions–2013 Report," October 2013, www.pbl.nl/en/publications/trends-in-global-co2-emissions-2013-report

32. NASA, "Global Climate Change," 2014; Environmental Protection Agency, "Climate Change Facts: Answers to Common Questions," 2014; J. C. L Olivier et al., "Trends in Global CO_2 Emissions–2013 Report," 2013.

33. NASA, "Global Climate Change," 2014.

34. Ibid; J. C. L. Olivier et al., "Trends in Global CO_2 Emissions-2013 Report," 2013.

35. Ibid; U.S. Environmental Protection Agency, "National Greenhouse Gas Emissions Data," April 2014, www.epa.gov/climatechange/ghgemissions/usinventoryreport.html

36. Ibid.

37. World Commission on Environment and Development, *Our Common Future* (Oxford: Oxford University Press, 1987): 27.

38. J. C. L. Olivier et al., "Trends in Global CO_2 Emissions–2014 Report," 2014.

39. Ibid.

40. Ibid.

41. Environmental Defense Fund, "Cap and Trade—How Cap and Trade Works, 2015, www.edf.org/climate/how-cap-and-trade-works

42. Ibid.

43. The Water Information Program, "Water Facts," June 2015, www.waterinfo.org/resources/water-facts

44. Ibid.

45. Pacific Institute, "Water Use Trends in the United States," April 2015, http://pacinst.org/wp-content/uploads/sites/21/2015/04/Water-Use-Trends-Report.pdf

46. Ibid.

47. Ibid.

48. The Water Information Program, "Water Facts," June 2015, www.waterinfo.org/resources/water-facts

49. Department of National Intelligence, "Worldwide Threat Assessment of the Intelligence Community," January 9, 2014, www.dni.gov/files/documents/Intelligence%20Reports/2014%20WWTA%20%20SFR_SSCI_29_Jan.pdf; Department of National Intelligence, "Global Water Security," February 2012, www.dni.gov/files/documents/Special%20Report_ICA%20Global%20Water%20Security.pdf

50. World Economic Forum, "Global Agenda Council on Water Security 2012–2014," June 2015, www3.weforum.org/docs/GAC/2013/Connect/WEF_GAC_WaterSecurity_2012-2014_Connect.pdf; Water Information Program. "Water Facts," 2015.

51. M. Kostich, A. Batt, and J. Lazorcheck, "Concentrations of Prioritized Pharmaceuticals in Effluents from 50 Large Wastewater Treatment Plants in the U.S. and Implications for Risk Estimation," *Environmental Pollution* 184 (2014): 354–59.

52. U.S. Geological Survey, "National Water Quality Assessment Program" June 2015, http://water.usgs.gov/nawga/

53. U.S. Environmental Protection Agency, "Advancing Sustainable Materials Management 2013 Fact Sheet—Assessing Trends in Material Generation, Recycling and Disposal in the United States," June 2015, www.epa.gov/epawaste/nonhaz/municipal/pubs/2013_advncng_smm_fs.pdf

54. Ibid.

55. Ibid.

56. U.S. Environmental Protection Agency, "Superfund: Superfund National Accomplishments Summary, Fiscal Year 2013," June 2014, www.epa.gov/superfund/accomp/pdfs/FY_2013_SF_EOY_accomp_sum_FINAL.pdf

57. U.S. Environmental Protection Agency, "Hazardous Waste," June 2015, www.epa.gov/osw/basic-hazard.htm; U.S. Environmental Protection Agency, "Household Hazardous Waste," 2014, www.epa.gov/osw/conserve/materials/hhw.htm

58. U.S. Nuclear Regulatory Commission, "Radiation Basics," 2014, www.nrc.gov/about-nrc/radiation/health-effects/radiation-basics.html

59. Ibid.

60. Reuters, "Factbox: Key Facts on Chernobyl Nuclear Accident," March 2011, www.reuters.com

61. International Atomic Energy Agency, "IAEA Issues Projections for Nuclear Power from 2020–2050," May 12, 2015, www.iaea.org/newscenter/news/iaea-issues-projections-nuclear-power-2020-2050; U.S. Energy Information Administration, "Independent Statistics and Analysis," 2012, www.eia.gov

62. National Institute for Occupational Safety and Health, "Workplace Safety and Health Topics: Noise and Hearing Loss Prevention," 2011, www.cdc.gov

Pulled Statistics:

Page 458, Population Reference Bureau, "2014 World Population Data Sheet," 2014, www.prb.org/pdf14/2014-world-population-data-sheet_eng.pdf

Page 467, EPA, "Advancing Sustainable Materials Management: 2013 Fact Sheet," June 2015, www.epa.gov/epawaste/nonhaz/municipal/pubs/2013_advncng_smm_fs.pdf

Chapter 16: Making Smart Health Care Choices

1. S. Collins, P. Rasmussen, and M. Doty, "Gaining Ground: Americans' Health Insurance Coverage and Access to Care After the Affordable Care Act's First Open Enrollment Period," July 2014, www.commonwealthfund.org/publications/issue-briefs/2014/jul/health-coverage-access-aca

2. M. A. Hillen et al., " How Can Communication by Oncologists Enhance Patients' Trust? An Experimental Study," *Annals of Oncology* 25, no. 4 (2014): 896–901.

3. The Joint Commission, "About The Joint Commission," 2015, www.jointcommission.org

4. J. James, "New Evidence-Based Estimates of Patient Harms Associated with Hospital Care," *Journal of Patient Safety* 9, no. 3 (2013): 122–28.

5. Consumer Health, "Patient Rights: Informed Consent," March 2013, www.emedicinehealth.com/patient_rights/article_em.htm#patient_rights

6. Centers for Disease Control and Prevention, "Therapeutic Drug Use," May 14, 2015, www.cdc.gov/nchs/fastats/drug-use-therapeutic.htm

7. W. Zhong et al., "Age and Sex Patterns of Drug Prescribing in a Defined American Population," *Mayo Clinic Proceedings* 88, no. 7 (2013): 697–707.

8. L. Gallelli et al., "Safety and Efficacy of Generic Drugs with Respect to Brand Formulation," *Journal of Pharmacology and Pharmacotherapeutics* 4, Supplement 1 (2013): S110–14.

9. Kaiser Family Foundation, "Total HMO Enrollment, July 2012," May 2014, http://kff.org/other/state-indicator/total-hmo-enrollment

10. Centers for Medicare and Medicaid Services, "National Health Expenditure Projections 2013–2023," 2013, www.cms.gov/Research-Statistics-Data-and-Systems/Statistics-Trends-and-Reports/NationalHealthExpendData/Downloads/Proj2013.pdf

11. National Committee to Preserve Social Security and Medicare, "Fast Facts About Medicare," February 2015, www.ncpssm.org/Medicare/MedicareFastFacts

12. U.S. Department of Health & Human Services, "2015 Poverty Guidelines," January 2015, http://aspe.hhs.gov/poverty/15poverty.cfm

13. Centers for Medicare and Medicaid Services, "National Health Expenditure Projections," 2013.

14. Centers for Medicare and Medicaid Services, "Children's Health Insurance Program," July 2015, www.medicaid.gov/chip/chip-program-information.html

15. National Conference of State Legislators, "Health Insurance: Premiums and Increases," June 2015, www.ncsl.org/issues-research/health/health-insurance-premiums.aspx

16. The Rand Corporation, "The Affordable Care Act in Depth," April 8, 2015, www.rand.org/health/key-topics/aca/in-depth.html

17. S. Collins, P. Rasmussen, and M. Doty, "Gaining Ground: Americans' Health Insurance Coverage," 2014.

18. American College Health Association, *American College Health Association–National College Health Assessment II: Reference Group Executive Summary. Spring 2014* (Hanover, MD: American College Health Association, 2014).

19. Bureau of Labor Statistics, U.S. Department of Labor, "Occupational Outlook Handbook: Physicians and Surgeons," January 2014, www.bls.gov/ooh/healthcare/physicians-and-surgeons.htm

20. American Hospital Association, "Fast Facts on U.S. Hospitals," January 2014, www.aha.org/research/rc/stat-studies/fast-facts.shtml

21. O. W. Brawley, *How We Do Harm: A Doctor Breaks Ranks about Being Sick in America* (New York: St. Martin's Press, 2011).

22. Centers for Medicare and Medicaid Services, "National Health Expenditure Projections 2013–2023," 2013.

23. Ibid.

24. America's Health Insurance Plans, "Fast Check: Administrative Costs," November 2012, www.ahip.org/ACA-Toolbox/Documents/Communications-Toolkit/Fact-Check-Administrative-Costs.aspx

25. Central Intelligence Agency, "Country Comparison: Life Expectancy at Birth. CIA World Factbook," June 2015, www.cia.gov/library/publications/the-world-factbook/rankorder/2102rank.html

26. Ibid.

27. Central Intelligence Agency, "Country Comparison: Infant Mortality Rate. CIA Factbook," June 2015, www.cia.gov/library/publications/the-world-factbook/rankorder/2091rank.html

28. Department of Health and Human Services, "Report to Congress: National Strategy for Quality Improvement in Health Care," 2011, www.ahrq.gov/workingforquality/nqs/nqs2011annlrpt.htm

Pulled Statistics:

Page 482, Centers for Disease Control and Prevention, "Hospital Utilization," 2015, www.cdc.gov

Page 492, J. John, "A New, Evidence-based Estimate of Patient Harms Associated with Hospital Care," *Journal of Patient Safety* 9, no. 3 (2013): 122–28.

Focus On: Understanding Complementary and Integrative Health

1. National Center for Complementary and Integrative Health, "Complementary, Alternative, or Integrative Health: What's in a Name?," March 2015, https://nccih.nih.gov/health/integrative-health#types
2. Ibid.
3. Ibid.
4. Ibid.
5. T. C. Clarke et al., "Trends in the Use of Complementary Health Approaches among Adults: United States, 2002–2012," National Health Statistics Reports, no. 79 (Hyattsville, MD: National Center for Health Statistics), February 2015. Available at www.cdc.gov/nchs/data/nhsr/nhsr079.pdf
6. Ibid.
7. National Center for Complementary and Integrative Health, "Traditional Chinese Medicine: An Introduction," October 2013, http://nccam.nih.gov/health/whatiscam/chinesemed.htm
8. National Center for Complementary and Integrative Health, "Ayurvedic Medicine: An Introduction," NCCIH Publication no. D287, January 2015, http://nccam.nih.gov/health/ayurveda/introduction.htm
9. Ibid.
10. Ibid.
11. National Center for Complementary and Integrative Health, "Homeopathy: An Introduction," NCCIH Publication no. D439, April 2015, http://nccih.nih.gov/health/homeopathy
12. Ibid.

13. National Center for Complementary and Integrative Health, "Naturopathy: An Introduction," NCCIH Publication no. D372, March 2012, https://nccih.nih.gov/health/naturopathy/naturopathyintro.htm
14. Ibid.
15. National Center for Complementary and Integrative Health, "Complementary, Alternative, or Integrative Health: What's in a Name?" 2015.
16. American Chiropractic Association, "About Chiropractic," Accessed June 2015, www.acatoday.org/level1_css.cfm?T1ID=42
17. NIH-National Center for Complementary and Integrative Health, "Spinal Manipulation," January 28, 2015, https://nccih.nih.gov/health/spinalmanipulation
18. Ibid.
19. National Center for Complementary and Integrative Health, "Massage Therapy for Health Purposes: What You Need to Know," NCCIH Publication no. D327, updated February 2014, http://nccih.nih.gov/health/massage/massageintroduction.htm
20. Ibid.
21. Ibid.
22. Bureau of Labor Statistics, U.S. Department of Labor, "Massage Therapists," *Occupational Outlook Handbook, 2012–2013 Edition,* January 2014, www.bls.gov/ooh/Healthcare/Massage-therapists.htm
23. National Center for Complementary and Integrative Health, "Acupuncture: What You Need to Know," NCCIH Publication no. D404, November 2014, http://nccih.nih.gov/health/acupuncture/introduction.htm
24. R. S. Hinman et al., "Acupuncture for Chronic Knee Pain. A Randomized Clinical Trial," *Journal of the American Medical Association* 312, no. 13 (2014): 1313–22.
25. A. J. Vickers and K. Linde, "Acupuncture for Chronic Pain," *Journal of the American Medical Association* 311, no. 9 (2014): 955–56.
26. National Center for Complementary and Integrative Health, "Acupuncture: What You Need to Know, 2014.
27. G. A. Kelley and K. S. Kelley, "Meditative Movement Therapies and Health-Related Quality-of-Life in Adults: A Systematic Review of Meta-Analyses," *PLoS ONE* 10, no.6 (2015): e0129181, doi: 10.1371/journal.pone.0129181

28. R. Hammerschlag, B. L. Marx, and M. Alckin, "Nontouch Biofield Therapy: A Systematic Review of Human Randomized Controlled Trials Reporting Use of Only Nonphysical Contact Treatment," *Journal of Alternative and Complementary Medicine* 20, no. 12 (2014): 881–92, doi: 10.1089/acm.2014.0017
29. Academy of Nutrition and Dietetics, "Position of the Academy of Nutrition and Dietetics: Functional Foods," *Journal of the Academy of Nutrition and Dietetics* 113, no. 8 (2013): 1096–1103.
30. A. Kerimi and G. Williamson, "The Cardiovascular Benefits of Dark Chocolate," *Vascular Pharmacology* 15 (2015), doi: 10.1016/j.vph.2015.05.011
31. National Center for Complementary and Integrative Health, "Oral Probiotics: An Introduction," NCCIH Publication no. D345, December 2012, https://nccih.nih.gov/health/probiotics/introduction.htm
32. Ibid.
33. U. S. Food and Drug Administration, "Questions and Answers on Dietary Supplements," April 2015, www.fda.gov/Food/DietarySupplements/QADietarySupplements/default.htm
34. Ibid.
35. Ibid.
36. Ibid.
37. National Center for Complementary and Integrative Health, "Alerts and Advisories," June 2015, https://nccih.nih.gov/news/alerts
38. National Center for Complementary and Integrative Health, "Using Dietary Supplements Wisely," NCCIH Publication no. D426, updated June 2014, https://nccih.nih.gov/health/supplements/wiseuse.htm
39. U. S. Pharmacopeial Convention, "Dietary Supplements," 2015, www.usp.org/usp-consumers/dietary-supplements-consumers

Pulled Statistics:

Page 495, T. C. Clarke et al., "Trends in the Use of Complementary Health Approaches among Adults: United States, 2002–2012," *National Health Statistics Reports* 79 (Hyattsville, MD: National Center for Health Statistics), February 2015. Available at www.cdc.gov/nchs/data/nhsr/nhsr079.pdf

PHOTO CREDITS

INDEX